WHITTINGTON POSTGRADUATE MEDICINE

WHITTINGTON POSTGRADUATE MEDICINE

EDITORIAL BOARD

BUTTERWORTHS

ENGLAND: BUTTERWORTH & CO. (PUBLISHERS) LTD.
                LONDON: 88 Kingsway, W.C.2B 6AB

AUSTRALIA: BUTTERWORTHS PTY. LTD.
                SYDNEY: 586 Pacific Highway, 2067
                MELBOURNE: 343 Little Collins Street, 3000
                BRISBANE: 240 Queen Street, 4000

CANADA: BUTTERWORTH & CO. (CANADA) LTD.
                TORONTO: 14 Curity Avenue, 374

NEW ZEALAND: BUTTERWORTHS OF NEW ZEALAND LTD.
                WELLINGTON: 26–28 Waring Taylor Street, 1

SOUTH AFRICA: BUTTERWORTH & CO. (SOUTH AFRICA) (PTY.) LTD.
                DURBAN: 152–154 Gale Street

Suggested U.D.C. Number 616 (075·8)

ISBN 0 407 93499 5 (Cased Edn)

0 407 93500 2 (Limp Edn)

Printed offset in Great Britain by
The Camelot Press Ltd, London and Southampton

Contents

Preface vii

1 — The Examination of the Cardiac Case 1
    E. Montuschi

2 — Ischaemic Heart Disease: Aetiology and Prevention . . . 21
    D. E. Sharland

3 — Cardiac Arrhythmias and Disorders of Conduction 45
    R. A. L. Sutton

4 — Growth Disorders in Childhood 75
    Max Friedman

5 — Chronic Complications of Diabetes 97
    Arnold Bloom

6 — The Diagnosis of Common Colonic Disorders 119
    Eric Beck

7 — Renal Glomerular Disease 143
    B. I. Hoffbrand

8 — Adverse Reactions to Drugs and Diseases of the Chest . . . 179
    P. D. B. Davies

9 — Some Aspects of Peripheral Neuropathy 199
    Peter Croft

10 — Co-ordinated Care of the Patient with Rheumatoid Disease . 221
    A. G. White

11 — The Bullous Dermatoses 253
    C. M. Ridley

12 — Serum Enzymes in Diagnosis 273
    T. L. Dormandy

13 — Multiple Choice Questions and Case Presentations 287

Index 315

Preface

Formal postgraduate lectures and bed-side teaching were started at Whittington Hospital just 25 years ago and hence the contributors to this book are experienced in clinical teaching and the needs of the postgraduate students. The book is not intended to be comprehensive but each chapter aims at providing a balanced and informed review of subjects of current interest.

The examination for the diploma of Membership of the Royal College of Physicians of the U.K. is in two parts. Part 1 consists of multiple choice questions. Part 2 now contains a written section with case histories and data interpretation. The last chapter of this book contains typical multiple choice questions, case histories and data interpretation, with appropriate answers and comments.

It is hoped that this book will prove of particular value to postgraduates working for a higher degree and will help them to gain a better understanding of the problems and attitudes in modern medicine.

Arnold Bloom

1

The Examination of the Cardiac Case

E. Montuschi

INTRODUCTION

The examination of a patient with cardiac disease or disorder presents a challenge to the young physician. This chapter has been written, not as a comprehensive survey of all possible physical signs, but in the hope that it may help in surmounting a number of difficulties which have been found to occur more frequently when teaching post-graduates.

The physician who, in the presence of a cardiac case, rushes immediately to his stethoscope in search of the murmur immediately displays a lack of understanding of what cardiology is all about. Even when a qualitative diagnosis is reached by such a rudimentary examination a full diagnosis, which must comprise an assessment of the severity of the lesion, requires careful observation of the effects that disordered action of the heart has on the arterial and venous circulation, both at systemic and pulmonary levels.

POINTS IN DIAGNOSIS

It should be remembered, first of all, that a diminished supply of fully oxygenated blood to the tissues during the years of growth leads to stunting of growth. This may be generalized, and of cardinal importance in paediatric cardiology, or localized, as in the failure of the lower limbs to match the development of the upper limbs in coarctation of the aorta. More commonly, a small aortic knuckle in mitral valve disease signifies that obstruction of blood flow at the mitral ring was already significant during the years of growth. A general examination might show developmental abnormalities such as Marfan and Down's syndrome which correlate with some forms of congenital heart disease. Recently, although as yet in a small number of cases, lentiginosis has

1

been found to correlate with hypertrophic obstructive cardiomyopathy. Adenoma sebaceum should raise a suspicion of a rhabdomyoma of the myocardium while macroglossia should point to the possibility of cardiac amyloidosis. Cardiac haemosiderosis should spring to mind in the presence of abnormal pigmentation. A premature arcus senilis, xanthelasma and xanthoma tendinosum indicate the likelihood of familial disorders of lipid metabolism and with it premature coronary artery disease. Disturbance of thyroid and pituitary function may prove to be the key to the aetiology of some cardiac disorders, as may signs of severe anaemia, always remembering that the clinical diagnosis of moderate anaemia can be excessively misleading. The stigmata of Paget's disease may explain a hyperdynamic circulatory state occasionally leading to failure. A nutritional history may be of considerable importance, with special reference to alcohol intake. One must not forget the recently described epidemic of cardiomyopathies due to cobalt contamination of beer described in Canada. Obviously a history of prolonged severe thiamine deficiency would suggest beriberi heart disease. The family history itself may point to the familial variety of hypertrophic cardiomyopathy and deafness, with a familial history of sudden death, may alert to a more careful observation of the Q–T interval in the electrocardiogram (ECG). This is found to be prolonged in the sordo-cardiac syndrome.

Familial neurological disorders such as Friedreich's ataxia and dystrophia myotonica are often accompanied by cardiomyopathies and disorders of conduction.

Epidemiology also has an important contribution if one recalls the African cardiomyopathies, the possibility that pulmonary hypertension may be due to schistosomiasis, and that disorders of rhythm and cardiomyopathies may be due to Chagas' disease.

The presence or absence of cyanosis must be noted and, if present, whether it be central or peripheral. Differential cyanosis, more marked in the lower than the upper limbs, is pathognomonic of patent ductus arteriosus with a reversed shunt. While a malar flush is characteristically found in mitral valve disease, which may still be in the presymptomatic stage, it is very common in advanced cardiac failure of whatever origin. It is then often associated with a mottled cyanosis of the extremities and with a peculiar yellowish tinge of the skin even in the absence of jaundice. These are the findings of a chronic low-output state.

Clubbing, when accompanied by central cyanosis, usually indicates a right-to-left shunt at cardiac or pulmonary level. Clubbing without cyanosis should raise a suspicion of bacterial endocarditis. The suspicion would be heightened by the findings of subungual splinter haemorrhages but these are not pathognomonic as they may also be found in the normal. Osler's nodes and the less commonly remembered Janaway's spots (0.5 cm macules on the palms and soles) and boat shaped fundal haemorrhages make the diagnosis of bacterial endocarditis nearly certain.

The patient's breathing and posture will then be observed. Orthopnoea is a sign of stiff lungs from pulmonary venous congestion. The patient's ability to lie flat in spite of signs of right ventricular (RV) failure (that is, a raised jugular venous pressure, a large liver with or without ascites and dependent oedema), should bring to mind the possibility of obstruction to RV inflow. The obstruction may be extracardiac (as in constrictive pericarditis) or at atrial level, as in the rare right atrial myxoma, or more commonly in tricuspid valve disease. When the obstruction is at RV level, the lesion may be due to failure of compliance of the right ventricle (as in cardiac amyloidosis) or to an obstructive cardiomyopathy involving the right ventricle, either primarily or because of bulging of the interventricular septum into the RV cavity, as in the disputed Bernheim Syndrome.

The Arterial Pulses

From the days of Hippocrates the peripheral pulse has been of prime importance in the diagnosis of circulatory states, and it remains so because it more accurately reflects the degree of altered haemodynamics at cardiac level than the findings at examination of the heart itself, especially when dealing with aortic valve disease. It is always wise to feel both radial pulses simultaneously. Inequality of these pulses may be due to local anatomical variants or to atheromatous narrowing or obstruction. However, in aortic stenosis (and particularly in the congenital supravalvular variety) the right radial and carotid pulses may be wider than the left. This is due to a jet effect from the stenotic orifice up to the innominate artery. Routine and simultaneous examination of the radial and femoral pulses will ensure against the clinical crime of missing the diagnosis of aortic coarctation. The presence of foot pulses does not guard against failure to make this diagnosis. Little will be said about the quality of the pulse, whether of full or small volume and whether collapsing or tardus or bisferiens, except to emphasize the importance of these observations and to warn that in minor deviations from the normal, observer error is high, even to the experts. One should not make a diagnosis on physical signs which are not clear-cut. Special mention is made of a flicking pulse because of recent interest in hypertrophic obstructive cardiomyopathies. Pulsus alternans, an important sign of early left ventricular (LV) failure, is easily missed by the palpating finger if alternation is less than 20 mmHg, and it is frequently missed at sphygmomanometry unless thought of and looked for. The same applies to the misnamed arterial pulsus paradoxus of Kussmaul. This sign is not pathognomonic of pericardial constriction or effusion — it may be present in the acute stages of obstructive airways disease, and with diminished RV compliance as in cardiac amyloidosis, and also with a very flabby myocardium. It has recently been described in acute pulmonary embolism.

Disturbances of rhythm are usually easily recognized if it is remembered that a compensatory pause is the hallmark of ventricular ectopic beats and that, with complete irregularity, the presence of two consecutive long pauses is the hallmark of atrial fibrillation. The ear is, however, much more sensitive than touch in detecting disorders of rhythm. When in doubt, auscultation should supplement and take precedence over palpation in the diagnosis of dysrhythmias. Auscultation also has the advantage of enabling the detection of very premature heart beats which may not reach the arterial pulses. It is slovenly to talk about a fibrillating pulse, as fibrillation obviously occurs at atrial level. The term 'completely irregular' seems preferable to the more pedantic one of 'irregularly irregular'. Sinus arrhythmia is rarely present in hyperdynamic circulatory states. In particular, it is excessively rare in thyrotoxicosis with its predominant sympathetic tone and is therefore a useful sign in the differential 'office' diagnosis between a nervous tachycardia and thyrotoxicosis.

In significant aortic regurgitation the arterial pulses can be seen in the neck (Corrigan's sign). The impulse may impart a synchronous nodding to the head (de Musset's sign) and may also cause an impulse to the retinal arteries. In order to detect this phenomenon the retinal arteries are best observed on a bend. A coarse arterial impulse is not infrequently observed at the root of the neck on the right and is usually due to kinking of the common carotid; it is not infrequently accompanied by a fixed distension of the left external jugular vein. This syndrome is usually found in middle-aged or elderly women. Foreshortening of the thoracic cage from post-menopausal osteoporosis with unfolding of the arch of the aorta, presses the innominate artery up into the neck; this leads to kinking of the right carotid and also causes mild pressure on the left innominate vein. It may also cause the aortic impulse to be easily seen and felt in the suprasternal notch.

The Venous Pulse

The behaviour of the jugular veins repays careful observation *(Figure 1.1)*. From a study of the jugular venous pulse James Mackenzie described accurately disorders of cardiac rhythm without the aid of the electrocardiograph. Observation must therefore comprise a study of the various components of the jugular venous pulse, when present, as obviously in atrial fibrillation there will be no A waves. Simple observational mistakes may be due to faulty posturing of the patient at an

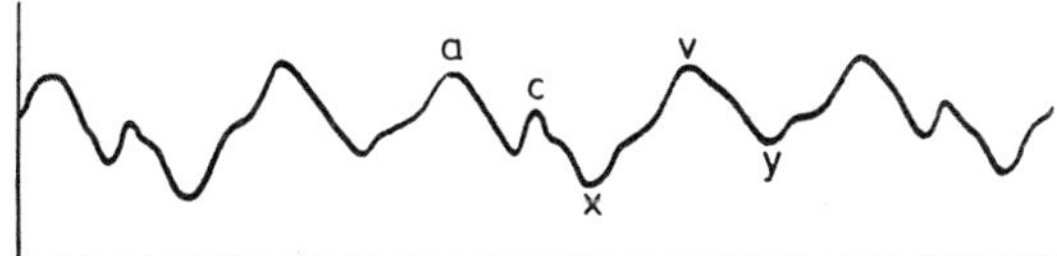

Figure 1.1. The normal jugular phlebogram

angle of less than 45 degrees and to the failure of distinguishing between a venous and an arterial pulsation in the neck. The latter transmits a clear impulse to the palpating finger and is not subject to variation with the manoeuvres which increase or decrease the venous impulse such as the phases of respiration, light pressure at the root of the neck, and abdominal compression, which increases central venous pressure. It cannot be too strongly emphasized that pressure over an enlarged liver in the right subcostal region, with a view to demonstrating a so-called hepato-jugular reflux, is a manoeuvre that should be relegated to the dustbin of oblivion. It offers no advantage over manual compression of the lower abdomen in increasing central venous pressure, and pressure over a large congested liver is known to cause unnecessary discomfort to the patient.

The most common error in the clinical study of the jugular venous pulse is to confine one's observation to the superficial veins, neglecting the deep ones. Deep vein pulsations are best observed in slanting light as a diffuse impulse which might well move the lower lobes of the ears. Indeed, the venous impulse may occasionally reach the temporal fossa, a phenomenon easily missed when the mind is unprepared to expect it. In severe congestive cardiac failure it is not infrequent to find an apparent discrepancy between the height of the superficial and the deep venous pressures, the pressures seeming to be lower in the superficial than in the deep veins. It has been shown that a considerable increase in venous tone occurs in congestive cardiac failure, presumably mediated through an increase in circulating catecholamines. Increased venous tone would more easily obstruct venous flow in the superficial than in the deep veins. The superficial veins are smaller in calibre and are also exposed to ambient temperature, while the larger deep veins are always at central body temperature. These comments may explain the apparent paradox of the difference in height of the venous column between the superficial and the deep veins.

When the A waves are present and clearly observable they may be useful in the diagnosis of disorders of rhythm such as atrial flutter and second and third degree heart block. Cannon waves occur when atrial contraction occurs against a closed tricuspid valve. They thus occur more frequently with junctional ectopic beats. In complete heart block cannon waves are not synchronous with cannon sounds as the latter occur when P–R interval is very short. Giant A waves may signify tricuspid valve stenosis where the gentle slope of the Y descent repays observation. They also occur with increased end diastolic pressure in the right ventricle either because of pulmonary valve stenosis or because of severe pulmonary hypertension. Large V waves are instead the hallmark of tricuspid regurgitation but deductions about the valvular or functional origin of tricuspid regurgitation cannot be made on this basis alone. The tricuspid ring is easily stretched with dilatation of the right ventricle, and it has been known for many years that tricuspid regurgitation is constantly present when there is congestive cardiac failure. However, in the presence of conspicuous V waves it is useful to notice whether or not the venous impulses are transmitted to the liver imparting an expansile pulse to it. This sign is reliable only if the impulse is felt on bimanual palpation of the right lower costal margin. Occasionally, the refluxing venous impulse reaches the lower limbs and can be observed in large venous varicosities. A rise instead of a fall in the venous pressure on inspiration is an important sign of constrictive pericarditis or cardiac temponade. As there is no obstruction, in early diastole, to venous inflow into the right heart, the Y descent will be precipitous if short, contrary to what happens in tricuspid stenosis. The venous pressure rises abnormally in expiration in obstructive airways disease because of the magnitude of the expiratory increase in intrathoracic pressure. It is therefore not a sign of congestive cardiac failure.

METHODS OF EXAMINATION

Inspection

Inspection of the anterior chest wall may show a generalized bulging on the left. When this can be shown not to be due to an asymmetry secondary to spinal deformity, bulging of the precordium indicates that significant enlargement of the heart was present during the years of growth. Systolic retraction of the intercostal spaces anteriorly indicates considerable cardiac enlargement and should not suggest adherent pericardium. Broadbent's sign of adherent pericardium also consists of systolic retraction of the intercostal spaces, but in the posterior axillary line. This sign must be comparatively rare.

An abnormal localized impulse may, rarely, be observed to the right of the sternum in aneurysms of the ascending aorta.

In ischaemic heart disease careful inspection of the chest wall on the left is well worth carrying out as it may give a first clue to the presence of an aneurysm of the left ventricle or to a large area of ventricular dyskinesia.

The apex beat may be visible. When forceful (because of LV hypertrophy) it might be observed to lift with a pre-systolic shudder which corresponds to the fourth heart sound. A forceful epigastric pulsation indicates RV hypertrophy. It can be a useful additional sign in the diagnosis of pulmonary embolism and in the assessment of pulmonary hypertension in mitral valve disease. It is often present in cor pulmonale.

Percussion

Percussion is of very limited value in assessing the size of the cardiac chambers because of the very wide observer error. It can be useful in determining the apex beat when this is neither visible nor palpable. An area of cardiac dullness external to the apex beat can suggest pericardial effusion. Dullness to the right in the third interspace may be due to aneurysmatic dilatation of the ascending aorta.

Palpation

While percussion rarely yields useful information, an examination of the heart without careful palpation of the precordium is necessarily incomplete. A general impression of tumultuous action of the heart confirms the impression of a hyperdynamic circulatory state suggested by the warmth of the hands and the rapid full pulse.

The apex beat should be felt both with the full palm of the hand, and, when lifting, with a slightly flexed index finger. With the palm of the hand a first appreciation will be gained of whether there is RV or LV hypertrophy as RV hypertrophy gives rise to a localized lift in only extremely rare instances. With the open hand a tapping apex beat can be appreciated. The word tapping describes a sharp localized tap which corresponds to the closing snap of the mitral valve. In pure mitral stenosis the right ventricle dominates over the left; therefore most tapping apex beats are RV in character. However, aortic valve disease or systemic hypertension can co-exist with mitral stenosis. The apex beat will then be LV in character but will retain its central tap. With the open palm the presence or absence of apical thrills will be noted.

Palpation of the apex beat with the flexed right index finger makes it easier to localize the impulse, to appreciate its force, and to note whether it is sustained, as in aortic valve stenosis and in systemic hypertension, or flicking, as in aortic regurgitation. Careful exmination of a lifting apex beat often demonstrates a hump in the ascending limb of the beat, this being due to the fourth heart sound.

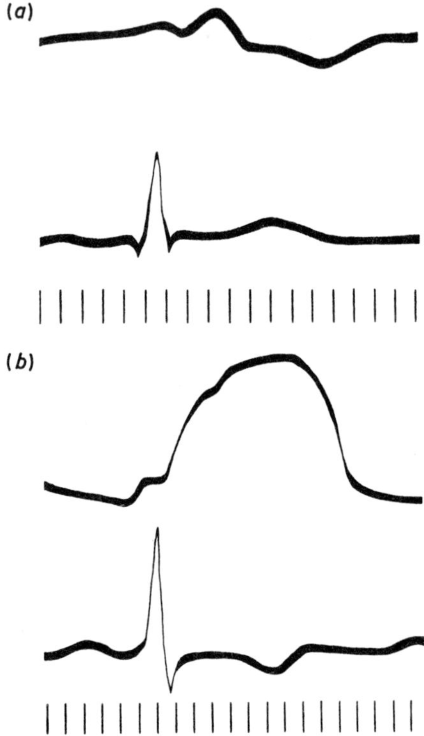

Figure 1.2. (a) Normal apex cardiogram with reference ECG. (b) Apex cardiogram in significant aortic stenosis. The atrial beat is clearly seen. Reference ECG.

Third heart sounds, normal and pathological, can rarely be appreciated by the examining finger but may be registered by the apex cardiogram. The same technique of examination should be applied to other visible impulses in the chest wall due to post-infarction ventricular aneurysm or large areas of ventricular dyskinesia. When present it is interesting to follow the impulse from the point of its maximal intensity along the rib which can be rocked so that a lift can be appreciated right up to the anterior axillary line.

Radiography and radioscopy show the classic appearances of LV aneurysm only in a minority of these cases although, of course, cine-angiography of the left ventricle more readily demonstrates areas of LV dyskinesia. Obviously, these investigations are only justified if aneurysmectomy or infarctectomy are envisaged.

Palpation of the left parasternal region is an obligatory step in the examination of the cardiac case. A sustained left parasternal heave is present when there is pulmonary hypertension although this might be masked by overlying lung in obstructive airways disease. In significant pulmonary hypertension the pulmonary component of the second may be felt. Systolic, and, much more rarely, diastolic, thrills may be felt in aortic and pulmonary valve disease but a systolic thrill does not necessarily denote a significant obstruction to ventricular outflow if the cardiac output is high.

Auscultation

Auscultation of the heart requires not so much exceptional qualities of hearing as the ability to concentrate the attention on what may be significant in the given case, ignoring at that moment other phenomena in the cardiac cycle. The data are always meaningful and must be interpreted in the light of haemodynamic events, even when the final diagnosis is that of normal variants or innocent murmurs. The word innocent is to be preferred to the word functional as the latter is equivocal in its meaning. A Graham Steell murmur, for example, does not signify organic disease of the pulmonary valve but pulmonary regurgitation actually takes place because of highly significant pulmonary hypertension: it is a functional but not an innocent murmur. From the viewpoint of mental discipline and training, and for clarity in the record, it is useful to make a graphic representation of the findings at auscultation.

It must be pointed out immediately that the classical areas of auscultation, the mitral, tricuspid, aortic and pulmonary areas, are distant from the heart valves which are bunched together at the centre of the heart. These areas represent only the loci where heart sounds and murmurs which originate from a given heart valve are usually best appreciated. Heart sounds which are due to valve closure in low pressure areas transmit poorly so that tricuspid valve closure cannot be heard at the base of the heart and pulmonary valve closure can only be appreciated at the apex when there is pulmonary hypertension. Sounds and murmurs transmit in the direction of the blood stream — hence the classical areas of auscultation. An aortic diastolic murmur may be heard only at the apex or might transmit to the sole of the foot. With dilatation of the ascending aorta, now more commonly of atheromatous than of luetic origin, it is not surprising that the murmur of aortic reflux should be heard maximally to the right of the sternum. Murmurs also transmit through bone, especially aortic ejection murmurs. These are best heard over the right clavicle with the diaphragm of the stethoscope and, when loud, they can be followed to the tip of the acromion, to the olecranon, and also to the styloid process of the radius. Even a loud mitral systolic murmurs rarely transmits to the clavicle. The loudness of the murmurs is related not only to the severity of the anatomical lesion but also to blood flow. This is best demonstrated by listening to an aortic ejection murmur in a patient with atrial fibrillation, when it will be easy to appreciate how the intensity of the murmur varies with the length of the preceding diastolic pause. The autopsy finding of a pinpoint aortic or mitral stenosis can cause an unpleasant shock to the clinician who had failed to diagnose the condition in life because the extreme poverty of blood flow did not give rise to a murmur. As an insurance against this it is wise to screen a patient with unexplained cardiac failure with the image intensifier which will reveal heavy calcification of the affected valve.

HEART SOUNDS

The key to ausculation is clear identification of the first and second heart sounds as such. At average heart rates and when there are no added sounds, little difficulty is experienced because of the difference in duration between the systolic and diastolic pauses between the heart sounds. At high rates it is useful to attempt to slow the heart with carotid sinus pressure. When this fails the advice commonly given is to time events in the cardiac cycle by simultaneous auscultation of the heart and palpation of the carotid or radial pulse. This advice is usually unhelpful and is based on the unsound comparison between instrumentally obtained simultaneous reference tracings such as a phonocardiogram and a carotid pulse tracing, with the clinical examination. In a difficult situation, when the clinician's ear (his most accurate timing device) gives rise to uncertainty, he is asked to perform an even more difficult task — that of splitting his attention between what he hears and what he feels, in order to clarify the situation. The examiner should instead inch his way with the stethoscope over the precordium and the various elective areas of auscultation. At some point, usually towards the base of the heart, the identification of the first and second sound as such will become clear and other added sounds and murmurs can be placed by inching back to the area of auscultation where they were noted at first. When the apex beat is thrusting and well localized, timing of the heart sounds can be helped also by watching the systolic lift imparted to the examiner's stethoscope. A fourth heart sound can also not infrequently be seen by this technique *(Figure 1.3)*.

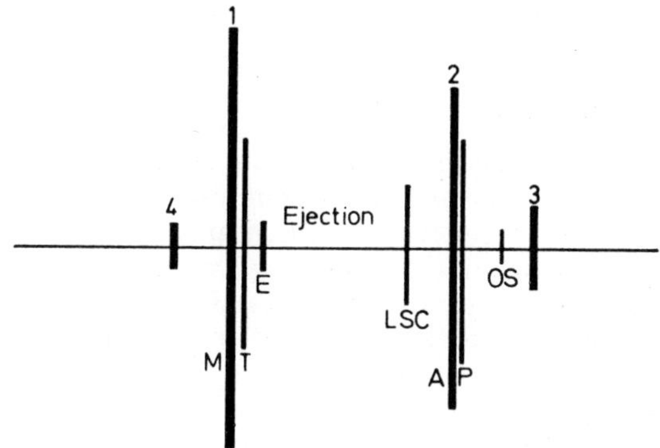

Figure 1.3. The normal heart sounds and possible added sounds

The First Heart Sound

This is mainly due to the closure of the mitral and tricuspid valves. It may be asynchronous, especially in the presence of right bundle branch block (RBBB). An unusually wide split of the first sound is characteristic of Ebstein's anomaly of the tricuspid valve with which there will also be splitting of the second sound giving rise to a characteristic quadruple rhythm. Tricuspid valve closure does not transmit widely except in organic tricuspid stenosis; therefore, splitting of the first heart sound should be diagnosed with considerable diffidence if it can be heard at the base of the heart. Some other explanation, such as an ejection click, will usually be found to be correct. A number of factors influence the intensity of the first heart sound, one particular factor being the thickness of the chest wall and the presence or absence of overlying lung; in severe obstructive airways disease the only profitable area of auscultation may be over the bare area of the xiphisternum.

Other factors being equal, the intensity of the first heart sound depends on the distance travelled by the valves in closing. An early atrial contraction will thrust the valves into the ventricular cavity and allow time for them gently to float upwards; the first heart sound will be soft. A late atrial contraction will thrust the valves deep into the ventricular cavity with little time for them to float upwards; the first heart sound will be loud. Therefore, when a study of a jugular venous pulse has not already given the clue, careful auscultation permits a diagnosis of a prolonged P-R interval and, more confidently, of a variable P-R interval. No magic, only a little care, is needed. The exceptionally loud mitral first sound found in mitral stenosis is due to the closing snap of the mitral valve and corresponds to a tapping apex beat.

The Second Heart Sound

The second heart sound is due to closure of the semilunar valves. As pulmonary valve closure is a low pressure event it is best heard parasternally at the third left interspace. It transmits widely and to the apex only when there is significant pulmonary hypertension. Careful study of the second heart sound, the identification of its components, and their behaviour with the phases of respiration, is extremely worthwhile. In the normal, the surge of blood into the RV cavities on inspiration delays pulmonary valve closure giving rise to an inspiratory split of the second sound. An RBBB will further widen the split which will then usually be accompanied by a split first sound. A wide fixed split of the second sound is the hallmark of atrial septal defect. Respiratory variations of blood flow through the RV cavity (and hence the pulmonary artery) are offset by variations in size of the interatrial left-to-right shunt of opposite sign as the left-to-right shunt diminishes in proportion to the inspiratory increase in venous return to the right atrium. A wide fixed split of the second sound has also been described in thrombo-embolic pulmonary hypertension. Here the pulmonary component of the second sound will be markedly accentuated. In significant pulmonary stenosis the pulmonary component of the second sound will be delayed and be considerably attenuated. As pulmonary systolic murmurs are common in young people with vigorous heart action and particularly in pregnancy (there are frequent referrals for a cardiological opinion from ante-natal clinics) a careful appraisal of the second heart sound usually permits the distinction between an innocent flow murmur and organic heart disease to be made with confidence on clinical grounds alone.

Whenever there is significant delay in activation of LV contraction, as in coarse left bundle branch block (LBBB) or when there is prolongation of LV systole, as in some cases of hypertensive heart disease, in aortic stenosis, in ischaemic heart disease and (because of volume overload) in some patients with patent ductus arteriosus, aortic valve closure may occur after pulmonary valve closure. There will then be reversed splitting of the second sound which is diagnosed clinically because the split is wider on expiration and closes on inspiration. This may be of interest in the assessment of early and yet nearly symptomless hypertensive heart disease and in intermittent LBBB.

Rapid Ventricular Filling Sounds

These comprise the third and fourth heart sounds and summation gallop. The terminology used leaves unjudged the still controversial question of whether the sounds are solely produced by rapid distension of the ventricular wall or whether vibration of the mitral and tricuspid valve leaflets, set in action by rapid ventricular filling, are necessary for their production. Rapid ventricular filling sounds are of low frequency and do not tend to transmit widely, but in summation gallop, when the third and fourth heart sound are added, the louder sound may occasionally transmit to the base. The third heart sound can frequently be heard in youths and men up to the age of 35, especially when the heart action is vigorous. It is rarely heard with the subject sitting and standing as in these postures venous return to the heart is diminished. A faint physiological third sound can be made louder by increasing venous return with elevation of the legs. These manoeuvres can be useful in identifying the third sound in cases of doubt. Significant mitral regurgitation, because of rapid ventricular filling, gives rise to a loud third sound beyond the age at which physiological third sounds are heard, without the grave meaning of a protodiastolic gallop from ventricular failure. As rapid ventricular filling is needed to produce the third sound it is incompatible with mitral stenosis. When found in a patient with pure mitral stenosis it must originate from the right ventricle because of severe pulmonary hypertension. Not unexpectedly, a loud third sound is found in constrictive pericarditis, there being no obstacle to the rapid inrush of blood from the systemic and pulmonary veins at the beginning of diastole. The pathological protodiastolic gallop is indistinguishable in timing and character from a physiological third sound. Atrial pressure must, however, be raised and we are dealing with a sick subject rather than with a healthy youth.

The fourth heart sound is inaudible in the normal. It becomes audible with increased force of atrial contraction because of raised end-diastolic pressure in the receiving ventricle. It is a very common abnormal physical sign in systemic and pulmonary hypertension, in ischaemic heart disease and in cardiomyopathies, and can occur at the stage when symptoms of ventricular failure are few. Not unexpectedly, a right atrial fourth sound is accompanied by a large A wave in the jugular venous pulse. We shall recall that a left atrial fourth heart sound cannot infrequently be felt by careful palpation of the apex and that

13

occasionally it can also be seen. In complete heart block with a slow ventricular rate the sound produced by independent atrial contraction may be audible. It is particularly loud when an independent atrial contraction occurs in early diastole thus summating an otherwise inaudible third and fourth sound *(Figure 1.4)*.

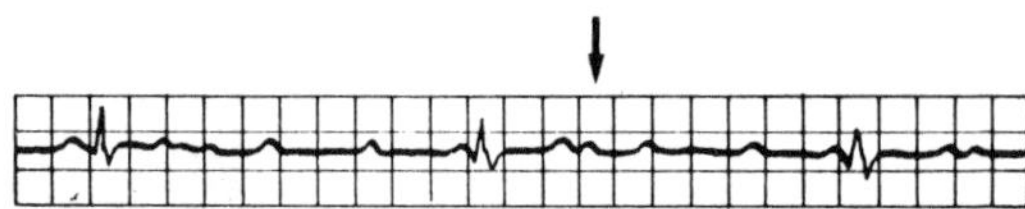

Figure 1.4. ECG of a patient with complete heart block. The arrow indicates the point at which an added sound is clearly audible due to summation of a third and fourth heart sound

At moderately high rates, and in particular when the P–R interval is prolonged, a third and fourth heart sound may summate, producing a loud triple rhythm. It is then useful to try to slow the heart rate by carotid sinus pressure. When this succeeds the added sound may disappear, thus proclaiming itself an innocent phenomenon; if it remains, the longer diastolic pause will permit its timing and identification as a third or fourth sound.

Snaps and Clicks

Snaps and clicks are the words we use to describe the quality of those added sounds which are high pitched and of brief duration, unlike the low pitched third and fourth sounds previously discussed. The opening snap of a thickened and stenosed mitral and tricuspid valve is a sign well known from the beginning of the century, but it came into its own with the advent of cardiac surgery when it was shown that its presence guaranteed that at least the anterior cusp of the mitral valve remained pliant. Its absence makes it likely that the valve is heavily calcified and unsuitable for a closed surgical approach. The opening snap is a very common physical sign in mitral stenosis and it is nearly always present when apex beat is tapping in quality and the first sound is loud. There is as yet excessive timidity in recognizing its presence, the most common error in diagnosis being a split second sound. However, the time interval is larger and the relation of the added sound to aortic valve closure is practically constant. Indeed, the opening snap is often a very loud sound which transmits even to the second right interspace, the so-called aortic area. When the snap is weak the point of election for auscultation is internally to the apex beat. With the heart in sinus

14

rhythm an opening snap can be diagnosed with certainty if, listening in the third left interspace, the second heart sound can be heard to split on inspiration, with the added sound remaining constant *(Figure 1.5)*. There is some relation between the height of the left atrial pressure and the timing of the opening snap, an early opening snap indicating a higher left atrial pressure than a late one; this becomes particularly clear after mitral commissurotomy which rarely obliterates the added sound.

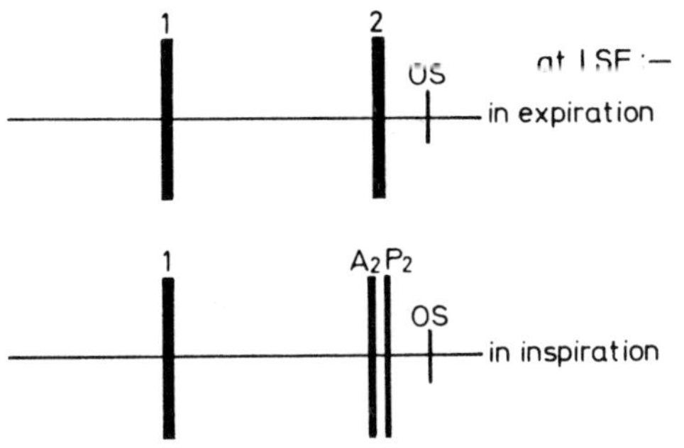

Figure 1.5. A demonstration of the inspiratory split which proves that the added sound is an opening snap

Ejection clicks are clicking sounds which occur very soon after the first heart sound and are due mainly to sudden distension of the aorta or the pulmonary artery in systemic or pulmonary hypertension, or when there is aortic or pulmonary valve stenosis. Ejection clicks are not present in supra- and sub-valvular stenosis. The added sound may be louder than the first sound; there is then a differential diagnosis with a split first heart sound and with an atrial sound followed by a first heart sound. Although, occasionally, the correct diagnosis can only be established by a phonocardiogram with a simultaneous carotid reference tracing, usually inching the stethoscope around the anterior chest wall permits an accurate identification of the findings. Mid and late systolic clicks were thought to be due to the snapping of a small pericardial adhesion. Occasionally this interpretation may be correct as when the clicking systolic noise can be observed to appear for the first time after a myocardial infarction. More commonly mid and late systolic clicks represent a congenital anomaly of the chordae tendineae of the mitral valve. When they are accompanied by a late systolic murmur there is usually minimal mitral regurgitation with ballooning of the posterior cusp of the mitral valve in the left atrium. Haemodynamically, the phenomenon is of no importance but cases of bacterial endocarditis have been described with the infection being implanted on this minor anatomical abnormality. Therefore, prophylactic protective action should be taken before dental extractions, etc. A late systolic click presents a problem in differential diagnosis with wide splitting of the second sound and with a second sound followed by an opening snap. These diagnostic errors will be avoided if the possibility of a late systolic click is kept in mind, and if correct timing of events in the cardiac cycle is sought by inching the stethoscope over the precordium and noticing the respiratory variations of the second heart sound.

HEART MURMURS

Systolic Murmurs

In the diagnosis of systolic murmurs attention should be focused mainly on the relation of the end of the murmur to the second heart sound. A murmur which runs up to the second sound must originate from a regurgitant mitral or tricuspid valve or from an intraventricular septal defect. Ejection systolic murmurs which end before the second heart sound, usually originate from the aortic or pulmonary valves. However, the murmur of VSD may be shortened by the development of a rise in pressure in the RV cavity (from pulmonary stenosis or pulmonary hypertension). It has also been shown that when mitral regurgitation arises from disease of the subvalvular apparatus it may cause an ejection rather than a pansystolic or late systolic murmur, thus making the diagnosis difficult. Late systolic murmurs have already been mentioned when discussing mid and late systolic clicks; they represent minimal mitral and occasionally tricuspid regurgitation. In deciding where a systolic murmur originates it is wise to follow it round from its area of maximal intensity in order, for example, better to appreciate the character of the second sound or to note the presence of an ejection click. It will be remembered that systolic murmurs from the aorta and pulmonary artery transmit readily to bone, while mitral and tricuspid murmurs do not. Pharmacological tests with drugs which cause a fall in intra-aortic pressure (for example, amyl nitrite) cause an increase in intensity of aortic ejection murmurs and a decrease in mitral regurgitant murmurs. Elevation of intra-aortic pressure, either with drugs or with a firm sustained hand-grip, have the opposite effect. This follows from the fact, already emphasized elsewhere, that the intensity and length of the murmur is related not only to the severity of the anatomical lesion but also to blood flow. However, in aortic and pulmonary valve stenosis there is a good correlation between the site of maximal intesity of the murmur in systole and the severity of the lesion, maximal intensity being early with little obstruction to ventricular outflow, and much later in systole with considerable valvular obstruction to ventricular outflow *(Figure 1.6)*.

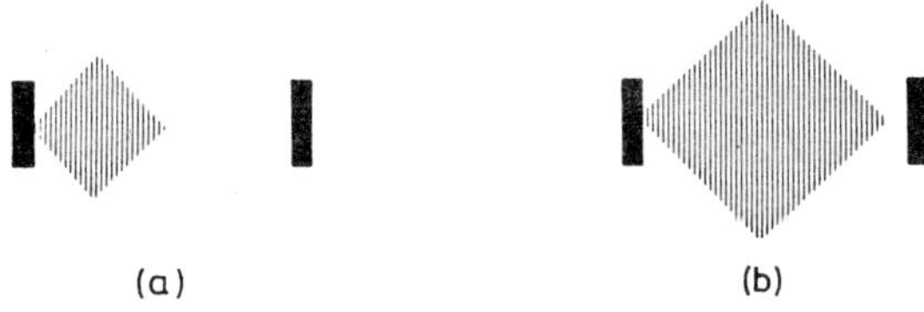

(a)　　　　　　　　　　(b)

Figure 1.6. Ventricular outflow with (a) no obstruction,
and (b) moderate obstruction

In hypertrophic obstructive cardiomyopathy the maximal intensity of the murmur will also be late in systole. The absence of obstruction to LV outflow in early systole will be revealed by the flicking character of the pulse. This again emphasizes that careful auscultation alone may not give a full diagnosis. As for tricuspid systolic murmurs, the inspiratory increase in blood flow to the RV cavity will increase the intensity of the murmur in inspiration except when tricuspid regurgitation is so severe that the right atrium and right ventricle form a practical continuum.

Diastolic Murmurs

These are due either to mitral and tricuspid stenosis or to aortic or pulmonary regurgitation. The frequency of the murmur (low pitched in stenotic murmurs; high pitched in regurgitant ones) and the timing of its maximal intensity (crescendo in stenotic and decrescendo in regurgitant murmurs) are useful in the differential diagnosis. The relation between the onset of the murmur and the second heart sound is the most important point in the differential diagnosis between a diastolic murmur of mitral stenosis and that of aortic regurgitation. There is an obligatory gap — often indicated by the opening snap, and due to the absence of blood flow at the time — between the second heart sound and the onset of the murmur of tricuspid and mitral stenosis. The term 'delayed diastolic murmurs' is more precise than the usually adopted appellation 'mid-diastolic murmurs'. Even when delayed diastolic murmurs are not due to organic valvular stenosis, but to torrential blood flow through the mitral and tricuspid valves, there is a delay in their onset which is often indicated by a loud third sound. To the auscultating ear there is no appreciable delay between the second heart sound and the onset of diastolic murmur of aortic and pulmonary regurgitation. Here again the appellation 'immediate' is preferable to the less definite but more commonly used 'early' diastolic murmur. Similarly, the word 'blowing' is a poor description of an aortic regurgitant murmur since this word describes a process of blowing out rather than of actual refluxing of blood into the ventricular cavity. The French 'souffle aspiratif' accurately describes both the acoustic and haemodynamic events. In this country we need only refrain from using a word which is both unnecessary and misleading. While the murmurs of aortic and pulmonary regurgitation are decrescendo, for obvious haemodynamic reasons*, the crescendo murmur of mitral and tricuspid stenosis frequently ends with a presystolic accentuation due to atrial systole. This atrial systolic murmur may be the only one present and, when doubtful, it is made more prominent by placing the patient in the left lateral position. A true atrial systolic murmur obviously cannot occur in the presence of atrial fibrillation. Recently, however, it has been shown that a true presystolic accentuation of the delayed diastolic murmur can occur with atrial fibrillation due to an increased telediastolic gradient between the atrium and the ventricles. Tricuspid and pulmonary diastolic murmurs increase in intensity on inspiration because of the inspiratory increase in blood flow through the right cavities of the heart. The tricuspid diastolic flow murmur found in large atrial septal defects is an exception to this rule because of equalization of blood flow through variations of the shunt at intra-atrial level of opposite direction.

Continuous Murmurs

These originate at the site of continuous blood flow throughout the cardiac cycle and have the quality of the sound produced by a humming top. They do not usually radiate widely. They are to be distinguished from to and fro murmurs which have distinct systolic and diastolic components. The best known of continuous murmurs is the Gibson murmur from patent ductus arteriosus but a continuous murmur can originate from an aorto-pulmonary window, from a sinus of Valsava rupturing into the RV cavity, or from a fistula between a coronary artery and a cavity in the right heart. A continuous murmur originates at the site of anastomosis between a subclavian and pulmonary artery after the Blalock operation; its disappearance should lead to a strong suspicion that the anastomosis is no longer functioning. The systolic

*An exception is the crescendo diminuendo diastolic murmur which may rarely be heard at the third left interspace in stenosis of the left coronary artery. This is due to coronary blood flow being maximal in diastole.

18

murmur found in arterial stenosis may also spill over in diastole; this is not infrequently observed in carotid and subclavian stenosis.

EXOCARDIAL SOUNDS

Best known of the exocardial sounds is a pericardial friction rub. It is not uncommonly described as being most easily heard at the base of the heart although it is often best audible over the bare area at the xiphisternum. Pressure over the chest wall with a stethoscope increases the intensity of the scratching sound which is not quite synchronous with the systolic and diastolic phases of the cardiac cycle. A pericardial rub does not exclude the presence of a significant pericardial effusion because of the tendency of pericardial effusions to accumulate at the back of the heart. In lean subjects with a flat chest wall, and especially when there is some degree of pectus excavatus, a systolic grating sound is not infrequently found over the mid and lower sternum. It is obviously of exocardial origin. In massive acute pulmonary embolism an exocardial sound may be appreciated, presumably due to the sudden blowing out of the main trunk of the pulmonary artery. It is always a transient phenomenon.

THE LUNGS AND PLEURA

Passive venous congestion from obstruction to outflow of the left atrium or from LV failure leads to pulmonary oedema which will not be described in detail, this being more appropriate to a textbook of cardiology. It is well to recall, however, that in acute pulmonary oedema there is a considerable outpouring of catecholamines with consequent pallor, profuse sweating and an acute rise in blood pressure. The bronchial mucosa may participate in the oedema, thus increasing the degree of ventilatory obstruction. In middle-aged and elderly patients who already have a degree of obstructive airways disease the bedside differential diagnosis between an exacerbation of true obstructive airways disease and added LV failure may be difficult. In these circumstances an emergency x-ray of the chest may be invaluable because a mistake in diagnosis and treatment can be fatal. In less acute cases, when there are only basal crepitations, radiography of the chest is also invaluable in the differential diagnosis. Heart failure is too frequently diagnosed because of the finding of basal crepitations which may be due simply to bronchial over-secretion, especially in chronic smokers. Routine daily radiographs of the chest in coronary care units have clearly shown a poor correlation between symptoms and signs with the degree of pulmonary oedema demonstrated on the x-ray films.

Pleural effusions complicate congestive cardiac failure and, when large, contribute to respiratory embarrassment, especially when left-sided. There is only a statistical correlation between the side of the pleural effusion and the cardiac chamber dominantly affected.

THE ABDOMEN

Passive venous congestion in the territory of the great veins leads to swelling of the liver which may become acutely swollen and tender and thus cause abdominal discomfort, anorexia and vomiting. In small children, vomiting may be an early symptom of heart failure. It will be recalled that expansile pulsation of the liver occurs in organic tricuspid disease and that it is best appreciated with bi-manual palpation of the right lower costal region rather than with abdominal palpation of the liver. Chronic passive venous congestion can also lead to moderate splenomegaly, clinically appreciable. In organic tricuspid valvular disease and in constrictive pericarditis, hepatomegaly and ascites may apparently dominate the clinical picture thus leading the unwary into a mistaken diagnosis of primary hepatic disease. Careful observation of the jugular venous pulse will help in avoiding this mistake. Because of the fall in cardiac output and passive venous congestion, cardiac failure leads to avid salt and water retention by the kidneys, thus causing oedema. In chronic severe cardiac failure wasting and anasarca also reflect protein malnutrition which may be a compound of low intake, deficient synthesis by the liver, increased catabolism and frank protein-losing enteropathy. It would be inappropriate to describe this here but a general warning is given that oedema is not due to cardiac failure unless there are other manifestations of the disease. Cardiac failure is too frequently diagnosed because of the finding of dependent oedema which is due to other causes.

ACKNOWLEDGEMENT

My thanks are due to Dr. Peter Gillam for permission to base *Figure 1.2a* and *b* on his slides.

2

Ischaemic Heart Disease: Aetiology and Prevention

D. E. Sharland

INTRODUCTION

The epidemic diseases of 50 years ago — diphtheria, tuberculosis and poliomyelitis, for example — have now been largely replaced as a cause of morbidity and mortality by ischaemic heart disease (IHD). In the U.K. in 1968 IHD was responsible for over 30,000 deaths occurring in men aged 35–64; these deaths all occurred in men at their most productive time of life. Both the numbers and the percentage of women of this age group dying from IHD are lower — about 7,500 out of approximately 57,000 deaths. Likewise, in the U.S.A. and Australia, deaths from IHD account for nearly one-third of all deaths in men aged 35–64. These figures take no account of the death rate in the 65-year-olds and over, in which group the rate continues to rise, especially in women. The financial cost to the U.S.A. has been estimated to run into billions of dollars a year (not to mention the emotional loss to the families concerned).

Just as the approach to the management of infectious diseases was preventative, so it will be shown that the management of IHD must be the same. Whatever the value of intensive coronary care, anticoagulants and cardiac surgery, the fact is that nearly one-third of cases first present as 'sudden death'. A large proportion of these will occur outside hospitals and many will never see a doctor. Hospital series of cases will tend to be biased by the absence of those patients presenting with 'sudden death' as the first manifestation of the disease.

The problem will be considered under three major headings:

(1)   Definition of IHD
(2)   Aetiology of IHD
(3)   Current attempts at prevention

DEFINITION OF IHD

An expert committee of World Health Organization put forward the following definition in 1962:

> 'IHD or coronary heart disease, is the cardiac disability, acute or chronic, arising from reduction or arrest of blood supply to the myocardium in association with disease processes in the coronary arterial system'.

It will be seen that IHD and coronary heart disease (CHD) are used interchangeably although etymologically they have slightly different meanings, common and widespread usage having resulted in their being regarded as synonymous. It is important, therefore, to note that coronary *heart* disease is not synonymous with coronary *artery* disease, which term should be reserved for the findings made at autopsy or on coronary angiography. Although coronary artery disease is almost universal, especially among adult men, IHD will probably affect about only one in four or five of those under the age of 65.

The World Health Organization also produced a clinical classification of IHD, but it is rather too cumbersome for most practical purposes. The various heart conditions grouped under the following four headings are suggested as being simpler and will cover about 95 per cent of cases seen.

Angina pectoris

In the classical case with chest pain or tightness which may radiate to one or both arms or up into the neck and may be related to physical or emotional stress, there is little dispute about the diagnosis. It is, however, subjective and dependent on the history given by the patient and the assessment of that history by the physician. This produces considerable problems when considering the incidence of angina pectoris as recorded by physicians in different countries or even by physicians in the same country. Objective evidence, as provided by the electrocardiogram (ECG) may range from a Q wave infarct, T wave changes only, ECG changes present only on exercise, and even a normal ECG. Angina has to be differentiated from chest pain arising from other sites such as the oesophagus and musculo-skeletal system. The presence of ischaemic changes in the ECG does not automatically rule out non-cardiac causes of the pain. The pathologist at autopsy is quite unable to say that the patient had angina during life.

Myocardial Infarction

Clinically, this is usually the most obvious form of IHD. Within a few hours the histological and later macroscopic findings in the myocardium are usually quite clear. The extraordinary rarity of these findings in autopsies before the twentieth century is one of the strongest indications that IHD is a disease of the twentieth century. Myocardial infarction may be fatal or non-fatal.

Sudden Death

This is a very important group making up nearly one-third of all cases of IHD. In many it will be the first manifestation of this disease and by its very nature will tend to be omitted from hospital series of cases. Many such patients will never see a doctor in life. The definition of 'sudden' varies with different authorities, some using it to mean death 'within minutes' and others for death occurring in 'up to 6 days'. Not all 'sudden deaths' are due to IHD. Other causes include aortic stenosis, ruptural aneurysm and cerebral haemorrhage. There is, however, an appreciable tendency of ascribing to IHD all cases of 'sudden death' where no cause is immediately apparent.

Cardiac Failure

Cardiac failure (either left or right) may follow one or more episodes of IHD. In some patients cardiac failure may be the first mode of presentation of IHD. This seems to be rather more common in the older age-groups, although it must be emphasized that *not all* cases of cardiac failure in the elderly are due to IHD. Other causes will include cardiac amyloid, cardiomyopathies, and beriberi.

AETIOLOGY OF IHD

Many factors are involved in the aetiology of IHD though they are not all of equal importance. Some factors (such as social class and the level of physical activity of work) are interlocked (Table 2.1).

Before considering each factor mentioned in the Table it is of interest to summarize the sources of the evidence.

(1) *Comparative studies of races with different prevalences of ischaemic heart disease.* The main difficulty is that the quality of data relating to the incidence of disease and causes of death varies greatly from country to country.

(2)　*A comparison of subjects suffering from IHD with subjects apparently free from IHD*. Only patients who survive their episode of IHD will be considered and the so-called 'controls' are all potential candidates for IHD.

TABLE 2.1

Major Causes of IHD

Irreversible	Potentially reversible
Major Factors	
Age	
Sex	Hyperlipidaemia
Race	Hypertension
Diabetes and potential	Cigarette smoking
diabetic states	Excess weight
Abnormal ECG	Social class and
Personality	physical activity
Family history	Diet
Minor factors	
Short stature in women	
Poor hand grip	
Low vital capacity	
Hyperuricaemia	

(3)　*Prospective studies based on groups of people free of IHD*. Usually various parameters, such as blood pressure and serum cholesterol, are measured at the commencement of the study and can then be reviewed retrospectively at convenient intervals. Thus, the serum cholesterol of those who are still free from IHD after 5 years can be compared with that of those who have been afflicted by IHD over the course of that 5 years. To get meaningful results the co-operation of a large number of fit people is required over the course of some years (at least 5 years).

Probably the most famous study was one carried out at Framingham in the U.S.A. in which over 5,000 men and women aged from 30 to 59 and initially free of IHD were followed for up to 12 years. A large amount of base-line clinical and biochemical data was collected and supplemented by re-examination every 2 years.

Various aetiological factors will now be considered starting with those which have been regarded as irreversible. It must be emphasized that other factors not mentioned will probably be found to be of importance.

MAJOR IRREVERSIBLE CAUSES

Age and Sex

Age and sex are best considered together In men, IHD is rare below the age of 30, but the incidence rises sharply after the age of 40. In women the incidence is very rare in the premenopausal years, but shows a sharp rise in the later fifties. In the sixties and seventies, the incidence is similar to that seen in men. However, while considerable reliability can be placed on the diagnosis of IHD in the under-60 age-group, over the age of 70 the diagnosis becomes less easy and is often only one facet of the problems facing the geriatric patient. In this age-group there will often be additional cerebrovascular, renal, and pulmonary disease.

Race

There is a monumental amount of literature on this subject, some of which is very dubious in value. Difficulties result from:

(1)   Varying criteria for the diagnosis of IHD. Some countries have a low death rate from arteriosclerotic and degenerative heart disease, but an unusually high death rate from 'other diseases of the heart'; this suggests differences in terminology rather than pathology.

(2)   Varying standards of medical care and diagnosis. It has been said that the incidence of IHD is directly related to the number of medical practitioners in a country!

(3)   Death certification. In some countries, death certification is not always carried out by a doctor.

(4)   Diagnostic fashions. These will result in the excessive application of certain diagnoses. Bronchopneumonia, for example, is commonly applied to the elderly when perhaps the diagnosis is really senility. In younger age-groups any unexplained death will tend to be labelled as being due to IHD.

(5)   Uncertain data. In many countries the background data on the population numbers and age structure are very uncertain.

(6)   The fact that even if the diagnosis of cause of death is correct there is no one group in the international classification of disease which includes all deaths from IHD and no other causes.

Despite these difficulties very striking facts stand out. Studies in South Africa have shown very marked racial differences in IHD. While the South Africans of European origin have a high incidence of IHD, the native Bantu have an extraordinarily low incidence based on clinical, ECG, and autopsy evidence. The Cape coloured, ethnically of mixed race and tending to occupy a social position intermediate between that of the Bantu and the European South African, similarly show an intermediate incidence of IHD. Possible explanations for these differences have excited considerable interest. The mean serum cholesterol levels are lowest in the Bantu, intermediate in the Cape coloured, and high in the European S.A. The dietary fat intake is lowest in the Bantu, intermediate in the Cape coloured and high in the European S.A. There are, of course, many other differences such as those in genetic, and socioeconomic structure and in the level of physical activity, to mention only a few.

The relative unimportance of genetic factors is indicated by the incidence of IHD in a homogeneous ethnic group (the Japanese), living in three different environments — workers in Japan, Japanese in Hawaii, and Japanese living in America. There is a gradation in incidence of IHD from a low level in Japan to intermediate levels in Hawaii and to relatively high levels in those domiciled in America. The importance of environmental factors is further emphasized by the fact that Japanese in the higher social classes in Japan (and also those in the higher social classes in countries normally having a low incidence of IHD) have a higher level of IHD.

Thus, surveys of the racial incidence of IHD show wide variation and suggest that increasing affluence is associated with a rising level of IHD. This may be due to a number of factors or a combination of factors, such as changing diet, smoking, decreasing physical activity, or to other factors as yet unrecognized.

Diabetes and Potential Diabetes

The presence of diabetes increases the liability of IHD and also eliminates the relative immunity shown by younger women. It has become increasingly apparent that a large proportion of sufferers from IHD show an abnormal carbohydrate tolerance. It might be argued that this disorder, or at least those with a tendency to diabetes, should be regarded as reversible. Studies are in hand at present to ascertain whether reduction of carbohydrate intolerance might reduce the liability to the various arterial complications of diabetes.

Abnormal Electrocardiogram

Many ECG abnormalities are associated with an increased incidence of IHD. The most common of these are the signs of left ventricular (LV) hypertrophy, often associated with hypertension, but not always so. Other ECG abnormalities include minor T wave changes such as undue T wave flattening in V_6, any type of conduction defect, and the presence of atrial fibrillation.

It may be argued that these changes indicate the presence of IHD and that the subsequent appearance of more florid forms of IHD is not surprising. This argument is difficult to refute — hence the use of the word 'association' in the opening sentence.

Personality and Mental Stress

While mental stress has been traditionally accorded an important position as a factor in the aetiology of IHD, objective studies of this have been few because of the difficulty in quantitating 'psychiatric' factors. A stress may produce very different psychological effects in different subjects. Retrospective studies are very suspect as it is not usually difficult to find some mental stress to blame for almost any illness. Nevertheless, objetive prospective studies have been carried out in latter years in a number of large American business organizations. Workers have been classified into ambitious 'go-getters' and more easy-going types and it has been shown that the former have a higher incidence of IHD.

Family History

It has been shown that the incidence of IHD is higher among close relatives of those with IHD than among controls. In one study it was shown that in the first degree relatives (that is, parents and siblings) of men who died from IHD under the age of 55 and of women who died from IHD under the age of 65, there was a seven-fold risk of developing IHD. None of the studies carried out so far seems to show whether this can be entirely accounted for by other known aetiological factors such as hyperlipidaemia or hypertension.

POTENTIALLY REVERSIBLE AETIOLOGICAL FACTORS

Hyperlipidaemia

Because of the obvious fatty constitution of the atheromatous plaques, abnormalities in the pattern of blood lipids have been sought for a long time. The earliest experimental work at about the time of World War I showed that an 'atheroma-like' lesion can be produced by feeding animals a diet high in cholesterol. The term 'atheroma-like' is used because the changes in animals are different in a number of essentials from those seen in men, notably in that cholesterol is deposited in tissues other than the arterial intima and IHD does not ensue.

In man the fat content of blood has been studied both in respect to its chemical make-up, that is, the amount of cholesterol, phospholipids, triglycerides and fatty acids present, and also in respect to its physical make-up — the lipoprotein complexes present. Lipids are, by definition, insoluble in water and, therefore, in plasma they have to be combined

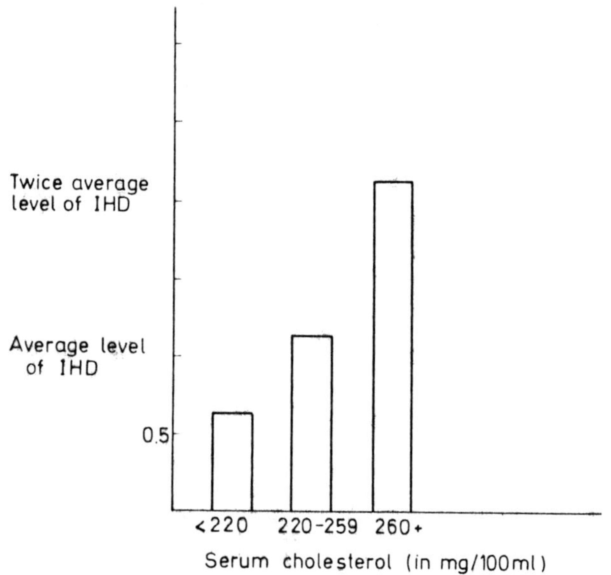

Figure 2.1. Risk of developing IHD in men aged 30–59 (derived from Framingham prospective study)

with proteins to form water-soluble lipoprotein complexes. These show variations in chemical content — for example, chylomicrons are predominantly made up of triglycerides, while low density β lipoproteins are made up mainly of cholesterol. They may also be classified on the basis of their physical properties. Thus, using electrophoretic techniques, they can be shown to be travelling with α or β globulins, or in a band just in front of the β globulins — in a pre-beta band. Differences in molecular density can be demonstrated using sophisticated ultracentri-

28

fugation; the units of measurement are named after the inventor, Svedberg.

To summarise a vast mass of data on lipids and IHD, the following points may be made:

(1)   The majority of studies have shown that serum cholesterol is the most important lipid related to IHD.

(2)   Racial groups with a high incidence of IHD show a high mean level of serum cholesterol, whereas racial groups with a low incidence of IHD show a low mean level of serum cholesterol. It should be said, however, with respect to *individual* patients, that a man with a normally low serum cholesterol can develop IHD while one with a customarily high cholesterol may remain free of disease for many years.

(3)   Within any population group, sufferers from IHD usually show a higher mean serum cholesterol than those apparently free of the disease.

(4)   Prospective studies of men and women free of IHD have shown that those with a higher serum cholesterol are more likely to develop IHD — this is particularly true of young men *(Figure 2.1)*. There is some evidence that in young women elevated serum triglycerides may also be of some value as a predictor of future IHD.

Familial Hyperlipoproteinaemia

Extreme abnormalities of serum lipids have been recognized for many years as a feature of this group. Intensive studies have been carried out into the chemical constitution of these lipids and into their distribution among various proteins. Fredrickson has proposed a classification into five groups which show certain characteristic chemical features and clinical courses. Each has to be distinguished from lipid abnormalities which occur secondary to certain other diseases such as diabetes and hypothyroidism.

Type 1 (familial hyperchylomicronaemia). — This is characterized by a deficiency of lipoprotein lipase so that the body has difficulty in disposing of ingested triglycerides. The excess of chylomicrons in which ingested triglycerides (TG's) are carried gives the plasma a milky appearance even in the fasting state. Chemical analysis confirms the marked elevation of TG's and there may also be some elevation of cholesterol. These will both fall rapidly to normal on elimination of fat from the diet.

Clinically, the patients may present with xanthomas which appear suddenly on the skin — eruptive xanthoma, bouts of abdominal pain and pancreatitis. It may be discovered accidentally by the unusual lactescence of plasma taken in the fasting state, or, rarely, may be seen on examination of the optic fundus when lipaemia retinalis may be seen. Premature vascular disease does not appear to be a feature of this condition.

Treatment, as has already been implied, is by dietary fat restriction supplemented by medium chain fatty acids which do not depend on chylomicrons for their transport.

Type 2 (familial or essential hypercholesterolaemia). — In this condition there is elevation of the low density lipoproteins and, therefore, elevation of the serum cholesterol. In contrast to the type 1 abnormality there will be no visible changes in the appearance of the plasma. The degree of clinical change will depend upon whether the subject is homozygous or heterozygous, the former producing more marked changes than the latter.

Clinically, the characteristic features are the appearance of xanthomas in relation to tendons, on the extensor surfaces of the skin and around the eyes (xanthelasma) with premature vascular disease. As with the chemical changes, the clinical features are more florid in the homozygotes and survival into the fifth decade is unusual. Those who are heterozygous show a high incidence of IHD, but its onset is usually delayed until the fifth or sixth decade.

Treatment consists of a diet in which the saturated fatty acids are reduced and the polyunsaturated fatty acids (PFA) increased, supplemented with drugs such as cholestyramine and clofibrate. In general this tends to be the most difficult form of hyperlipidaemia to deal with. Although correction of the serum lipid abnormalities may lead to slow regression of the xanthomas, evidence as to whether any benefit is produced in retarding the development of IHD is not yet clear.

Type 3 (broad beta disease). — An abnormal low density B-lipoprotein is present on paper electrophoresis as a broad band covering both the 'beta' and 'pre-beta' regions, and associated with a variable rise of the serum cholesterol and triglycerides.

Clinically, there may be xanthomatous deposits on the palms of the hands and over the elbows and buttocks. There may be evidence of IHD and peripheral vascular disease. Treatment is by weight reduction since lipid changes are very sensitive to changes in dietary carbohydrate intake. Changes in the nature of the dietary fat and supplementation by clofibrate may be necessary. Correction of the serum lipids is followed by fairly rapid regression of the xanthomas and there may possibly be improvement in the vascular disease.

Type 4. – In this condition there is an increase in the very low density lipoproteins and therefore a rise in the level of triglycerides (TG's). As the TG's are not contained in chylomicrons there are no visible changes in the appearance of the plasma. The serum cholesterol may be elevated in some cases. Clinically, diabetes or an abnormal glucose tolerance test is a common finding and the patients may suffer from xanthomas or IHD.

Treatment is by reduction of the dietary carbohydrate and sometimes clofibrate and nicotinic acid may be used.

Type 5. – The abnormalities in this form are very similar to those in type 4 except that there is also an increase in the chylomicrons. Chemical analysis, therefore, will show raised TG's and cholesterol.

Clinically, an impaired glucose tolerance may be found in over 75 per cent of cases and there may be xanthomas and episodes of abdominal pain. Vascular disease is not conspicuous and in this respect it resembles type 1 hyperlipoproteinaemia.

Treatment is by reducing both the dietary carbohydrate and fat, supplemented with nicotinic acid (3–6 g daily).

Fredrickson's classification is not absolute or final. These familial hyperlipoproteinaemias provide extreme examples of lipoprotein abnormalities and, in practice, they are uncommon. Only 5 cases were found in over 5,000 surveyed at Framingham. It is not clear at present whether the commonly found hypercholesterolaemia is due to dietary or genetic factors or to a mixture of both. Undoubtedly, in a population habitually consuming a high fat diet the resultant serum cholesterol levels will show wide variation.

In summary, it can be stated that innumerable studies have agreed on the important association between elevated serum cholesterol and the subsequent development of IHD. They have indicated that many of the so-called normal levels of serum cholesterol given in books and laboratory 'hand-outs' are grossly abnormal and will lead to an increased incidence of IHD. Although there is some suggestive data, it remains to be proved that reducing the serum cholesterol of an individual (or a group of individuals) will reduce the risk of subsequent IHD. It must be emphasized that those with an habitual low serum cholesterol do not have a 'nil' risk of IHD, but only a lower risk than those with a high cholesterol.

Hypertension

The higher the blood pressure, the greater the risk of IHD. Much of the information on this has come from prospective studies such as that at Framingham on individuals initially free of IHD. These studies have shown:

(1)   As a predictor of IHD a casual systolic blood pressure is the most useful measurement *(Figure 2.2)*.

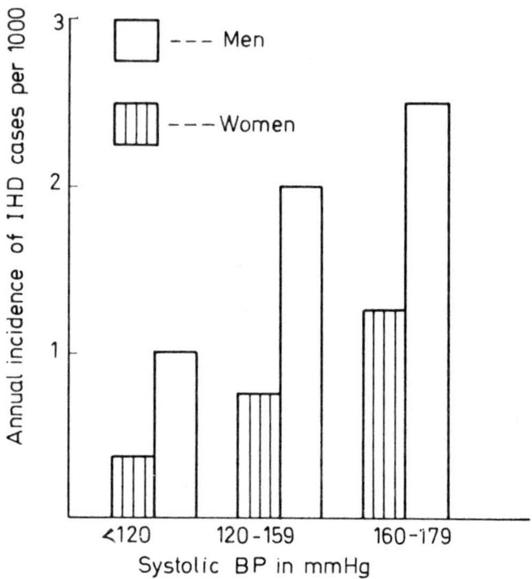

Figure 2.2. Annual incidence of IHD in men and women aged 45–64 (derived from Framingham prospective study)

It will be noted that the levels of blood pressure involved are at first sight quite modest; for example, those with a systolic pressure of 160 mmHg have a significantly higher risk than those with a casual systolic pressure of 120 mmHg.

(2)   The diastolic blood pressure does not produce a better indicator and nor does the pulse pressure.

Cigarette and Other Smoking

In this context cigarette smoking produces the greatest danger, while cigar and pipe smoking appear to be relatively benign. This is similar to the findings in respect to carcinoma of the bronchus and chronic bronchitis where again cigarette smoking seems to be the important aetiological factor.

A number of prospective studies have shown that cigarette smoking increases the risk of myocardial infarction and sudden death by up to 2–3 times in the younger smoker or by about 1½ times in the older smoker. Surprisingly, smoking shows no relation to angina pectoris. These studies have also shown that prolonged cessation of smoking is followed within a year by a reduction in the incidence of IHD, and those who have abandoned the habit for 10 years or more are subject to the same risks as non-smokers. The causative factor in the tobacco has not as yet been identified although variations in its composition might account for the observation that smoking has less effect on the incidence of IHD in certain countries.

Excess Weight

One of the earliest harmful factors to be recognized was obesity and this emerged from the statistics of insurance companies. In latter years the importance of this factor has become less clear as it was often found to be associated with other factors such as hypercholesterolaemia and hypertension. Nevertheless, prospective studies have confirmed that excess weight itself, even when independent of such factors as hypercholesterolaemia, is associated with increased incidence of IHD.

Social Class and Physical Activity

Classification by the Registrar General on the basis of social class divides the population into 5 groups with members of the major professions in class 1, craftsmen and skilled workers in class 3, and completely unskilled manual workers in class 5 (classes 2 and 4 lie in intermediate positions). The higher incidence of IHD in class 1 has been noted from very early times. Osler commented in the early part of this century that he did not see his first case of angina until he was a Fellow of the Royal College of Physicians — and the case was seen in private practice! There are probably many explanations for these differences, but one appeared to be related to the physical activity of the patient's usual occupation. Classification of patients according to the amount of their usual physical activity which will usually be greater in the less skilled shows a better correlation with the incidence of IHD. The hypothesis has, therefore, been put forward that those who are normally physically active have a lower incidence of IHD and, in these, when IHD does occur it is more likely to be in a more benign form with symptoms of angina rather than sudden death. Not all studies have come to the same conclusion. A notable exception is provided by the lumbarjacks of Finland who habitually undertake very heavy work and yet have a high incidence of IHD. The possible beneficial effects of exercise on those who have already suffered from cardiac infarction have been given increasing recognition by the development of carefully graded programmes of gymnastics for such patients.

The last word on the relationship of physical activity to IHD has not yet been said. Studies are at present in hand to assess the possible relationship of leisure physical activity and IHD.

Diet

The relation of diet to IHD has been much disputed. When first postulated by Ancel Keys in 1953 the relationship between the percentage of calories provided by dietary fat and the incidence of IHD in men aged 45–49 and men aged 55–59 in 6 countries seemed clear and impressive. When this hypothesis was extended to include many other countries the relationship was less clear (there being a wide variation in IHD in those countries with a high dietary fat intake) and the original hypothesis appeared to be discredited. However, more recent studies show a reasonably close association between the average national dietary consumption of saturated fatty acids (and not just the total fat) and the national death rate from IHD.

In summary it may be said that:

(1)   Those countries or racial groups with a low intake of saturated fatty acids have a low incidence of IHD. However, these races or groups show many differences other than those associated with their diet.

(2)   Within a racial group there is no evidence that those with IHD follow a diet different from those without IHD.

(3)   Within a population with a habitually high fat intake the reason for the large individual variations in serum cholesterol is not clear. Nevertheless, whatever the cause of the high serum cholesterol it can be lowered by diet or drugs in the vast majority of cases.

(4)   Certain racial groups are often cited as being exceptions to the general rule put forward in (1). The Eskimos, for example, enjoy a high fat intake and a low incidence of IHD. However, it can be pointed out that the average life span of the Eskimos is much shorter than that of people in Europe or the U.S.A. and the details of the causes of death are by no means complete.

Certain East Afican tribes are also cited as having a high fat intake, but with a low mean level of serum cholesterol. However, while percentage of fat is relatively high the mean calorie intake is very low and at some times of the year the tribesmen are near to starvation.

These two groups cannot, therefore, be regarded as providing exceptions to the general rule.

(5) The relationship between carbohydrate intake and serum cholesterol is slight. Likewise, the evidence that IHD is related to the intake of refined carbohydrates is tenuous. It is true that those countries whose people have a high fat intake also, in general, tend to have people with larger intakes of sucrose. Several studies based on Yudkin's postulate that IHD is related to the intake of refined carbohydrates have failed to confirm this.

MINOR FACTORS

Among the other interesting data which came out of the Framingham prospective study was evidence that short stature in women was associated with an increased level of IHD; other associations noted were a weak hand grip, a low vital capacity, and hyperuricaemia. The significance of these is obscure and it is not wished to exaggerate their importance — they merely indicate that there are further ramifications to the aetiology of IHD which are as yet untouched.

CONCLUSIONS

So far a mass of factors associated with IHD have been cited. Such associations, though suggestive, do not prove a cause and effect relationship. By looking for subjects possessing a number of adverse features — for example, serum cholesterol of over 260 mg/100 ml, systolic blood pressure of 160 or over, and cigarette smoking at the rate of 20 or more a day — it is possible to identify groups whose risk of developing IHD is ten or more times that of the normal. Conversely, subjects showing few adverse features have a much lower incidence of IHD although it must be stressed that even these subjects are not entirely free from the risk of IHD.

CURRENT ATTEMPTS AT PREVENTION

Prevention is either *secondary* or *primary*. Secondary prevention consists of methods used to reduce the recurrence rate in those with established IHD, principally by anticoagulants and cholesterol-lowering agents. The results of these treatments have ranged from 'no apparent benefit' to marginal reduction of the number of episodes of ischaemic heart pain (but no significant changes in death rate). By and large they have been abandoned and current hopes are pinned on the used of methods of primary prevention, which aims at the prevention of IHD in men who are currently free of IHD.

As is obvious from the list of known aetiological factors, only some are potentially reversible. Here the effects of lowering serum cholesterol, stopping smoking and reducing blood pressure will be considered. It is only the cessation of smoking which has so far produced clear beneficial effects on the development of IHD. In the case of serum cholesterol lowering, there are some very suggestive but, as yet, inconclusive results.

SERUM CHOLESTEROL REDUCTION

Serum cholesterol may be reduced in the majority of patients by means of a diet or the use of the drug clofibrate (Atromid-S).

The principle involved in all diets is a reduction in the intake of saturated fatty acids which are mainly but not exclusively animal in origin. The addition of polyunsaturated fatty acids (PFA), which are largely but not exclusively vegetable in origin, produces a further fall and also renders the diet more palatable. The dietary cholesterol is not such an important influence on serum cholesterol in man, but in any case a diet such as has been described will be low in cholesterol (Table 2.2). It must be emphasized that diets need tailoring to suit the patients' individual habits and success is only likely if a dietitian is involved.

In one dietary experiment in the U.S.A. there appeared to be a rather larger proportion of cases of malignant disease in those on PFA diet and the possibility that such diets might be carcinogenic was raised. However, reviews of the combined results of five diet studies did not produce any confirmation of this.

Many drugs have been used to reduce serum cholesterol. Some of them bring about unpleasant side effects, such as flushing from nicotinic acid, and a few such as Triparanol are positively dangerous. The most effective drug available (and to date remarkably safe) is clofibrate (Atromid-S). This drug produces the following effects:

    (1)   Lowers serum cholesterol
    (2)   Lowers serum triglycerides
    (3)   Lowers other serum lipids – for example, phospholipids
    (4)   Lowers platelet stickiness
    (5)   Decreases platelet turnover.
    (6)   Reduces the dosage requirements of oral anticoagulants such as

phenindione (dindevan) and warfarin, the practical implication of this being that patients who are already on oral anticoagulants will need a smaller daily does if they are also given clofibrate.

TABLE 2.2

Cholesterol-Lowering Diet

Obligatory	Soya bean oil (85 g per day)
Allowed	Lean meat (85 g); all fish
	skimmed milk
	Polyunsaturated margarine (15g); skimmed milk
	Cheese; clear soups; bread; cereals
	Sponge cake (fat-free)
Not allowed	Butter; other margarine
	Cooking fat
	Other oils; pork and other fat meat
	Whole milk; cheese
	Eggs; most biscuits
	Bought cakes

Side effects are few and consist of occasional mild gastrointestinal upsets. The dose is one 0.5 g capsule 4 times daily, and it appears to work by increasing the excretion of cholesterol via the bile. Drug reduction of serum cholesterol has the advantage of producing the minimum disruption of the patients' normal way of life. Nevertheless, while there are still so many unanswered questions on its value, or its mode of action and possible long-term effects (clofibrate was introduced in the late 1950's) it should be confined to those who are experienced in its uses and should not be prescribed in a haphazard fashion.

Whichever method of serum cholesterol reduction is used the net effect is about the same, that is, about a 10—20 per cent reduction from the base-line cholesterol level. With high base-line serum cholesterol, the reduction will usually be greater than in those with a lower base-line. It has been shown that these reductions can be maintained for years; for example, for up to 6 years in the Medical Research Council trial of polyunsaturated fatty acids on men who had survived one cardiac infarct *(Figure 2.3)*.

There is no evidence that either diet or clofibrate loses its effect over the course of time, although co-operation probably does become strained. Nevertheless, a large-scale study carried out in the U.S.A. using fit volunteers has shown that it is possible to produce considerable changes

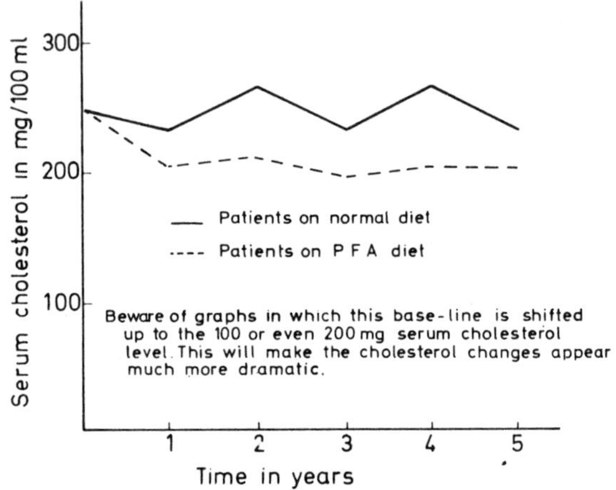

Figure 2.3. Serum cholesterol changes on polyunsaturated fatty acid (PFA) diet

in the type of most dietary fats so that the serum cholesterol is reduced with minimal changes in the appearance and taste of such foods. If the value of such dietary fat changes could be established without reasonable doubt, there could be a great stimulus for industry to produce such modified foods.

Three major studies of the effects of the lowering of serum cholesterol on the subsequent development of IHD will now be described and discussed — these were carried out in the U.S.A., in Finland and in Scotland, respectively.

United States of America

One of the first experiments in prevention was started in New York and was known as the 'anti-coronary club'. It was first set up to study the feasibility of making long-term dietary changes and thus producing a reduction in serum cholesterol over a long time. The study was concerned with fit men and, therefore, attracted a highly motivated and selected group. When this project was found to be practical, a similar group of motivated men was sought who were not on a cholesterol-lowering diet. For this the co-operation of men attending a cancer prevention clinic was obtained. Although it was shown that this body of men were very similar to those on the cholesterol-lowering diet, they cannot be truly called a 'control' group as they did not enter the study at the same time and their allocation to diet was not carried out randomly. The term 'control' is much abused in medical literature and should only be used for patients obtained by the method just cited. A group of 941 men, initially free of IHD, were entered into the experimental diet group and the later 'so-called' control group was made up of 457 men free of IHD. The experimental group showed a 13 per cent fall in serum cholesterol level and this was maintained for up to 7 years while the control group only showed a minimal fall of about 2 per cent. In the analysis of the clinical progress, those on the experimental diet were classified into two groups: active participants (those who co-operated fully) and inactive participants (those whose co-operation was not complete). However, even in this latter group minimal contact was kept and an annual check-up was carried out. The occurrence of new 'coronary events' in the control group was approximately double that of the active participants in the diet group, while the inactive diet participants showed an intermediate position, the figures being 1.025 events per 100,000 person years of experience, 430 events per 100,000 person years of experience, and 748 events per 100,000 person years of experience respectively.

Comment

(1) As has already been indicated, the non-diet group are not a true control group and it is, therefore, difficult to be certain that they are in every way comparable to the dietary group.

(2) Comparison of the known risk factors shows that if there is any bias it is against the experimental group; for example, base-line cholesterol was a little higher at 260 mg/100 ml compared with 250 mg/100 ml in the control group (no account can be taken of unknown or unrecognized risk factors).

(3) The inflation of the number of new coronary events to numbers per 100,000 person years experience tends to exaggerate the differences.

Notwithstanding the above remarks the results of the anti-coronary club are of considerable interest.

Finland

A fascinating study carried out over the course of 12 years on the inmates of two mental hospitals in Finland has just been completed. During the first 6 years of this experiment the diet of all inmates in one hospital (hospital A) was changed to a high polyunsaturated fatty acid diet, while in the second hospital (hospital B) it was left as the usual high satufated fatty acid diet. The subjects studied were men aged 34–64 at the beginning of the trial, there being 327 men in hospital A and 254 in hospital B. As might have been anticipated there was a significant fall in the mean serum cholesterol levels in hospital A of about 10 per cent. The clinical progress was based on annual ECG's and on mortality. The ECG evidence of new 'coronary events' was significantly lower in the hospital on the polyunsaturated fatty acid diet and the death rate from coronary disease was lower, but in this case the difference was not significant.

In 1965 (after 6 years of the above experiment) the diets were reversed so that hospital A now had the normal diet while hospital B had the polyunsaturated fatty acid diet. This was followed by the expected changes in serum cholesterol levels and also, in the longer term, in the constitution of the adipose tissue. Long-term changes in the nature of dietary fats (as occurs in those on polyunsaturated fatty acid diets) are eventually followed by changes in the pattern of tissue fatty acids.

At the end of the second 6-year period it was possible to show that the death rates from IHD in both hospitals and in both sexes were lower during the dietary period.

Comment

(1)   The cross-over design compensates in many ways for the fact that the patients were not allocated randomly — compensates, that is, for the absence of a true control group.

(2)   The experiment was carried out on a shifting population and not on the same group as was admitted at the commencement. In fact, quite appreciable shifts of certain chronic patients appear to have occurred during the second 6-year period in one hospital.

(3)   There appears to have been an appreciable difference in the age structure and rate of 'turnover' of patients in the two hospitals.

(4)   It is surprising that progress of the patients in the second 6-year period was not followed by regular ECG'S — this method is objective and appeared to produce some quite suggestive results in the first 6-year period.

While this study has once again confirmed the efficiency of dietary methods of producing changes in serum and tissue lipids, the clinical effects are only suggestive.

Edinburgh

A promising prevention programme based on the use of clofibrate (Atromid-S) was started in 1965. For this, all blood donors were classified on their serum cholesterol levels into three equal groups — a low, a medium, and a high cholesterol group. All those with a high cholesterol and half of those in the low cholesterol groups were invited to enter an experiment calculated to reduce the incidence of IHD. Those with a high cholesterol were randomly allocated to treatment with Atromid-S (1.5 g daily) or a placebo, providing therefore, a true control group. Those with a low cholesterol were all given placebo; thus two groups of men on placebo were provided. The cholesterol status of the patients was not known by the physicians concerned and the patients were followed-up every 6 months for the first 2 years and thereafter annually. Over 2,000 men had been collected after 2 years and those on Atromid-S had shown an average fall of 16 per cent in the mean serum cholesterol levels. No further results are available, though it is estimated that an intake of about 15,000 men followed for about 5 years will be necessary.

Comment

(1)   This is a proper controlled trial — a trial, that is, in which the treated and non-treated subjects are allocated at random at the onset of the study.

(2)   It is a double blind trial in that the physicians following the progress do not know the serum cholesterol status of the patient. It will be noted that one-third of the patients are taken from the low cholesterol group.

(3)   No further details are available, but it may be noted that it has now been spread to two further centres — one in Prague and the other in Budapest. This suggests that the concept and technique of the trial is working satisfactorily.

Preliminary experiments in reducing serum cholesterol appear to support the hypothesis that this is a significant (and potentially reversible) factor in the development of IHD, but final proof is still awaited.

CIGARETTE SMOKING

The association between cigarette smoking and IHD has already been reviewed. Many prospective studies have confirmed these observations which show that heavy cigarette smoking (20 or more a day) increases the risk of IHD two- or three-fold among younger men and to a lesser extent in older men. There is also evidence from these studies that those who give up smoking show a reduced incidence of IHD so that after about 10 years without smoking the risk of ex-smokers is comparable with that of non-smokers. Likewise in the prospective studies of British doctors it was shown that those who gave up smoking showed a small reduction in death from IHD (6 per cent) while the mortality of the ordinary population of comparable age rose by about 10 per cent. These changes indicate that cigarette smoking and the appearance of IHD are not each linked to a third factor such as heredity. Thus, the case for abandoning smoking would seem indisputable.

BLOOD PRESSURE

Although it has been demonstrated that quite modest elevations of blood pressure (for example, a systolic pressure of 160 mmHg), are associated with significantly increased liability to IHD, none of the trials of hypotensive drugs have demonstrated any reduction in the occurrence of IHD. In fact, with the amelioration of the cerebrovascular and renal complications of hypertension, deaths from IHD become more conspicuous. All the controlled trials of hypotensives have been on rather small numbers and the significance of these observations is very difficult to assess. Nevertheless, they do not negate the obvious value of hypotensives in the management of hypertension.

PHYSICAL ACTIVITY

Despite the somewhat confusing views concerning the relationship of IHD and exercise, most agree that physical activity is of benefit in this respect. Indeed, the increasing use of the motor car shows a crude relationship with the incidence of IHD! Apart from generous proferred advice no serious attempts have been made to use exercise prophylactically, although a number of studies of graduated exercises in patients with established IHD have been published. These have shown subjective benefits and also some improvement in the circulation as shown by the rise in heart and respiratory rate on graduated exercise.

CONCLUSION

A large number of factors have now been identified which appear to predispose to IHD. By combining two or more adverse factors, it is possible to identify groups with very much greater liability to the condition. While there is no doubt about the value of permanent cessation of cigarette smoking, the benefits from other changes still must be regarded as being sub judice. While elimination of IHD by prophylactic methods is unlikely to be seen, a 10–20 per cent reduction in its occurrence might be possible by the means described.

REFERENCES

Friedberg, C. K. (1966). *Diseases of the Heart.* 3rd edition. London: W. B. Saunders and Co.

Meade, T. and Chakrabarti, R. (1972). 'Arterial disease research: Observation or intervention? *Lancet,* **2,** 913

Morgan Jones, A. (1970). *Modern Trends in Cardiology.* Vol 2., London: Butterworths

Simborg, D. (1970). 'The status of risk factors and C.H.D.' *J. chron. Dis.* **22,** 515

Stanbury, J. B., Wyngaarden, J. B. and Fredrickson, D. S. (1966). *Metabolic Basis of Inherited Disease.* 3rd edition. Maidenhead: McGraw-Hill

3

Cardiac Arrhythmias and Disorders of Conduction

R. A. L. Sutton

These two motions, one of the ventricles, another of the auricles, take place consecutively, but in such a manner that there is a kind of rhythm or harmony preserved between them (chapter V).

Whilst the heart is gradually dying, it is sometimes seen to reply after two or three contractions of the auricles, roused as it were to action and making a single pulsation (chapter IV).

William Harvey (*De Motu Cordis*, 1628).
Translated by Robert Willis

INTRODUCTION

Within the past 10 years there has been a rapid increase in our knowledge and understanding of disorders of the heart beat. This has resulted especially from painstaking histological studies of the cardiac conducting system, and from the application of new techniques in clinical medicine including particularly cardiac monitoring, transvenous endocardial pacing and intracardiac electrocardiography (ECG).

This chapter reviews the diagnosis and management of the commoner cardiac arrhythmias and it places particular emphasis upon these recent advances. An account of the anatomy and physiology of the conducting system is followed by a brief description of some of the techniques used in the diagnosis of arrhythmias. In the remainder of the review the commoner disorders of the heart beat are considered individually.

ANATOMY OF THE CONDUCTING SYSTEM

The anatomical arrangement of the conducting system ensures that the normal impulse, arising in the sino-atrial node, is conducted to all parts of the atrial and ventricular muscle. The special properties of the different parts of the conducting system result in a co-ordinated contraction of the heart. The conducting system consists of specialized cardiac muscle fibres which receive innervation from the autonomic nervous system.

The Sino-atrial (SA) Node

This lies in the wall of the right atrium close to its junction with the superior vena cava. It is a cylindrical structure which surrounds its own special sinus node artery, a branch of the right coronary artery, in about 60 per cent of subjects, and the left coronary artery in the remaining 40 per cent. The segment of the artery which penetrates the SA node is particularly thin-walled, perhaps making the pacemaker cells more susceptible to the influence of its pulsatile blood flow. Microscopically, the SA node contains large numbers of small pacemaker cells.

Until recently, it was considered that conduction from the SA node to the atrio-ventricular (AV) node, which lies in the inter-atrial septum, resulted from diffuse spread of activity through unspecialized atrial muscle. However, it is now recognized that there are specialized inter-nodal conduction paths. Three rapidly-conducting inter-nodal tracts have been defined — anterior, middle and posterior — which connect the SA and AV nodes and which also send branches to the left atrium (via the anterior tract). Part of the posterior tract (the James bypass) may terminate in the lower AV node, providing a possible bypass to this slowly conducting region. These tracts provide for rapid and reliable conduction from the SA to the AV node and from the SA node to the remote parts of the atria. Theoretically, they might also permit direct spread of the sinus impulse to the AV node and ventricles when the unspecialized atrial muscle is paralysed. This is believed to be the mechanism whereby sinus rhythm may persist despite loss of P waves in hyperkaliaemia.

The Atrio-ventricular (AV) Node

This lies on the right side of the atrial septum close to the orifice of the coronary sinus. This junctional region is complex, both anatomically and physiologically, and has been the subject of particularly intensive recent study. It now appears that specialized junctional tissue is considerably more extensive than the original microscopic description suggested. The AV node is supplied by a special artery, the ramus septi fibrosi, which arises from the right coronary artery in over 90 per cent

46

of subjects. This artery also supplies the bundle of His and the first part of both bundle branches.

The junctional region is continuous with the bundle of His, which is normally the only conducting tissue connecting atria with ventricles. The bundle of His, which averages about 2 mm in width and 20 mm in length, penetrates the central fibrous body to reach the superior border of the muscular intra-ventricular septum, where it divides into right and left bundle branches. The bundle of His lies close to the mitral, tricuspid and aortic valves and is vulnerable to injury during operations on these structures. Direct connections (Mahaim fibres) arise from the bundle of His to supply the muscular septum. The right bundle branch (RBB) proceeds down the right side of the ventricular septum to supply the right ventricle (RV), while the left bundle branch (LBB) soon divides into a fine anterior and a broad posterior division which run towards the anterior and posterior papillary muscles respectively to supply the left ventricular (LV) muscle. The blood supply to the RBB and anterior division of LBB is from the anterior descending branch of the left coronary artery, while the posterior division of the LBB is supplied by the posterior descending branch of the left coronary artery.

The conducting system receives sympathetic and parasympathetic innervation. The SA node is supplied mainly by the right vagus and the AV node by the left vagus nerve.

PHYSIOLOGY OF THE CONDUCTING SYSTEM

The cardiac impulse is normally generated in the SA node and conducted thence into the atria and to the AV node and then down the bundle of His to the ventricles. As a result of the orderly spread of the impulse, the atria contract first, giving a final boost to ventricular filling. A short pause then occurs, due to slow conduction through the junctional region, and this allows the AV valve cusps to approximate. Ventricular contraction then follows in a peristaltic fashion commencing at the apex and expelling blood into the aorta and pulmonary artery. Simultaneous contraction of the papillary muscles maintains the competence of the AV valves. The specialized tissues of the heart generate and conduct impulses. The property of impulse generation (automaticity) is possessed by cells in the SA node, the inter-nodal pathways, parts of the junctional region, and in the His—Purkinjé system of the ventricles. Intracellular microelectrode recordings from these cells show a characteristic spontaneous slow diastolic depolarization. When the transmembrane potential reaches a certain threshold, rapid depolarization occurs which initiates a propagated impulse. The gradient of the slow diastolic depolarization determines the rate of firing, which is normally most rapid in the SA node (60–80/min), slower in the junctional pacemakers (40–60/min) and slowest in the His–Purkinjé system (less than 40/min). The lower pacemakers normally fail to generate impulses since they are prematurely discharged by the conducted impulses from the SA node. If, however, an impulse fails to arrive from above, the lower pacemakers assume control of the ventricles (escape rhythm).

Conduction is normally rapid through the specialized tissues of atria and ventricles (more than 1,000 mm/sec) but is very slow (20–200 mm/sec) in part of the junctional region (the AV node proper). Intracellular recordings from this area show a slow upstroke of the action potential which results in progressive slowing and attenuation of the impulse in the junction. It is now believed that impulse generation does not occur in the AV node proper, but in other parts of the junctional region, either above or below the slow conducting region. Such rhythms are better termed junctional than nodal. Another important characteristic of junctional cells is the prolonged persistence of refractoriness, up to 200 msec after repolarization has occurred. This property prevents the propagation of a second impulse too soon after the first, thus limiting the ventricular rate in conditions such as atrial fibrillation. There is considerable experimental evidence of longitudinal dissociation in the junction — that is, there appear to be two or more functional components which can act as separate pathways in both forward and retrograde directions.

Disturbances of impulse conduction may occur at any level in the conducting system, and may be of first, second or third degree. First degree block indicates delayed conduction. Second degree block is of two types, the Wenckebach phenomenon (Mobitz type I), and Mobitz type II block *(see Figures 3.2 and 3.9)*. The Wenckebach phenomenon consists of repeated cycles in which there is progressively increasing delay in conduction followed by a dropped beat. In Mobitz type II second degree block, there is no progressive change in conduction but instead there is an intermittent failure of conduction. In third degree block there is complete failure of conduction of all impulses.

TECHNIQUES USED IN THE DIAGNOSIS OF ARRHYTHMIAS

Conventional Electrocardiography

The ECG characteristics of the commoner arrhythmias will be considered later. Certain conduction disturbances, however, are manifested principally as abnormalities of the mean frontal plane QRS axis (axis deviation) and it is therefore necessary to recognize pathological right and left axis deviation on the standard ECG. *Figure 3.1* shows the axes of the three standard leads and the three unipolar leads together with their polarities. An impulse directed towards the positive pole of any of these leads results in a positive deflection in that lead, while an impulse directed towards the negative pole results in a negative deflection. *Figure 3.1* also shows (shaded) the normal range for the mean frontal plane QRS vector (− 30° to + 90°). A mean QRS vector directed within this range results in net deflections in leads I and II which are zero or positive (deflections above the base-line equal to or greater than deflections below the base-line) while the net deflection in lead III may be positive or negative. Right axis deviation (mean QRS vector greater than 90°) is recognized on the standard leads by a net negative deflection in lead I together with a net positive deflection in lead III. Pathological left axis deviation (mean QRS vector more than − 30°) is recognized by a net positive deflection in lead I together with a net negative deflection in both lead II and lead III. The mean frontal plane

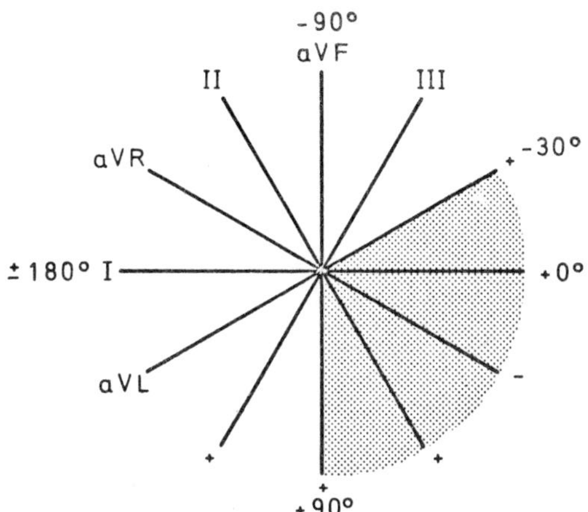

Figure 3.1. The electrical axis of the heart. The axes of the 3 standard leads and the 3 unipolar leads are shown, together with their polarities. The mean frontal plane QRS vector normally lies within the shaded range (− 30° to + 90°).

QRS axis is normally determined largely by the direction of spread of activation through the left ventricle. When both divisions of the left bundle are intact, the mean vector is between − 30° and + 90°. However, if either division of the left bundle is interrupted, the vector is grossly shifted. Left axis deviation results from block of the left anterior division (left anterior hemi-block — *see Figure 3.4*) while right axis deviation is produced by block of the left posterior division (left posterior hemi-block). LV hypertrophy alone, without a conduction disturbance, is associated with a normal axis. RV hypertrophy, however, may produce right axis deviation without an associated conduction disturbance, since the axis of the RV, unlike that of the LV, lies outside the range of the normal mean QRS vector.

Intra-cardiac Electrocardiography

The conventional ECG normally records the electrical activity of the atria and of the ventricles. The spread of the impulses through the intervening conducting tissue is not, however, recorded on surface leads. Where atrial activity is not clearly demonstrated by conventional leads, special leads may help, including right chest leads, and the oesophageal lead *(Figures 3.7c and 3.7d)*. Much more information can, however, be obtained by recording from intra-cardiac catheter electrodes. These may be positioned within the atrium at different levels, giving information on the presence and direction of spread of the atrial impulse *(Figure 3.2)*. In addition, records may be obtained of activity in the bundle of His, the junctional region, and the bundle branches. The technique of His bundle recording involves the introduction of a multipolar electrode catheter from the femoral vein into the right atrium and across the tricuspid valve. If recordings are taken from the catheter tip as it is withdrawn across the tricuspid valve (close to the septal leaflet of which the bundle of His lies) it is usually possible to record the potential produced by passage of the impulse down the His bundle *(Figure 3.2)*.

Potentials may also be recorded from the AV node and the RBB, and catheters have been inserted into the LV to record from the LBB. These potentials may be recorded during the patient's normal rhythm, and also during artificial atrial or ventricular pacing, and this technique has yielded much now information about conduction disorders and arrhythmias. Conventional ECG leads are recorded simultaneously with the His electrogram and this permits subdivision of the P–R interval. The A–H interval (normally 80–160 msec) is measured from the commencement of atrial activity to the His potential, and presumably represents mainly delay in the junctional region. The H–V interval (normally 30–50 msec) is measured from the His potential to the onset of ventricular activity, and represents the conduction time in the ventricular specialized tissue. The only important part of the cardiac conducting system which is now inaccessible to recording in the intact human subject is the SA node itself.

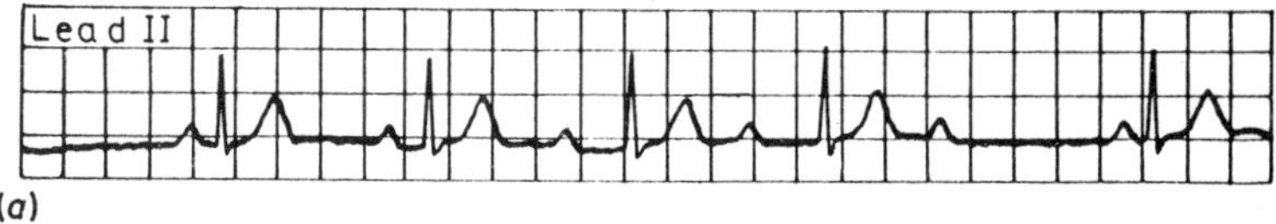

(a)

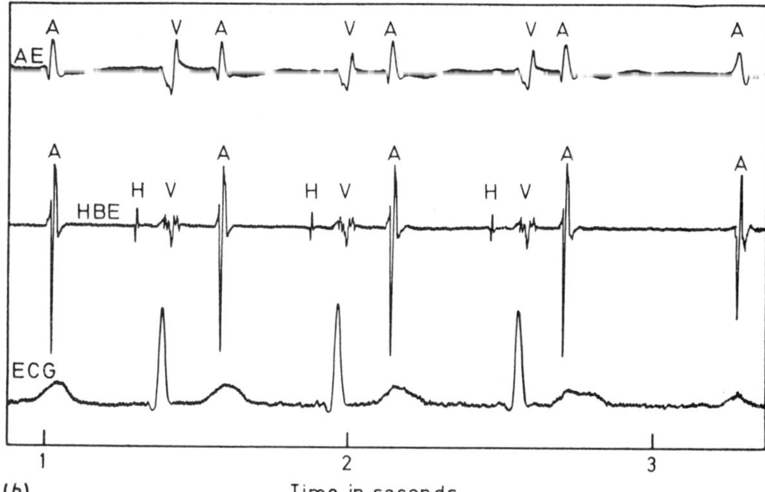

(b)   Time in seconds

Figure 3.2. The Wenckebach phenomenon. (a) Lead II from a conventional ECG (time intervals are 0.20 sec on all diagrams unless otherwise stated). (b) Top – the atrial electrogram (AE); middle – the His electrogram (HBE); and bottom – the surface ECG. The P waves are not easily identified on the surface ECG as they are almost superimposed on the T waves; atrial potentials are, however, shown on the intracardiac electrograms (A). The P–R interval increases progressively from first to third beat; the fourth atrial potential is not conducted to the ventricle. The His electrogram shows progressive lengthening of the A–H time, whilst the H–V time remains constant, indicating that the progressive delay is in the junctional region (above the His bundle). The fourth atrial potential is not followed by a His potential, confirming the site of block as the junctional region. This record is from a 21-year-old nurse, who suffered from transient loss of consciousness and was found to have intermittent second degree heart block on the conventional ECG (shown above).

Cardiac Monitoring

This has now become routine, especially in patients who have suffered a recent myocardial infarction. Monitoring equipment is constantly being improved, an important recent advance being the 'memory' oscilloscope which displays the past 5–10 seconds of the patient's ECG as a tracing moving slowly across the screen. This allows the individual watching the monitor to avert his gaze for a few seconds without missing important information, and some observers find this form of presentation easier to watch than the conventional monitor. Unfortunately, these machines are at present appreciably more expensive than standard oscilloscopes.

Much information on the diagnosis of cardiac arrhythmias is based on standard ECG leads, and for the identification of P waves and the recognition of certain conduction disorders lead V_1 is particularly useful. However, it is impracticable to monitor lead V_1 permanently since it necessitates leads on all four limbs. A useful alternative lead system for long-term monitoring known as the modified chest left arm lead, consists of a positive electrode in the normal V_1 position (right fourth interspace) and a negative electrode beneath the outer end of the left clavicle. The earth electrode is beneath the outer end of the right clavicle. This lead (MCL_1) gives complexes resembling those in V_1 while having the added advantage of not interfering with the application of defibrillator paddles, should the need for these arise.

DISORDERS OF THE HEART BEAT

Sinus Irregularities

The rate of discharge of the SA node is mainly influenced by its autonomic nerve supply. The SA node may be responsible for cardiac irregularities either because its discharge is irregular (sinus arryhthmia) or because not all sinus impulses are conducted onwards to the atria and AV junction (SA block). Sinus arrhythmia is most commonly associated with respiration, inspiration being associated with acceleration of rate, and expiration with slowing. This phenomenon is more marked in the young, and is said to be absent in the presence of a large atrial septal defect. Non-respiratory sinus arrhythmia may be produced by drugs such as opiates and digitalis. In the condition known as 'wandering pacemaker' there is a sudden change in the configuration of the P waves and usually in the P–R interval; this indicates a shift between the SA node and another atrial pacemaker. SA block may be partial or complete, but may be difficult to recognize as the activity of the SA node cannot be directly recorded. Intermittent 2:1 SA block causes a sudden halving of the rate of the P waves in the ECG. When prolonged SA block or sinus arrest occurs, a junctional pacemaker usually assumes control of the ventricles, producing an escape rhythm with a slower rate than that of the normal SA node. There may be some delay before such a rhythm commences, sufficient to cause transient loss of consciousness (Stokes—Adams attack). In the so-called sick sinus syndrome, sinus bradycardia or arrest may alternate with supraventricular tachyarrhythmias. Such arrhythmias may need to be treated by artificial pacing.

Ectopic Beats

The term ectopic beat implies an impulse arising in a site other than the SA node. Most such beats are premature, appearing before the next sinus beat is due, but escape beats are an exception, being characteristically post-mature. Most ectopic beats bear a constant time relationship to the previous normal beat; however, in parasystole (*see* page 57) this 'coupling interval' is variable.

Escape Beats

The cells of the specialized tissues below the SA node, which possess automaticity, normally fail to initiate impulses because they are constantly prematurely discharged by impulses arising in the SA node. If an impulse fails to arrive from above, the lower pacemaker with the most rapid intrinsic rate assumes control, producing an escape beat, and this is usually a pacemaker in the junctional region or the His—Purkinjé system. The delay before the first escape beat is often longer than the subsequent interval between beats. Escape beats occur with sinus bradycardia, SA block and AV block, and they may also be seen in atrial flutter *(see Figure 3.5)* and atrial fibrillation, in which they terminate particularly long diastolic pauses. Escape beats arising in the junctional region or the bundle of His closely resemble sinus beats in their QRS configuration, while those arising more peripherally produce more bizarre complexes.

Extrasystoles

The term extrasystole is used here to describe ectopic beats other than escape and parasystolic beats. The term is not ideal, since there is commonly a premature beat, followed by a compensatory pause, and not a true extra systole. These are usually premature beats arising in the atria, the junctional region or the ventricles. Their precise pathogenesis is controversial, but any theory attempting to explain them must account for their (usually) constant time relationship to the previous beat. They may result from the discharge of an ectopic pacemaker, or from the phenomenon of re-entry (*see* below). Their significance depends very much upon the clinical setting in which they are noted;

much effort is currently directed towards the suppression of ventricular extrasystoles in the first few days following a myocardial infarct as these may precipitate ventricular fibrillation, while on the other hand many healthy individuals without evidence of heart disease have frequent extrasystoles. It is probably not correct, however, to regard these latter extrasystoles as entirely benign. In the Tecumseh epidemiological study from the U.S.A., subjects showing ventricular extrasystoles on a routine ECG had an incidence of coronary heart disease of 3 times, and an incidence of sudden death over the next 6 years of 6 times, that of subjects without ventricular extrasystoles. Extrasystoles only have clinically important haemodynamic consequences if they are very frequent, but they may be noticed by the patient and are an important cause of cardiac neurosis.

Atrial extrasystoles. – These are premature beats arising from an ectopic atrial site. The P wave so produced is different in shape from that of the normal sinus beat. The fate of such an impulse on reaching

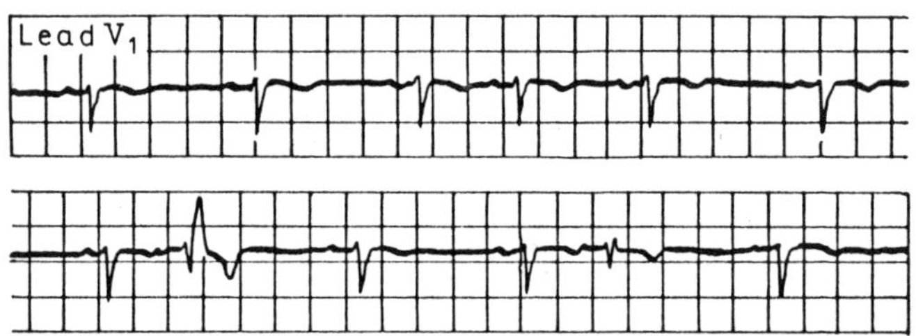

Figure 3.3. Atrial extrasystoles. The lower strip is a continuation of the upper strip. The fourth, eighth and eleventh complexes are atrial extrasystoles. Each of these QRS complexes is preceded by a premature P wave. The fourth QRS complex is identical with those of the sinus beats, the eighth shows the pattern of RBBB with an RSR₁ configuration in V₁ (indicating aberrant conduction), and the eleventh again shows an RSR₁ pattern, but the QRS complex is narrower than that of the eighth beat. The degree of aberration appears to be related to the prematurity of the atrial extrasystole; the P–P intervals of these 3 extrasystoles are 0.56, 0.40 and 0.46 sec respectively.

the AV junction depends upon its degree of prematurity. If very premature, it may fail to be conducted, producing a blocked atrial extrasystole. If less premature, it may be conducted to the ventricle, but may find part of the conducting system still refractory. If the junctional region is partly refractory this atrial extrasystole will be conducted with an abnormally long P–R interval. If part of the His–Purkinjé system is refractory, the atrial extrasystole may be conducted with a bundle branch block (BBB) pattern *(Figure 3.3)*. Such aberrantly conducted atrial extrasystoles are easily confused on the ECG with ventricular extrasystoles unless the P wave is identified. Careful studies have shown, however, that the majority of atrial or junctional beats conducted with aberration show RBBB with a triphasic RSR_1 pattern in lead V_1, whereas ectopic beats arising in the LV, and having a RBBB pattern, usually have a monophasic (R) or biphasic (Q–R) pattern in lead V_1. Finally, atrial extrasystoles arising later in diastole may be conducted normally. Runs of three or more atrial extrasystoles are conventionally classed as atrial tachycardia.

Atrial extrasystoles are of little pathological significance but may precede (and initiate) atrial fibrillation. Atrial extrasystoles require treatment only if they are causing distressing palpitations and in this event they may be best treated with mild sedatives or with adrenergic beta-blockers such as practolol.

Junctional extrasystoles. – The terminology of what were formerly called nodal extrasystoles and tachycardias is undergoing revision now that it is believed that the AV node proper does not possess automaticity. Junctional beats probably arise either above the slow-conducting N region of the junction (in which case abnormal (inverted) P waves precede the QRS complex) or below it, between the N region and the upper His bundle, in which case inverted P waves may be buried in (or follow) the QRS complex, or there may be a failure of retrograde conduction into the atria. The clinical significance and management of junctional extrasystoles does not differ from that of atrial extrasystoles.

Ventricular extrasystoles. – These arise from a site between the upper His bundle and the peripheral Purkinje fibres; their QRS configuration on the ECG depends upon their site of origin. They are not preceded by a P wave unless they happen to fall very late, interrupting the P–R interval of the next conducted beat. Those arising in the His bundle or proximal parts of the main fascicles may have QRS complexes of normal width differing little from those of normal beats, while those arising more peripherally have a widened QRS complex, with a LBBB configuration when arising in the RV, and a RBBB configuration when arising in the LV *(Figure 3.4)*. There may be retrograde conduction of ventricular extrasystoles into the atria (recent evidence suggests that this may occur in about 50 per cent of ventricular extrasystoles) and, if so, the SA node will be discharged and its rhythm interrupted. Ventricular extrasystoles may be interpolated between two normal sinus beats; this usually occurs where the sinus rate is slow. Frequently the P–R interval of the following

55

sinus beat is prolonged owing to penetration of the ventricular extrasystole into the junctional region rendering it partially refractory (concealed conduction).

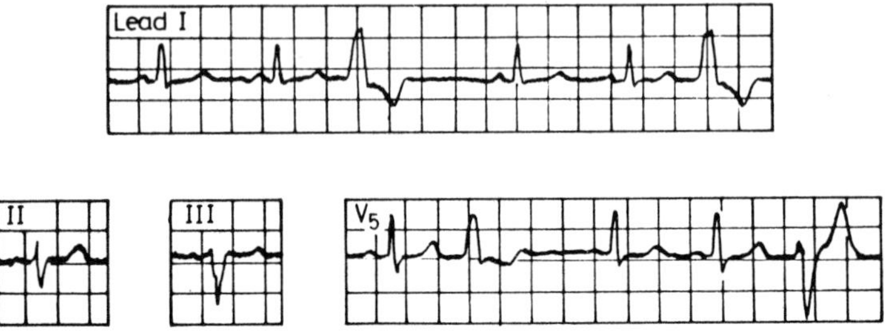

Figure 3.4. Left anterior hemiblock; ventricular extrasystoles. The net deflection is negative in leads II and III and positive in lead I, indicating left axis deviation. Lead I shows ectopic beats following the second and fourth sinus beats. These are premature and show the pattern of LBBB, and no preceding P waves. They are therefore probably ventricular extrasystoles arising in the RV, with a constant coupling interval (R−R = 0.48 sec). Lead V_5 also shows a second type of ectopic beat (the last complex) with RBBB morphology and a longer coupling interval (0.52 sec), probably arising from a different focus situated in the LV. This ECG, therefore, shows multifocal ventricular extrasystoles and left anterior hemiblock. The patient was a 45-year old woman with severe progressive systemic sclerosis, but no cardiac symptoms.

The main ECG problem in diagnosing ventricular extrasystoles is to distinguish them from supraventricular extrasystoles with aberrant conduction, where the preceding P wave is not apparent or the patient is in atrial fibrillation. As stated above, an RSR_1 pattern in lead V_1 is usual in supraventricular extrasystoles but rare in ventricular extrasystoles. An ECG recorded with an oesophageal lead may reveal P waves which are not apparent on the conventional ECG. A His electrogram will also permit a distinction between ventricular and supraventricular extrasystoles since in the latter case a His potential will be seen preceding ventricular activity.

We have already seen that the clinical significance of ventricular extrasystoles depends upon the clinical setting. Neither their configuration nor their frequency is any guide to the existence or absence of serious underlying heart disease. Where the heart is otherwise normal, treatment is only required if the ventricular extrasystoles are causing the patient distress. The patient himself may recognize precipitating factors such as alcohol, fatigue or cigarettes and should avoid these. Mild exertion may abolish ectopic beats occurring at rest. If drug treatment is required, sedation or adrenergic beta-blockers such as practolol may be effective. In the patient who has recently suffered a myocardial infarction ventricular extrasystoles are currently treated if they are frequent (more than 5/min), multifocal, occurring in runs, or if they are very early in diastole, interrupting the T wave of the previous beat, where there is an increased risk of precipitation of ventricular fibrillation (the R on T phenomenon). Intravenous lignocaine is the current drug of choice, in an initial dose of 50–100 mg, followed by an infusion of 2–4 mg/min. Those patients whose ventricular extrasystoles are not suppressed by lignocaine present a difficult problem; many other drugs including procainamide, diphenylhydantoin, bretylium tosylate and beta adrenergic blocking drugs have been used in an attempt to suppress the extrasystoles.

Parasystole

This is an uncommon but interesting arrhythmia which usually originates in the ventricles. The condition has distinctive ECG but not clinical features; unlike simple extrasystole it is usually associated with organic heart disease. The ECG features which permit the diagnosis of parasystole are:

(1)   Unifocal extrasystoles with varying coupling intervals to the preceding normal beat.

(2)   A mathematical relationship between the inter-ectopic intervals. These are all multiples of a single common denominator.

(3)   The occurrence of fusion beats, intermediate in form between sinus beats and the extrasystoles.

The arryhthmia is believed to originate from a protected ectopic pacemaker which discharges regularly. The pacemaker is only able to initiate beats when its discharge falls outside the refractory period of the surrounding tissue. By protected is meant the property of being uninfluenced in its regular discharge by impulses conducted from above. The common denominator of the inter-ectopic intervals represents the cycle length of the parasystolic pacemaker. Occasionally, a parasystolic ventricular focus may discharge more rapidly than the SA node, and it then assumes complete control of the ventricles, producing a parasystolic ventricular tachycardia (*see* page 63). Fusion beats occur when both the conducted sinus impulse and the parasystolic impulse reach the ventricles simultaneously, so that parts of the ventricles are activated from each pacemaker. Fusion beats also occur in several other arrhythmias including AV dissociation and ventricular tachycardia. There is no specific treatment for parasystole.

Supraventricular Tachycardias

Tachycardias arising from sites other than the SA node may be paroxysmal or sustained. Conventionally, runs of more than three ectopic beats represent a paroxysmal tachycardia; it is suggested by Stock (1970) that such rhythms persisting beyond 24 hours should be termed sustained ectopic tachycardias. Supraventricular tachycardias originate above the junctional region. They include atrial and nodal tachycardia, atrial flutter and atrial fibrillation.

Atrial Tachycardia

Paroxysmal atrial tachycardia is a common rhythm disturbance, frequently occurring in otherwise normal hearts. The frequency and duration of attacks is extremely variable, but they commonly last from a few minutes to a few hours. The heart rate is usually between 100 and 200/min in adults. With atrial rates exceeding 200/min, there is usually some degree of AV block so that the ventricular rate is slower. The symptoms of atrial tachycardia include palpitations, dyspnoea and polyuria; if there is co-existent heart disease, or the ventricular rate is very rapid, the tachycardia may cause angina and heart failure.

The ECG characteristics include P waves which differ in shape from those of the patient's normal sinus beats, and may be hard to identify if superimposed on T waves. The QRS complexes may be identical with those of the sinus beats or may show aberration. In the latter case they usually show a RBBB pattern with an RSR_1 configuration in lead V_1. Oesophageal or intracardiac ECG's will usually clarify the origin where this is in doubt. Usually every beat shows aberrant conduction of a constant type, presumably because the part of the His–Purkinjé system which does not conduct the impulse forwards, is depolarized in a retrograde direction from the periphery with each impulse, and is therefore always refractory when the next impulse arrives from above.

There has been a prolonged controversy regarding the pathogenesis of paroxysmal atrial tachycardia, which has been variously attributed either to a rapidly firing ectopic atrial pacemaker, or to the phenomenon of re-entry. Re-entry was first suspected as underlying the paroxysmal tachycardia of the Wolff–Parkinson–White (WPW) syndrome (*see* below). This mechanism involves forward conduction from the atria to the ventricles via the His bundle, with retrograde conduction back to the atria via an abnormal pathway, resulting in a continuous circus pathway involving the AV node, with a rapid ventricular response. Recent elegant studies (Goldreyer, 1972) using His electrograms and atrial pacing, strongly suggest that a similar re-entry mechanism may underlie paroxysmal atrial tachycardia which is not associated with the WPW syndrome. These studies involved the delivery of a premature stimulus to the atria. The more premature the stimulus, the slower its conduction through the junctional region (longer A–H time). In patients prone to spontaneous atrial tachycardia, when this A–H interval exceeded a particular threshold, the tachycardia was provoked, whereas in subjects not prone to spontaneous tachycardias, this did not occur. It appears likely, therefore, that delayed conduction in the junctional region allows the atrium to recover its excitability by the time the impulse reaches the lower junctional region, so that the impulse can re-enter the atrium as well as going forwards to the ventricle, thus initiating the tachycardia. The spontaneous onset of the paroxysm, commencing with an early premature atrial extrasystole, conducted with a long A–H interval, has been documented. Paroxysmal junctional tachycardia is probably the same arrhythmia as paroxysmal atrial tachycardia, differing only in the velocity of conduction through the AV junction.

Non-paroxysmal atrial tachycardias, for example in heart disease and digitalis overdosage, may arise from an ectopic atrial focus rather than being due to a re-entry mechanism. The spontaneous onset of such an atrial tachycardia with a premature beat late in the atrial cycle and conducted with a normal A–H interval has been documented (Goldreyer, 1972).

Non-paroxysmal atrial tachycardia with AV block commonly results from digitalis intoxication, and under these circumstances should be treated by withdrawal of the digitalis, potassium replacement, and if necessary an adrenergic beta-blocker. When this rhythm is not due to digitalis intoxication, it may be treated with digitalis, which will slow the ventricular response, or with a beta adrenergic blocker, or alternatively by d.c. cardioversion.

The treatment of paroxysmal atrial tachycardia should be conservative, since the attacks rarely last as long as 24 hours. The attacks may be stopped by carotid sinus pressure (the patient must be taught how to do this), by taking a deep breath and then straining or leaning forwards, or by swallowing ice cream or ice cold water. Many drugs have also been used, including digitalis, pressor amines, neostigmine, beta adrenergic blocking drugs and, recently, verapamil. This latter drug is a derivative of papaverine, originally introduced for the treatment of myocardial ischaemia, and subsequently shown to have anti-arrhythmic properties. In refractory cases synchronized d.c. shock and even endocardial pacing may be required. In the prophylactic treatment of paroxysmal atrial tachycardia the traditional drug has been quinidine (conveniently given as a sustained release preparation) but beta adrenergic blockers such as practolol may be more effective therapy.

Atrial Flutter

Atrial flutter consists of rapid (250–350/min) atrial contractions, usually recorded on the ECG as a characteristic saw-tooth deflection in leads II, III, and aVF. An isoelectric base-line may be seen in some leads. The ventricular response is commonly 2:1 giving a regular tachycardia at about 150/min. In this situation, and where there is a 1:1 conduction, the nature of the arrhythmia may not be obvious on the ECG, especially if there is aberrant conduction into the ventricles. Under these circumstances, it is helpful to apply carotid sinus pressure while running the ECG, as this will often increase the degree of AV block and reveal the characteristic flutter waves *(Figure 3.5)*.

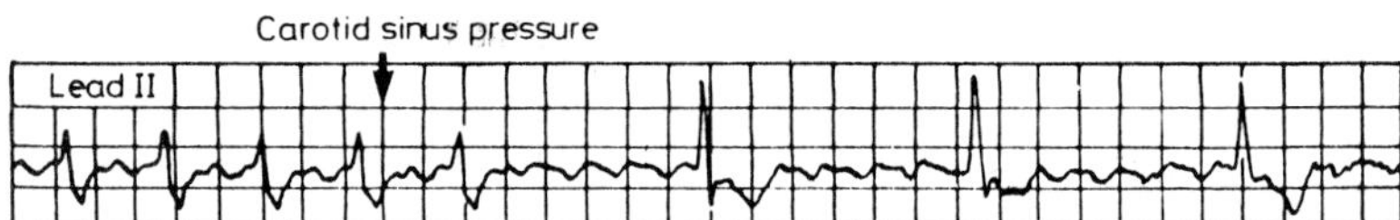

Figure 3.5. Atrial flutter with 2:1 block; carotid sinus pressure. The initial rhythm could not be confidently diagnosed as atrial flutter. The QRS complexes show the pattern of RBBB which antedated the arrhythmia. Carotid sinus pressure exposes a longer segment of the base-line, in which the flutter waves are clearly seen. The QRS complexes which appear during this period are of different morphology from the conducted beats, and show no fixed relationship to the flutter waves, suggesting that they are not conducted complexes, but that they arise independently in a lower pacemaker, probably below the bundle of His. If this interpretation is correct, carotid sinus pressure has resulted in a prolonged period of complete A–V block, associated with the appearance of an idio-ventricular escape rhythm at about 45 beats/min.

Atrial flutter is believed to result from an intra-atrial re-entrant circuit, not involving the AV node. Like atrial fibrillation, it may be associated with many different varieties of heart disease. Treatment may be by synchronized d.c. cardioversion (which can usually be achieved with a small shock) or with digitalis and/or adrenergic beta-blocking drugs.

Atrial Fibrillation

Atrial fibrillation is characterized by rapid electrical activity of the atria (fibrillary waves on the ECG) at a rate exceeding 350/min, in which there are no co-ordinated atrial contractions and the conducted ventricular response is quite irregular. The pathogenesis of atrial fibrillation has been debated since the days of Sir Thomas Lewis, but it is now believed to involve multiple micro re-entry circuits in the atria. The fibrillary waves tend to be larger in patients with left atrial hypertrophy and in cases where the onset of atrial fibrillation has been recent. The irregularity of the ventricular response probably results from conduction of the atrial impulses to varying depths into the junctional region (concealed conduction) resulting in variable refractoriness of the region. At irregular intervals occasional fibrillary waves succeed in being conducted to the ventricles. The mechanism of acceleration of ventricular rate on exercise in atrial fibrillation presumably involves an autonomically mediated decrease in refractoriness of the junction, while slowing with digitalis results from increased refractoriness.

Atrial fibrillation may be sustained or paroxysmal, and may be associated with almost any type of organic heart disease, but it is relatively uncommon in otherwise normal hearts. Lone atrial fibrillation does, however, occur (especially in males), and the spontaneous ventricular rate is usually relatively slow. The possibility of thyrotoxicosis should always be considered where the aetiology of atrial fibrillation is obscure. The symptoms of atrial fibrillation may range from none to severe heart failure, depending upon the ventricular rate and the associated heart disease. Apart from the impairment of cardiac output which results from loss of a co-ordinated atrial contraction, the other major complication of this condition is the formation of thrombus in the atria, with embolization especially into the systemic circulation. This is commoner where there is significant associated mitral valve disease, and such patients should usually be treated with anticoagulants, which effectively reduce embolization.

The choice of treatment for atrial fibrillation depends upon the clinical circumstances. Most patients receive digitalis in order to control ventricular rate. Where toxic doses fail to control the rate, thyrotoxicosis or pulmonary embolism should be suspected, and the addition of a beta adrenergic blocker (for example, practolol) may help. Verapamil appears to be rather effective in reverting atrial fibrillation to sinus rhythm, as well as in slowing the ventricular response. Synchronized d.c. cardioversion may be employed, with the usual precautions (including anticoagulation), in an attempt to revert atrial fibrillation, but there is a high incidence of relapse in most series, and there is a need for a reliable method of predicting the likelihood of a sustained remission. Good candidates are patients with atrial fibrillation following a recent myocardial infarct, and those with underlying causes which have been corrected such as post-operative mitral valve disease and atrial septal defect, and treated thyrotoxicosis. Conversion tends to be easier when the fibrillary waves are coarse.

Junctional Tachycardias

We have already seen that paroxysmal nodal tachycardia is the same arrhythmia as paroxysmal atrial tachycardia. Non-paroxysmal junctional tachycardias occur when junctional pacemakers accelerate so that the rate exceeds that of the SA node. This type of rhythm is frequently seen following recent inferior myocardial infarction, when no treatment is usually required, and may occur in digitalis overdosage. Retrograde

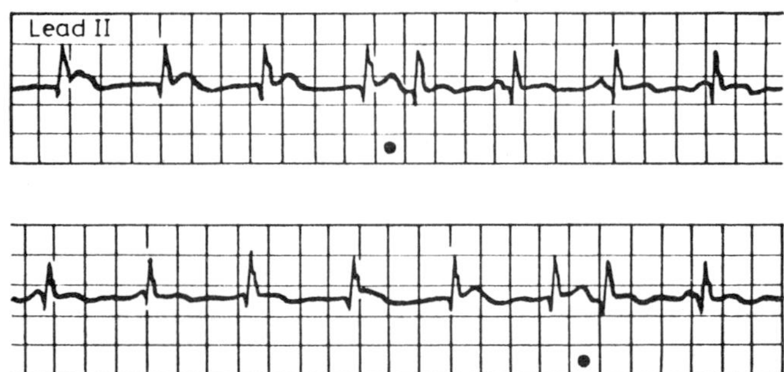

Figure 3.6. Junctional rhythm with AV dissociation (upper and lower strips are continuous). The QRS complexes are of normal width and the ventricular rate about 86/min. The P waves are independent of the QRS complexes and at a slightly slower rate. They can be seen in the upper strip deforming the ST segments. Occasionally (see marks) the P wave falls at a point where the junctional region is able to conduct, and the resulting QRS complex interrupts the regular rhythm (capture beat). The basic rhythm is junctional with no retrograde conduction into the atria. The atria are independently driven at a slightly slower rate by the SA node. This tracing was taken from a 58-year-old woman admitted to hospital 3 days previously with an inferior myocardial infarction.

conduction into the atria may be blocked so that the atria are driven at a slower rate than the ventricles by their separate pacemaker, producing the phenomenon of A–V dissociation. This dissociation may be incomplete, with forward conduction into the ventricles of occasional atrial impulses (capture beats) which happen to reach the junctional tissue outside its refractory period (Figure 3.6).

Where retrograde conduction occurs, in paroxysmal or non-paroxysmal junctional tachycardia, atrial contractions may coincide with ventricular systole giving rise to regular cannon waves. By convention, rhythms in which the retrograde P waves precede the QRS complex by more than 0.12 sec have been classed as coronary sinus rhythms, whereas those with a P–R interval of less than 0.12 sec have been called nodal rhythms. It may be preferable, however, to replace this arbitrary classification by one distinguishing prenodal junctional rhythms (with retrograde P waves preceding QRS complexes) from post nodal junctional rhythms in which there are either dissociated P waves or retrograde P's buried in or following the QRS complexes.

Ventricular Tachycardia

Ventricular tachycardias arise from ectopic pacemakers in the wall of the ventricles. They are usually associated with organic heart disease, and, perhaps owing to the uncoordinated ventricular contractions which occur, tend to impair cardiac function more than supraventricular tachycardias with a similar heart rate. The ECG features include bizarre widened QRS complexes at a rate usually between 120 and 200/min. The complexes are not preceded by P waves. If retrograde conduction occurs, inverted P waves are usually buried in the QRS complexes *(Figure 3.7c)*; if retrograde conduction does not occur, P waves are unrelated to the QRS complexes (dissociation) (*see Figures 3.7a* and *3.7d*), and occasional capture beats may be seen when atrial impulses reach the His-Purkinjé system at a time when it is not refractory. Such conducted beats may be of normal, narrow, QRS configuration and, if observed, provide valuable evidence that the arrhythmia is a ventricular tachycardia. The most difficult differential diagnosis from ventricular tachycardia is supraventricular tachycardia with aberrant conduction. Some valuable differentiating features (on ECG) are listed in Table 3.1.

Ventricular tachycardias may be divided into several types:

(1)   The common, extrasystolic ventricular tachycardia, usually initiated by a ventricular ectopic beat and either paroxysmal or sustained *(Figure 3.7a)*.

(2)   Parasystolic ventricular tachycardia (*see* page 57). Fusion beats are common in this variety, which may be intermittent.

(3)   Accelerated idioventricular rhythm *(Figure 3.7b)*. This variety is analogous to non-paroxysmal junctional tachycardia and also may occur following myocardial infarction and in digitalis overdosage. A

TABLE 3.1

Ventricular Tachycardia and
Supraventricular Tachycardia with Aberrant Conduction –
Some Valuable Differentiating Features on ECG

	Ventricular tachycardia	*Supraventricular tachycardia with aberrant conduction*
Rate	120–200/min	150–240/min
Regularity	50 per cent of cases show slight variation in cycle length of 0.02–0.03 sec	Regular except with second degree AV block or atrial fibrillation
QRS showing RBBB pattern	Rare	85 per cent
Relation of P waves to QRS	Dissociated or retrograde P waves	1:1 relationship or occasional second degree AV block
Capture and/or fusion beats	Diagnostic	Not seen
Relation of QRS to that preceding or following arrhythmia	May resemble ventricular extrasystoles, if present	(1) Identical if BBB precedes or follows the arrhythmia (2) May resemble aberrant supraventricular extrasystoles, if present
His electrogram	His potential buried in ventricular impulse	His potential precedes ventricular impulse

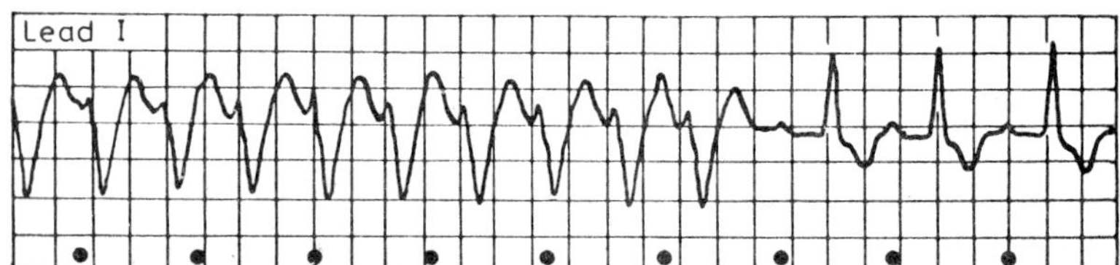

Figure 3.7a. Extrasystolic ventricular tachycardia, terminated by intravenous lignocaine. The first 10 complexes represent the end of a paroxysm of ventricular tachycardia, and are followed by sinus beats with a long P–R interval (0.22 sec). Dissociated P waves can, with difficulty, be identified deforming the complexes of the ventricular tachycardia at the points marked. For example, they coincide with the T waves of beats 6 and 9 and the R wave of beat 5, making them taller, and with the S wave of beat 8, which is less deep than its neighbours. The patient, a 76-year-old man, had suffered a recent inferior myocardial infarct which was complicated by recurrent paroxysms of ventricular tachycardia.

ventricular pacemaker acquires an accelerated discharge rate exceeding that of the SA node, and assumes control of the heart, periods of idioventricular rhythm usually alternating with periods of sinus rhythm. The rate tends to be slow for a ventricular tachycardia (between 60 and 100/min). Capture beats frequently occur. This variety is relatively harmless and rarely progresses to ventricular fibrillation.

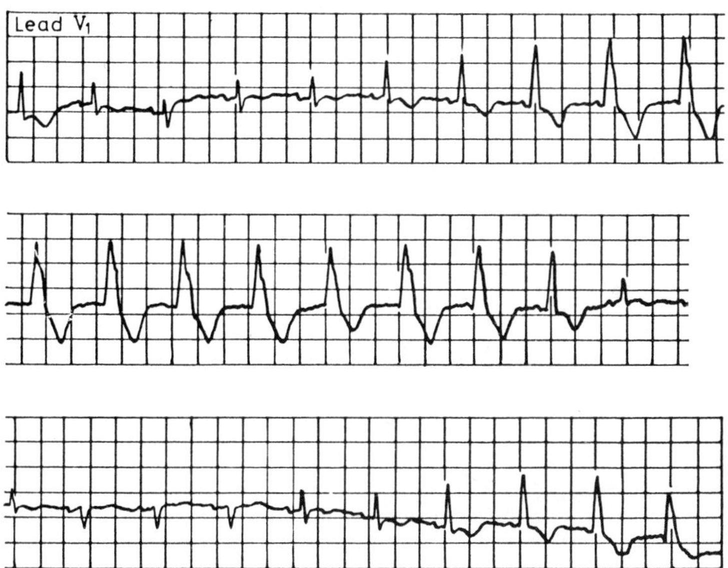

Figure 3.7b. Accelerated idioventricular rhythm (the three strips are continuous). A ventricular pacemaker is firing at a rate very close to that of the SA node. Normal sinus beats are seen in the bottom strip (beats 2–4); the last complex at the end of the upper strip and the first 6 complexes of the middle strip arise from the ventricular pacemaker. The remaining complexes are fusion beats showing varying degrees of activation of the ventricles from both pacemakers, with variation in the P–R interval. This tracing was taken from a 62-year-old man with a recent inferior myocardial infarction

(4) Repetitive paroxysmal ventricular tachycardia *(Figure 3.7c)*. This rare arrhythmia consists of groups usually of 3–6 ventricular extrasystoles following most or all sinus beats. When it occurs in otherwise normal hearts it is surprisingly well tolerated and has a good prognosis.

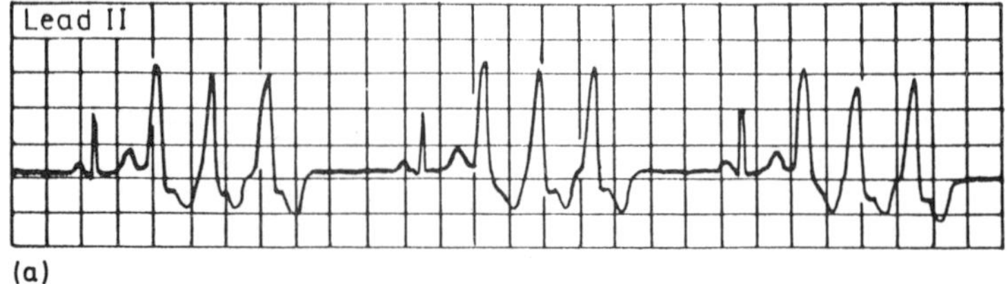

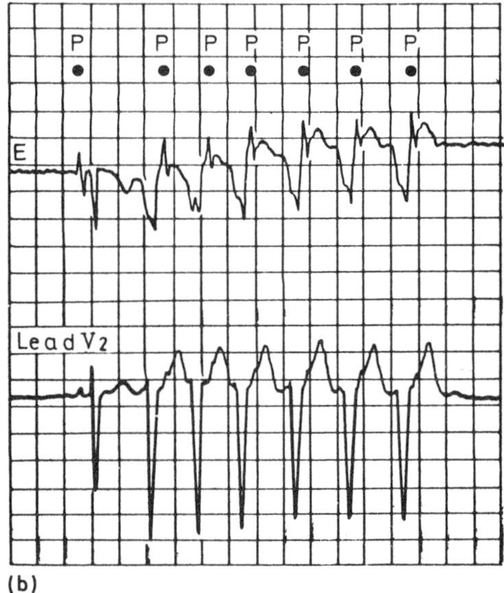

Figure 3.7c. Repetitive paroxysmal ventricular tachycardia. The patient was a 31-year-old woman. (a) Lead II. Each sinus beat is followed by a run of 3 ventricular extrasystoles. (b) Lead V_2 with simultaneous oesophageal lead (E). Here a paroxysm of 6 ventricular extrasystoles has occurred. The P waves are not clearly seen in leads II and V_2 during the paroxysms, but the oesophageal lead shows that there is retrograde conduction into the atria, with a P wave superimposed on the ST segment of each ventricular extrasystole (see marks). The slight irregularity of this brief ventricular tachycardia is clearly seen.

The clinical characteristics of ventricular tachycardia may include wide splitting of the first and second heart sounds and, if dissociated atrial contractions are present, varying intensity of the first sound and occasional cannon waves. Carotid sinus pressure, which may halt a supraventricular tachycardia, does not affect the heart rate in ventricular tachycardia.

66

The treatment of extrasystolic ventricular tachycardia is either by d.c. cardioversion (the method of choice in most cases) or with the same drugs as are used to abolish ventricular extrasystoles (*see* page 57).

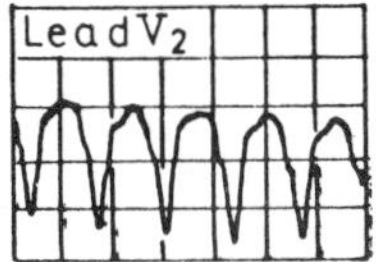

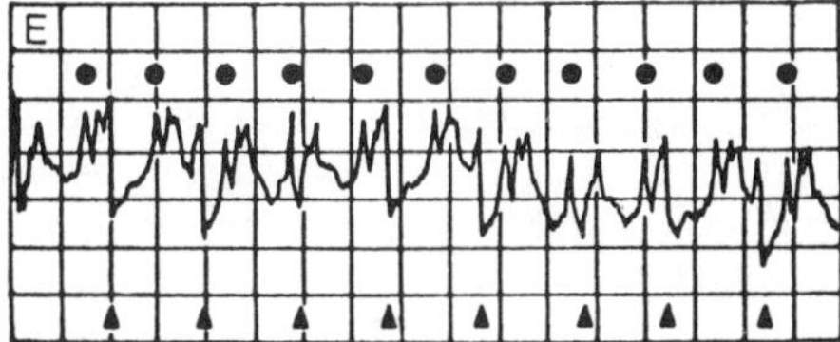

Figure 3.7d. Ventricular tachycardia; oesophageal lead. Lead V_2 (above) shows a tachycardia at about 210 beats/min with no identifiable P waves. The oesophageal lead (E) (below), which is not recorded simultaneously with V_2, shows QRS complexes (marked above) which are bifid in this lead, at about 210/min, while the unrelated P waves (marked below) are at a rate of about 150/min. The oesophageal lead proves that this is a ventricular tachycardia. The record is that of a 20-year-old man who had experienced several similar paroxysms during the previous 2 years.

Occasional refractory cases require pacing for their control. Parasystolic ventricular tachycardia, if recognized, should not be treated with an electric shock, since the parasystolic pacemaker is likely to resume activity at once. Accelerated idioventricular rhythm requires no special treatment. Repetitive paroxysmal ventricular tachycardia, if causing symptoms, may respond well to adrenergic beta-blocking drugs.

Ventricular Flutter and Fibrillation

These are ventricular rhythms analogous to atrial flutter and fibrillation, associated with an ineffective cardiac action, and producing rapid loss of consciousness. If transient, they produce Stokes—Adams attacks; if more prolonged, resuscitative measures and defibrillation are required if the patient is to survive.

Pre-excitation Syndrome

The first variety of pre-excitation to be described was the WPW syndrome, but other varieties have now been recognized. The essential characteristic is an abnormal conduction pathway between atria and ventricles which effectively bypasses the slowly conducting part of the AV junction and causes premature excitation of all or part of the ventricles. The abnormality may be congenital or acquired and is recognized on the ECG by a short P—R interval and/or delta waves *(Figure 3.8)*. The appearance of the ECG depends upon the anatomy of the abnormal pathway and, in particular, whether it bypasses part or all of the AV junction, and which part of the ventricles it prematurely excites. The common (WPW) variety results from a bundle of Kent, anatomically separate from the AV junction; in the other varieties the James and Mahaim fibres (*see* pages 46 and 47) close to (or within) the AV junction, may participate.

The condition is important for several reasons. The ECG in the WPW syndrome may resemble more serious conditions and result in an inappropriate prognosis being given. For example, negative delta waves may be produced in either anterior or inferior leads, leading to an erroneous diagnosis of myocardial infarction. Type A WPW syndrome, in which there are tall R waves in the right chest leads, may be confused with RV hypertrophy or RBBB. A second reason for recognizing the WPW syndrome is that some 80 per cent of patients with this abnormality suffer from paroxysmal supraventricular tachycardias. These include paroxysmal atrial tachycardia, in which re-entry due to retrograde conduction via the abnormal pathway is the usual underlying mechanism, with forward conduction down the His bundle. In this event the short P—R interval and the delta wave disappear during the tachycardia. Patients with pre-excitation are also prone to atrial fibrillation *(Figure 3.8)* perhaps provoked by the retrograde arrival of an impulse up the abnormal pathway during the vulnerable phase of atrial repolarization (analogous to the ventricular R on T phenomenon). With forward conduction down the abnormal pathway, rates may be very rapid owing to bypassing of the junctional region (with its long refractory period), and delta waves are seen. The His bundle may conduct occasional beats and these do not show the delta wave *(Figure 3.8)*.

These supraventricular arrhythmias in the pre-excitation syndrome

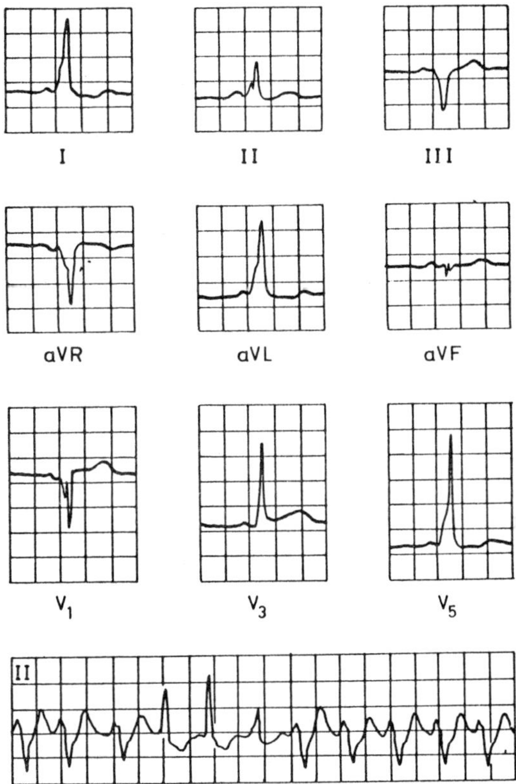

Figure 3.8. WPW syndrome, type B. This tracing shows the short P–R interval and the widened QRS complex associated with a delta wave characteristic of the WPW syndrome. Deep S waves in the right chest leads (V_1) are seen in type B WPW syndrome. This patient, a 59-year-old man, had suffered from disabling paroxysmal tachycardias, associated with angina, for some years. His recorded paroxysms were of atrial fibrillation, as shown in the rhythm strip above, with conduction to the ventricles either through the abnormal (Kent) pathway, giving 'total delta waves' as in the last 5 beats, or via the His bundle, giving normal, narrow complexes without delta waves (as in the fourth and fifth complexes). The resting ECG shows complexes which are, in effect, fusion beats between these two types of complex. Atrial fibrillation is a less common cause of the paroxysms in the WPW syndrome than reciprocating paroxysmal atrial tachycardia.

may respond to conventional drug therapy (adrenergic beta-blocking drugs are perhaps the treatment of choice) but are sometimes highly refractory. Such patients should be investigated in specialized centres, since in several patients it has proved possible to locate and divide the bundle of Kent at thoracotomy. Other refractory cases have been successfully treated with various forms of pacemaker, together with, if necessary, division of the bundle of His.

Intraventricular Conduction Disturbances Including AV Heart Block

Detailed pathological studies (and their correlation with ECG patterns) has made it possible to recognize lesions involving any one or more of the three fascicles into which the bundle of His divides. These are the RBB and the two divisions of the LBB. We have already seen above that an isolated lesion of the anterior division of the LBB produces left axis deviation. An isolated lesion of the posterior division produces right axis deviation, but this lesion is uncommon, as this division is fairly robust, and in order to diagnose it, other causes of right axis deviation, such as RV hypertrophy, must be excluded. The ECG appearances of a lesion of the RBB are well known. Combined lesions of more than one fascicle may also be recognized; for example, it is fairly common for the RBB and the left anterior division to be damaged, leaving only the left posterior division intact. This combination produces the ECG pattern of RBBB associated with left axis deviation *(Figure 3.9a)*.

The recording of the His potential in patients with various degrees of AV block allows localization of the lesion to the region above the bundle of His (the junction) in which case the A–H interval is affected, or to the region below the bundle of His (the fascicles) in which case the H–V interval is affected.

First Degree AV Block

In this condition there is abnormal prolongation of the P–R interval. It is usually due to disease in the junctional region, with prolongation of the A–H interval. This may occur in many types of heart disease — for example, acute rheumatic fever and acute inferior myocardial infarction. Usually the only abnormal physical sign is a very soft first heart sound, owing to the AV valve cusps having closed prior to the onset of ventricular systole. Prolongation of the A–H interval can be produced in normal hearts by rapid atrial pacing.

70

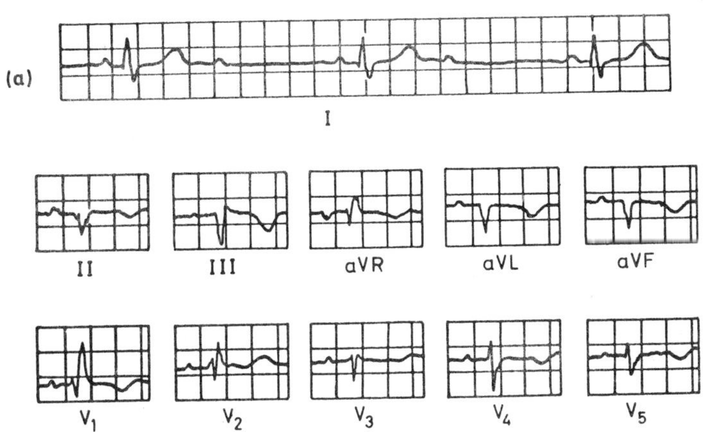

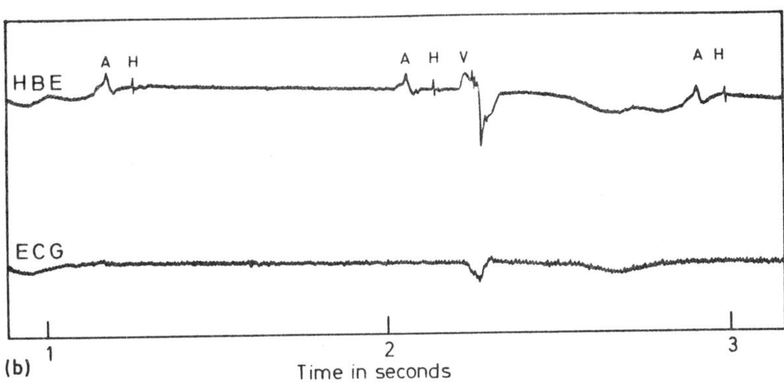

Figure 3.9. Mobitz type II second degree block. Permanent block of RBB and anterior division of LBB; second degree block of posterior division of LBB. (a) The conventional ECG. Lead I shows 2:1 A–V block; the conducted QRS complexes show RBBB (M-shaped complexes in V_1) with LAD (net negative deflections in leads II and III), indicating RBBB and left anterior hemiblock. (b) The His bundle electrogram (HBE) shows that a His potential follows each atrial potential, indicating that alternate beats are blocked below the His bundle (that is, in the fascicles, of which only the left posterior is functioning). The H–V time is prolonged in the conducted beats (86 msec) indicating abnormally slow conduction in the left posterior fascicle.

Second Degree AV Block

(1)   Mobitz type I (the Wenckebach phenomenon). This is also usually due to disease in the junctional region, producing progressive prolongation of the A–H interval with successive beats, until finally the H spike fails to follow the P wave of the dropped beat *(see Figure 3.2)*.

(2)   Mobitz type II. In this less common variety of second degree heart block the His impulse is occasionally absent in the non-conducted beats, but much more commonly the block occurs between the bundle of His and the ventricles, that is, in the fascicles, so that all P waves are followed by an H spike but in some no ventricular activity occurs. In this variety there is often complete block of two fascicles, with intermittent failure of the third, so that the conducted beats show a BBB pattern *(Figure 3.9)*.

Third Degree AV Block

In this condition there is a complete failure of forward conduction from atria to ventricles, which may be due to block in the junctional region, the bundle of His, or in all three fascicles. The last is now recognized as the most common variety in elderly patients presenting with complete heart block, in whom the underlying process is an idiopathic fibrosis of the conducting system and not, as was formerly thought, ischaemic damage to the bundle of His. In congenital complete heart block and in complete heart block complicating acute inferior myocardial infarction, the lesion is usually in the junctional region or upper His bundle; the ventricular rate is relatively rapid and may increase slightly on exertion, and the QRS complexes are usually of normal width and configuration. His potentials precede the ventricular complexes in this variety of complete heart block, since the pacemaker is above the site at which these potentials are recorded. In trifascicular block, the QRS complexes are usually wider and the rate slower. His potentials follow each P wave, as the block is below the site of recording from the bundle of His. Many of these patients with idiopathic fibrosis of the conducting system may be seen to develop consecutive block of the fascicles, beginning, for example, with simple RBBB, followed by the development of RBBB with left axis deviation indicating additional block of the left anterior fascicle, and finally progressing to complete heart block. Other sequences have also been recorded. The left posterior fascicle, being the least vulnerable, is frequently the last to be blocked. Patients may remain in sinus rhythm for long periods after the other two fascicles have become blocked. Similar bi-and tri-fascicular block may be seen in acute anteroseptal myocardial infarction, and in this situation the combination of RBBB with left axis deviation has been regarded by some cardiologists as an indication to insert a transvenous pacemaker, lest complete heart block should develop, since the prognosis, when anteroseptal infarction is complicated by complete heart block, is poor.

The physical signs of complete heart block are well known, and include bradycardia, a large volume pulse, and, if the atria continue to beat normally, a first heart sound of varying intensity and occasional cannon waves in the neck. These latter signs are absent if the atria are fibrillating. The symptoms of complete heart block may include tiredness, Stokes—Adams attacks, and the symptoms of congestive cardiac failure. Cardiac monitoring in complete heart block has shown that Stokes—Adams attacks may be due either to extreme bradycardia or asystole (if the idioventricular pacemaker fails, there may be a long interval before another pacemaker assumes control) or to ventricular tachyarrhythmias (transient ventricular tachycardia and ventricular fibrillation). Drug treatment aimed at helping one type of attack may provoke the other type; hence chronic pacing is becoming the treatment of choice for most cases. Stokes—Adams attacks or resistant heart failure are usually regarded as absolute indications for pacing. The technique most commonly employed at the present time is transvenous endocardial pacing using an electrode catheter with its tip impacted in the apex of the RV. This catheter may be connected to an external pacemaker, or, when chronic pacing is required, the pacing device may be implanted subcutaneously, usually in the axilla. Pacemakers may be of the fixed-rate or demand type; the latter are prevented from delivering an impulse by spontaneous ventricular potentials and are especially valuable in patients with intermittent complete heart block, in order to avoid the risk of delivering an impulse in the vulnerable phase of repolarization of the ventricles and precipitating ventricular fibrillation. Many more refined designs of pacemaker have been tried — for example, those stimulating both atria and ventricles in the desired sequence, and those which detect the patient's own P waves and insert a ventricular pacing impulse after an appropriate delay. These electronic *tours de force* are not, however, necessary for most cases of simple complete heart block, in which the prognosis has been greatly improved in the decade since the introduction of permanent pacing. Before the introduction of pacing, the chance of survival for 5 years was about 25 per cent, whereas with permanent pacing it may be 60 per cent or better.

ACKNOWLEDGEMENTS

My thanks are due to Dr. Arthur Hollman for *Figures 7a, b, c* and *d*; to Dr. R.L. Woodhead for the oesophageal leads in *Figures 7c* and *d*; to Dr. R.A.J. Spurrell for *Figure 2b*; and to Dr. A.M. Harris for *Figures 9a* and *b*.

REFERENCES

Bellet, S. (1971). *Clinical Disorders of the Heart Beat;* 3rd edition. Philadelphia: Lea and Febiger.

Brest, A. N. (1970). 'Arrhythmias', Vol 2, No. 2. In *Cardiovascular Clinics.* Philadelphia: F. A. Davis and Co

Goldreyer, B. N. (1972). 'Intracardiac electrocardiography in the analysis and understanding of cardiac arrhythmias.' *Ann. intern. Med.* **77**, 117

Schamroth, L. (1971). *An Introduction to Electrocardiography,* 4th edition. Oxford and Edinburgh: Blackwell Scientific Publications.

Stock, J. P. P. (1970). *Diagnosis and Treatment of Cardiac Arrhythmias,* 2nd edition. London: Butterworths

– (1971). 'New frontiers in arrhythmias.' *Br. Heart J.* **33**, 809

4

Growth Disorders in Childhood

Max Friedman

DISORDERS OF GROWTH AND DEVELOPMENT

Growth is a sensitive index of health in a child. Normal growth is resultant of a number of interrelating factors, some genetically determined, and others purely environmental. Endocrine disease, bone disease, malabsorption, malnutrition, chromosomal diseases and systemic diseases, may all affect normal growth. Children may be brought to the physician with a history of growth retardation, or during the course of an examination growth may be found to be abnormal. This may be the first clue to the diagnosis of an important disorder. The causes of growth retardation are shown in Table 4.1.

ASSESSMENT OF GROWTH AND DEVELOPMENT

During infancy and childhood the body increases in height and weight. The bony skeleton develops with an orderly sequence of calcification of the epiphyseal cartilages. As puberty unfolds, a growth spurt occurs, secondary sex characteristics appear, and the gonads increase in size. It is of some importance to be able to compare the different aspects of growth and development, in order to assess whether or not these are taking place in a normal and orderly fashion. In the full grown adult it is possible, by observation, to pass judgement on the relative height and weight of an individual, often without recourse to measurement or tables. It is often not possible to do this in the growing child, even for the experienced observer working with children. It is necessary to refer to percentile charts which show the range of variations of normal children in relation to age and sex. The deviations from the mean or average are expressed as percentiles. The fiftieth percentile indicates the mean

TABLE 4.1

Causes of Short Stature

General cause	Specific diseases or reasons for short stature
Nutritional	Deficient intake, for economic, social or psychological reasons Malabsorption syndrome Conditions giving rise to excessive thirst – e.g. diabetes insipidus
Systemic disease	Chronic pulmonary disease Congenital heart disease Prolonged anaemia Chronic renal glomerular disease Chronic liver disease Chronic infections
Chromosomal disorders	Gonadal dysgenesis (Turner's syndrome) Down's syndrome
Skeletal abnormalities	Primary disease affecting bone Osteogenesis imperfecta Achondroplasia Metatrophic dwarfism Diastrophic dwarfism Thoracic asphyxiating dystrophy Metaphyseal dysostosis Diseases of the spine – e.g. tuberculosis; scoliosis Diseases affecting the bone in addition to other tissues Mucopolysaccharide disease – e.g. Hunter's syndrome, Hurler's syndrome, and Morquio's disease Pseudo-hypoparathyroidism Ellis Van Creveld X-linked hypophosphataemic vitamin D resistant rickets Hypophosphatasia
Endocrine disorders	Hypothyroidism Hypopituitarism Isolated growth hormone deficiency Biologically inactive growth hormone production

TABLE 4.1 (*cont.*)

General cause	Specific diseases or reasons for short stature

Endocrine disorders (*cont.*)	Pan-hypopituitarism
	  Primary
	  Secondary
	    Tumours in region of hypothalamus
	    Fractured base of skull
	    Tuberculous meningitis
	    Encephalitis
	    Hand–Christian–Schüller disease
	
	Glucocorticoid excess
	  Administration of glucocorticoids in
	    pharmacological concentrations for
	    prolonged periods of time
	  Cushing's syndrome
	
	Diabetes
	
	Sexual precocity with premature fusion
	  of epiphysis

Constitutional delay in growth and puberty	
Familial and racial short stature	
Miscellaneous disorders giving rise to growth retardation	

or average; this means that 50 children in 100 are above or below the particular characteristic being assessed. If a child falls on the ninetieth percentile then 10 children in 100 would be larger, and 90 children in 100 would be smaller, matched for age and sex, for that particular characteristic. For a child falling on the third percentile there would be 97 children in 100, matched for age and sex, who were larger, and 3 in 100 smaller, for a particular characteristic. It will be seen that the percentile chart gives information about the development of a particular child in relationship to other children. Percentile charts are constructed by obtaining either cross-sectional measurements (the measurement of children of different ages) or longitudinal measurements (measurement of the same group of children and assessment of their development over a number of years).

In order to evaluate the growth of a child a number of parameters are useful and these will now be discussed.

Height

Percentile charts relating to height are available in various types. In the U.K. those produced by Tanner and Whitehouse are the most suitable. The percentile charts used should, if possible, be constructed from data obtained from the population in which they are used. This is important because of differences in genetic and nutritional backgrounds of different populations. A normal child falling on a particular percentile will continue to grow on that percentile for the rest of the growth period, unless something either retards or accelerates growth. A single reading of linear height of a child gives information of the height of that child in relation to the rest of the population of children of the same age and sex. A number of measurements taken over a period of time will show whether or not the child is 'falling off' the height percentiles, or if height is accelerating and the child is crossing the percentiles. A single measurement may show that a particular child is either well below the third percentile or above the ninety seventh percentile, indicating that there may be an abnormality which requires further investigation. The height measurement obtained on a single observation may still be within the normal range, but may be abnormal. For example, a child who is on the fiftieth percentile at 4 years of age may develop a malabsorption syndrome — when seen at 5 years of age that child may not have grown at a normal velocity for the past year, and may be on the twenty fifth percentile, that is, well within the normal range. If only the height at 5 years is known, the failure of growth over the preceding year may not be apparent.

The parental height is of some importance when assessing the height of a child. A child growing on the third percentile and having short parents may be completely normal. However, a child growing along the third percentile, whose parents are both very tall, may require further investigation to exclude an abnormality of growth. Charts relating mid-parental height (the average height of both parents) to the height of the child, can give some indication of whether or not a child is shorter or taller than would be expected.

Weight

Weight can be assessed by plotting on percentile charts in a similar fashion to that for height percentile charts. Weight, however, is much more variable and less constant than height. Fairly large fluctuations may occur, which are influenced by many factors. Weight may be affected by over-nutrition, or by under-nutrition due to lack of food, or a disease process interfering with absorption or utilization of food. This may affect both linear growth and weight.

Bone Development

Bone age is an objective assessment of the maturation of a series of selected centres of the skeleton. For most purposes an x-ray of the hands and wrists will give a reasonably accurate assessment of bone maturation. In some instances it may be necessary to obtain x-rays of other centres of bone maturation. The most commonly used means of assessing bone maturation is by reference to the publications by Greulich and Pyle (1959). Their atlas gives x-rays of the hands and wrists of normal children of both sexes, at different ages, and acts as a reference standard. There is a variety of tables which give the mean and 95 per cent confidence limits for the appearance of epiphyseal centres.

Skeletal Proportions

Comparison of upper segment length (crown–pubic length) to lower segment length (pubis–heel length) may be useful in assessment of abnormal stature. At birth the upper segment to lower segment ratio is 1.7:1, but by the age of 10 years the ratio is 1:1. In dwarfism due to hypothyroidism, the body proportions remain infantile, whereas in pituitary dwarfism the proportions of the upper segment in comparison to those of the lower segment are in keeping with the chronological age. In various abnormalities of skeletal growth associated with dwarfism, disturbance of the relation between the upper segment and the lower segment occurs. For example, in sex-linked dominant hypophosphataemic vitamin D resistant rickets, the upper segment may be normal, whereas the lower segment is greatly reduced, due to shortness of the limbs giving rise to total short stature.

Sexual Development

The degree of sexual development, and the time and order of the appearance of the various secondary sex characteristics in both boys and girls, has been studied by Turner, who described 5 stages of sexual development, beginning in the pre-adolescent stage, and going through to the mature adult. In boys, these stages are assessed by the changes in the penis and scrotum, whereas in girls they are best assessed by changes in breast development (Table 4.2). Pubertal changes can also be assessed in both sexes by examination of the pubic hair. These pass from the pre-adolescent stage where there is no pubic hair, to sparse, slightly pigmented downy hair at the base of the penis, or along the labia. This hair develops into darker, coarser hair, which spreads to

TABLE 4.2

Stages of Puberty

Boys — genital development	*Girls — breast development*

Stage 1
    Pre-adolescent.
    Testis, scrotum and
    penis are the same size
    as in early childhood
	Stage 1
	    Pre-adolescent.
	    Elevation of papilla
	    only

Stage 2
    Enlargement of the scrotum and
    testis.
    Skin of scrotum reddens and
    changes in texture.
    Little or no enlargement of
    the penis at this stage
	Stage 2
	    Breast bud stage.
	    Elevation of breast and
	    papilla as small mound.
	    Enlargement of areolar
	    diameter

Stage 3
    Enlargement of the penis,
    especially in length.
    Further growth of testis
    and scrotum.
	Stage 3
	    Further enlargement and
	    elevation of breast and
	    areola, with no separation
	    of their contours

Stage 4
    Increased size of penis
    with growth in breadth
    and development of the glans.
    Testis and scrotum larger,
    and scrotal skin darkened.
	Stage 4
	    Projection of areola and
	    papilla to form a
	    secondary mound above the
	    level of the breast

Stage 5
    Genitalia adult in size
    and shape.
	Stage 5
	    Mature stage. Projection
	    of papilla only, due to
	    recession of the areola
	    to the general contour
	    of the breast.

cover a larger area, when reaching the mature adult state. During puberty a growth spurt occurs. The time of onset of puberty is variable — the first signs of puberty may occur in entirely normal boys and girls, at any time between the ages of 9 and 17 years. The time taken to go through all the stages of puberty may be variable.

CONDITIONS ASSOCIATED WITH SHORT STATURE

Nutritional Dwarfism

Under-nutrition is by far the most common cause of growth retardation in the world today. This is a purely adaptive response to lack of nutriment needed for growth. A deficiency of an endocrine factor has not been established to account for the growth retardation which occurs in malnourished children. It has been shown that children with severe malnutrition have normal or elevated growth hormone levels. Both economic and political solutions are necessary for dealing with this problem adequately.

A syndrome of maternal deprivation has been described in which children are markedly stunted. The mechanism of growth failure in this condition is not clearly understood or resolved. Some investigators have found a diminished growth hormone secretion in these children, but this has not been confirmed by other investigators. When the children are removed from the home environment they grow normally, often having a relapse when returned to the parental home. The cause of growth retardation is in many cases due to under-nutrition. However, there is some evidence that in these children with emotional deprivation, there may be some abnormality of the hypothalamic–pituitary axis. Teenagers with anorexia nervosa may fail to grow, and often have delayed pubertal development.

A malabsorption syndrome must be excluded in a child with short stature, particularly if the child is falling off its percentiles. A history of frequent, pale, bulky stools may be an indication of the presence of steatorrhoea, although the absence of such a history does not exclude a malabsorption syndrome. Two relatively common causes of malabsorption in children are coeliac disease, and fibrocystic disease. In the former a history may be obtained of the onset after the introduction of gluten into the diet. Anorexia and abdominal distension are common features. In fibrocystic disease there may be a history of chest infections, and possibly a family history as this condition is an inherited autosomal recessive characteristic. However, some children with fibrocystic disease may present with a malabsorption syndrome and growth failure, without ever having given a history of respiratory problems.

Infants with diabetes insipidus either due to posterior pituitary insufficiency, or nephrogenic in origin, may not be able to feed adequately because of excessive thirst, and may be unable to communicate the need for fluid. These infants often refuse milk because of its high solute load, whereas they readily accept water. Following this they will take both liquid and solid foods. The recognition of this condition is important, as these children may become hypernatraemic and dehydrated, and may sustain serious irreversible brain damage.

Systemic Disease

Growth is a sensitive index of disease in children. Most severe diseases of a major organ will interfere with growth. Episodes of serious illness in children are often reflected radiologically as 'Harris lines'. These are transverse bands seen on the shaft of long bones, and indicate periods of growth arrest and deceleration. Cyanotic heart disease will frequently cause growth retardation, and catch-up growth may occur when the heart lesion is corrected surgically. In severe anaemia growth arrest may occur, and catch-up growth takes place when the anaemia is corrected. This is seen in severe iron deficiency anaemia of long standing, as well as in patients with thalassaemia. In the latter condition children often grow much better when managed on a high transfusion regime. In chronic renal and liver disease growth retardation may be a feature, though some children with chronic glomerular disease may be tall for reasons which are not clearly understood. Children with severe asthma may be retarded, and this is probably due to defective intake. When the obstructed airways are relieved children often display a dramatic improvement in their appetite, with an increase in growth.

The mechanism of growth retardation in major system disease is multifactorial. It is probably due to a combination of deficient intake and defective utilization of consumed nutriment. In some cases tissue anoxia and systemic acidosis may play a part. Recognition and management of these children depends on the underlying disease process and if possible, its treatment.

Chromosomal Disorders

Turner's syndrome, sometimes referred to by other names including gonadal dysplasia, ovarian agenesis, and Bonnevie—Ulrich syndrome, is associated with short stature. The usual case is a phenotypic female with absent or hypoplastic ovaries, shield-shaped chest and wide-spread nipples, a wide carrying angle, hyperteliorism, webbing of the neck, low-set ears, a low hair-line, and tendency to keloid formation. These children are of normal intelligence. Cardiac malformations are common, the most frequent lesion being coarctation of the aorta, occasionally associated with aortic stenosis or pulmonary stenosis. Lymphoedema

82

may occur in early infancy. Turner's syndrome is due to the lack of a second X chromosome in females. Some cases are due to the absence of a short arm of the X, or a mosaic chromosomal pattern. Phenotypical males may show all the features of Turner's syndrome, and on chromosomal analysis usually show an XY chromosomal constitution, though some have a mosaic pattern. Females with Turner's syndrome have streak ovaries and are infertile. They have a normally developed mullarian duct system, with a normal vagina, tubes and ovaries. They do not develop secondary sex characteristics, but respond normally to oestrogen substitution therapy, which should be administered at the time of expected puberty. Cyclical oestrogen therapy can produce vaginal withdrawal bleeding which may be desirable for psychological reasons. These girls can lead a normal sex life. Girls with Turner's syndrome do not usually exceed 152 cm (5 ft) in height, and any attempt to influence their final height with therapy has been disappointing. The incidence of Turner's syndrome is about 1:2500 live female births, though it is thought that it may be much commoner at conception, but the spontaneous abortion rate is very high. There is no correlation between the chromosomal abnormality and maternal age.

Another chromosomal abnormality associated with short stature is Down's syndrome, which is due to the presence of an extra 21 chromosome, giving a total chromosome complement of 47. The risk of a woman having an affected child rises with maternal age, and this is due to non-disjunction. In a lesser number of infants with Down's syndrome, especially those born to younger mothers, the abnormality of the chromosomes is due to translocation. These infants have a normal number of chromosomes; one chromosome, however, is abnormally large, and incorporates part of a third 21 chromosome. The clinical appearance of a child with Down's syndrome is characteristic, and presents little difficulty in recognition, except in the early neonatal period when the diagnosis may be missed. However, signs at this stage are floppiness and hypotonia, together with flatness of the face, a third fontanelle, and brushfield spots in the iris, a single palmer crease, and inturning fifth finger. Short stature is invariably present in this condition, and this causes little difficulty in establishing the cause. Other chromosomal abnormalities, including various trisomies, give rise to short stature, but these are associated with severe abnormalities which make diagnosis a relatively simple matter.

Skeletal Abnormalities

Disorders of the skeleton frequently affect stature. They are usually easily recognized because of the characteristic clinical and radiological picture. Primary diseases of bone, and diseases in which skeletal involvement is part of the overall disease, will affect stature. In most of these conditions treatment of the short stature is unsuccessful. An accurate diagnosis is necessary for appropriate genetic counselling because many of these conditions are hereditary.

In diseases affecting mainly long bones — for example, X linked hypophosphataemic vitamin D resistant rickets — the lower segment will be markedly affected, with the upper segment normal, whereas in those conditions in which the spine is affected (scoliosis of the spine, for example), the upper segment will be reduced and the lower segment normal.

Endocrine Disease

Hypothyroidism

Hypothyroidism during the growing period of life leads to severe growth retardation if treatment is delayed. The earlier the onset, the more marked the growth retardation. The clinical picture varies according to the time of onset and the period during which it remains untreated. Congenital hypothyroidism (cretinism) produces a most severe and serious developmental retardation. Delay in the diagnosis and treatment leads to permanent brain damage. Most babies with hypothyroidism look normal at birth. The classical signs of congenital hypothyroidism develop 6 to 8 weeks after birth. It is important to make the diagnosis before these signs develop as irreversible brain damage may already have occurred by that time. The earliest clinical sign of hypothyroidism is prolongation of physiological jaundice in the newborn period. Physiological jaundice usually lasts up to 10 days, and is due to immaturity of the gluconyl-transferase system in the liver. In congenital hypothyroidism the induction of the enzyme system is delayed, and jaundice is prolonged for up to 6 weeks. Screening of all babies with prolonged jaundice will pick out those with congenital hypothyroidism and allow early treatment.

Hypothyroidism gives rise to physical and mental torpor, circulatory impairment, with cold mottled extremities, a slow pulse rate, and a small pulse pressure. Muscle tone is poor, leading to abdominal distension and the presence of an umbilical hernia. The face is puffy, the tongue is thick, and there is a hoarse cry. A supraclavicular pad of fat is a frequent finding. In addition to short stature, infantile skeletal proportions persist, and delayed bone maturation is present. Epiphyseal dysgenesis may be present in long-standing cases of hypothyroidism, giving a crenated appearance to the epiphysis. This is best demonstrated

84

in the upper femoral epiphysis. Occasionally signs of hypothyroidism may be minimal in young children. Mental impairment may be absent, and failure to grow may be the presenting sign of the deficiency of thyroid hormone.

Hypothyroidism may be due to a congenital absence of the thyroid gland, to lack of thyroid stimulating hormone from the anterior pituitary, to lymphocytic thyroiditis, or to an enzyme defect in the synthesis and release of thyroxin. The diagnosis is established by measurement of the protein bound iodine (PBI) which will be low in most cases of hypothyroidism. In certain types of enzymatic defect (absence of the de-iodinating enzyme), the PBI will be normal or raised, and may give rise to an incorrect diagnosis. In these instances the measurement of thyroxin levels in the blood will elucidate the diagnosis. Serum cholesterol is of little value under the age of 2 years, but may be elevated after this age and used as an additional confirmation of evidence for the diagnosis.

Therapy consists of replacement of thyroid hormone. L-thyroxin is the preparation of choice. Replacement therapy should start with small doses of thyroxin which should be built up gradually. The initial dose should be 25 μg increasing by 25 μg at 2-weekly intervals, until the final required dose is achieved. The administration of adequate amounts of thyroxin should lead to the disappearance of the signs of thyroid insufficiency, normal growth and advancement in bone age. Some catch-up growth may occur, but if the period of thyroid deprivation has been prolonged, catch-up growth may not be sufficient to give normal adult height.

Hypopituitarism

Growth hormone deficiency leads to retardation of growth and bone age. Hypopituitarism may be due to a primary abnormality of the anterior pituitary glands, or to an organic lesion in the sella turcica or the suprasellar regions. Tumours, encephalitis, tuberculous meningitis, fractured base of skull, or infiltrations such as Hand—Christian—Schüller disease may all cause destruction of the anterior pituitary. These patients often have symptoms and signs related to the lesion and causing destruction of the pituitary. Headaches, visual field defects, and neurological signs may be present. In these conditions diabetes insipidus due to posterior pituitary insufficiency may occur. X-ray of the pituitary fossa may show an abnormality of the sella turcica or the clinoid processes.

Primary or idiopathic hypopituitarism is commoner than the secondary variety and may involve all the functions of the anterior pituitary.

Children with this disorder are usually of normal birth weight, and growth may proceed normally during the first year of life. They then start falling off the percentiles, growth and skeletal bone maturation proceding at a diminished rate. Growth retardation is usually marked. Their general appearance is that of a normal child, except that they look younger than children of their own age. Dentition is retarded, and sexual development is infantile. The body proportions are in keeping with their chronological age. They may have a tendency to hypoglycaemia. The diagnosis is established by finding low levels of immunoreactive growth hormone which do not rise following insulin-induced hypoglycaemia, or following the administration of an amino acid load such as arginine. Further evidence for the diagnosis can be produced by establishing absence of other pituitary trophic hormones, or the hormonal products of their target glands. Thus, thyroid-stimulating hormone or PBI may be low, but the thyroid gland will respond with a rise in the output of thyroxin following the administration of thyroid-stimulating hormones. Similarly, ACTH and cortisol levels are low, while the adrenal gland will respond with an output of cortisol following appropriate stimulation of the gland with ACTH. Measurement of gonadotrophin levels in children is not of any diagnostic value at the pre-pubertal stage.

Isolated growth hormone deficiency, without involvement of other trophic hormones of the anterior pituitary, may occur sporadically, or may be inherited, occasionally as an autosomal recessive condition. Untreated children are markedly dwarfed, often only reaching a height of 140 cm (4ft 7in). A rare form of dwarfism has been described, similar clinically to an isolated growth hormone deficiency, but with normal circulating levels of immunoreactive growth hormone. It has been postulated that the growth hormone produced by these children is biologically inactive. This abnormality is inherited as an autosomal recessive characteristic.

Administration of human growth hormone to children with growth hormone deficiency produces acceleration of growth velocity and catch-up growth. Unfortunately, growth hormone is only effective in producing growth if growth hormone deficiency exists. The use of growth hormone in other forms of dwarfism has been disappointing; doses of human growth hormone (5–10 mg given intramuscularly, twice weekly), appear to be sufficient to produce a growth spurt. Unfortunately, human growth hormone must be used, as growth hormone derived from other species appears to be ineffective in producing growth in humans. This limits the supply of growth hormone available for therapy, since it has to be extracted from human pituitary glands. Following the administration of growth hormone, growth over the first year of therapy is much greater than in subsequent years. In some cases this is due to the development of antibodies to growth hormone, which interferes with the activity of the administered hormone. If deficiencies of the other trophic hormones of the pituitary exist, these or the products of their target gland must be replaced.

Glucocorticoid Excess

Glucocorticoids are administered to children in pharmacological amounts for prolonged periods of time for the treatment of a variety of disease processes. They are very effective in controlling severe asthma, idiopathic nephrotic syndrome of childhood, and Still's disease, etc. Unfortunately, the side-effects of steroids are undesirable in the paediatric age-group. In addition to the usual undesirable effects which occur in adults, such as Cushingoid facies, osteoporosis, oedema, hypertension, reduced glucose tolerance, etc., corticosteroids administered during the growing period of life lead to growth retardation. Whatever the mechanism, the end result of glucocorticoid administration produces a marked stunting effect on growth. Bone maturation is also retarded. Glucocorticoids should be avoided during the growing period of life, if at all possible. Where pharmacologically effective doses of glucocorticoids are required, ACTH should be used as an alternative. In the doses required to control the signs and symptoms of the disease that requires treatment, this produces a therapeutic effect on the disease process, without causing stunted growth.

Endogenous excess glucocorticoid production is relatively rare in childhood. Tumours of the adrenal gland causing Cushing's syndrome are more common than bilateral adrenal hyperplasia or adenoma. Clinically these children present with moon facies, truncal obesity, buffalo hump, and striae. Hypertension, hirsutism, and glycosuria may be present. The diagnosis is established by finding a high 9 a.m. plasma cortisol level, and loss of the normal diurnal rhythm, the midnight levels being high. Urinary 17-hydroxycorticosteroids are raised; urinary cortisol levels are elevated. Cortisol production rate is increased. The differentiation of bilateral adrenal hyperplasia and adrenal adenoma or carcinoma often presents difficulties. Adrenal tumour cannot be suppressed by high doses of dexamethasone, whereas the child with bilateral adrenal hyperplasia will show a fall in both plasma cortisol levels and urinary 17-hydroxycorticosteroid levels. Metapyrone administration will increase urinary 17-hydroxycorticosteroids in hyperplasia, but will not effect urinary secretion of glucocorticoid metabolites in a tumour.

Treatment is directed at the removal of the adrenal tumour or adenoma. Bilateral total adrenalectomy is probably the treatment of choice in bilateral adrenal hyperplasia. Unfortunately, this is frequently followed by the development of a pituitary tumour which presents clinically with increasing pigmentation due to excess **ACTH** production and neurological signs. The pituitary then requires irradiation or radioactive implants.

When the source of excess glucocorticoids is removed, growth resumes and catch-up growth occurs. It may take up to 6 months for growth to recommence. If growth stunting has been severe and present for a long period of time, catch-up growth may be inadequate to give a socially acceptable adult height. For practical purposes growth stunting to any degree occurs only in glucocorticoid administration. In Cushing's syndrome the associated problems usually lead to early diagnosis and treatment.

Diabetes

Most investigators have found that there is a tendency for children at the onset of diabetes, to be taller and have a slightly more advanced bone age, than children in the general population. Poor control of diabetes may lead to growth retardation. However, when adequate control of the diabetes is established, normal growth resumes.

Sexual Precocity with Premature Fusion of Epiphyses

Sexual precocity due to precocious puberty or excess sex hormone production from the ovary, testes or adrenal may cause a growth spurt and increased maturation of the bone. This gives rise to premature fusion of the epiphyses. The final adult height of these children will be retarded. If seen at an early stage they present as problems of increased stature, and only at a later stage do they present as problems of growth retardation. This situation is discussed fully under the heading 'Conditions associated with tall stature' (page 90).

Constitutional Delay in Growth and Puberty

A large group of children who present with short stature have no physical or endocrine abnormality, but are subject to significant delay in maturation and growth. Apart from the growth factor they are healthy and normal in all other respects. Their bone age is delayed often by as much as 2–4 years. Throughout the growing period of life their linear growth may lag a number of years behind the average for their age. Puberty is frequently delayed in these patients, and this may often be the presenting complaint. There is frequently a history of delayed growth at puberty in one or other of the parents. If left untreated they generally have a normal puberty and adolescent growth spurt, and achieve a normal adult height. Puberty may only occur at the age of 17–20 years.

It is often not possible to differentiate these children from those with isolated growth hormone deficiency on clinical grounds alone. Measurement of growth hormone levels after insulin-induced hypoglycaemia does, however, readily differentiate the two conditions.

This condition is probably a variant of the normal pattern of growth development. The mechanism by which growth and development takes place is obscure. There are probably inborn differences in the rates of maturation of the hypothalamic–pituitary–gonadal axis.

There is no specific treatment which will hasten growth and bone maturation at the same rate. The administration of androgens to boys will produce secondary sex characteristics and a growth spurt. However, bone maturation will occur at a faster rate than linear growth, and final height will be compromised. A similar state will be produced by the administration of oestrogens to females with this condition. The pressure on the physician to administer these drugs is often very great and should be resisted. These children often have psychological problems. Their short stature, youthful appearance, and lack of secondary sex characteristics is a grave disadvantage. They require careful management and much reassurance.

Familial and Racial Short Stature

The height of the child is, to a great extent, determined by the height of the parents. The growth of the foetus is determined by the intra-uterine environment and maternal height, and not the paternal height. However, after birth there is a strong correlation between the child's height and that of the mid-parental height. The height of the child may be determined by factors other than those which are purely genetic. Genetic and environmental influences on growth can rarely be separated, since they interact on each other. Parents may be short for environmental reasons, and these same factors may influence the height of the children. The average height in children in the U.K. has increased considerably over the past 25 years, and similarly the height of Japanese immigrants to the U.S.A. is far greater than that of their parents, and greater than a group of children studied in Japan. This is due to a number of factors, including optimal dietary intake, and decreased incidence of infection.

Children with familial short stature have a normal bone age, and normal onset of puberty at the appropriate time. There is no form of treatment which will increase final adult height in these children. Growth hormone is ineffective, while sex and anabolic hormones will be deleterious and decrease the final adult height, though there may be a spectacular growth when first administered.

Certain racial groups such as the pygmies are dwarfed by most standards. There is some evidence that the pygmies do not respond normally to injected biologically-active growth hormone, and that they may have an end organ resistance to growth hormone.

Miscellaneous Disorders Giving Rise to Growth Retardation

In a number of disorders growth retardation is only one aspect of a generalized disorder. Growth retardation, in many of these conditions is present from an early stage of development, and patients first present as being shorter and lighter in weight, at birth, than would be expected for the period of gestation. In some of these a definite aetiological factor is present — for example, an intra-uterine infection such as rubella or syphilis — but in others no such factor is apparent. Severe CNS defects may be associated with growth failure from birth. The cause of this is unknown.

A number of specific and easily recognized syndromes such as Silver's syndrome, Cockayne's syndrome, Donahue's syndrome, bird-headed dwarfism, progeria, etc., have been described. Frequently, children with a combination of various abnormalities and short stature, are seen, who cannot be classified into a specific described syndrome.

In most of these cases the diagnosis is purely of academic interest, as no treatment is available for the growth failure. An accurate diagnosis may be of great importance, for genetic counselling, in some of these cases. Until more is known regarding the causation and the basic defects in the growth failure in this heterogeneous group, little is to be gained from trying to classify and segregate each individual child into a specific diagnostic category.

CONDITIONS ASSOCIATED WITH TALL STATURE

Excessive growth is a much rarer cause of growth abnormality than short stature. The most important causes are shown in Table 4.3.

HORMONAL CAUSES

Sexual Precocity

Sexual precocity gives rise to excess growth, with advance in the bone age, and premature fusion of the epiphyses. The child may present either as a problem of excess growth, or as growth retardation, depending on the stage at which the disease process is first seen. Most of these children present in the first instance with excess growth. The short stature is due to the effect of androgens which accelerate the growth and lead to excess bone maturation. Sexual precocity may be due to precocious puberty, that is a normal puberty starting before the age of

TABLE 4.3

Causes of Tall Stature in Children

Hormonal	Sexual precocity
	    Precocious puberty
	    Excess sex hormone production

	Pituitary gigantism Thyrotoxicosis
Miscellaneous conditions associated with excess growth	Cerebral gigantism Marfan's syndrome Homocystinuria
Constitutional	

9 years. The hypothalamic—pituitary—gonadal axis is activated at an earlier age than normal. Gonadotrophins are produced, which stimulate gonads to develop and mature. This, in turn, produces secondary sex characteristics, a growth spurt, and advanced bone age, maturation and development of spermatogenesis and ovulation (Table 4.4). The sexual development is complete.

In the female child 90 per cent of cases of precocious puberty are idiopathic, whereas in the male only 50 per cent of cases are idiopathic. The mechanism by which a normal pubertal process is initiated, is not clearly understood, and likewise why this should start at an earlier age than normal, is equally obscure. In the remainder of cases puberty appears to be initiated by lesions in the area of the hypothalamus, and these include brain tumours, mid-line hamartomas such as that which occurs in Von Recklinghausen's disease, following encephalitis and tuberculous meningitis. Albright's syndrome or polyostotic fibrous dysplasia is a syndrome of sexual precocity, skin pigmentation and bone changes and is due in part to a disorder of the hypothalamus. A number of rare tumours secreting gonadotrophin have been recorded as causing sexual precocity. In these cases gonadotrophin levels have been raised to mature adult level.

Excess production of oestrogens and androgens from the ovaries, the testes or the adrenals, leads to some of the signs of sexual precocity, but differs in a number of important aspects from precocious puberty in that the hypothalamic–pituitary–gonadal axis is not involved. Spermatogenesis, ovulation and normal menstrual cycles do not occur.

TABLE 4.4

Sexual Precocity

Precocious puberty – true or complete sexual precocity

Premature activation of the hypothalamic–pituitary–gondadal axis (that is, normal ovulatory menstrual cycles and spermatogenesis)

Aetiology	Lesion
Neurogenic	Brain tumour Encephalitis Tuberculous meningitis Albright's syndrome Obscure lesion of the hypothalamus
Gonadotrophin-secreting tumour	Hepatoma (rare) Teratoma (rare)
Idiopathic	None known

Excess or premature sex hormone secretion

Pseudo-sexual precocity; no ovulation or normal menstrual cycle; no spermatogenesis; secondary sex characteristics only

Aetiology	Lesion

Gonadal	Granulosa cell tumour
	   of the ovary
	Leydig cell tumour of
	   the testis
	Leuteoma

Adrenal	Feminizing adrenal tumour Virulizing adrenal tumour Adreno-genital syndrome

Gonadotrophin levels are not elevated. Secondary sex characteristics *only* develop. Oestrogen withdrawal bleeds may occur. A growth spurt and epiphyseal maturation take place. In the female the granuloma cell tumour of the ovary is the tumour which most commonly produces this condition, but other tumours of the ovary and adrenal may produce the same effect. In the male, adrenal tumours and, rarely, tumours of the testes, will produce excess androgens, and similarly give rise to increased growth and secondary sex characteristics.

Undiagnosed or inadequately treated adreno-genital syndrome may give rise to excessive growth and bone maturation, with premature fusion of the epiphyses. This is due to the production of steroids with androgen-like activity proximal to the enzymatic block. The administration of hydrocortisone in physiological replacement dosage will inhibit excess ACTH secretion and depress the formation of these androgen-like compounds. If too little cortisol is administered, ACTH suppression will be incomplete and excess steroid with androgen-like activity will be produced, giving rise to increased growth and enhanced bone maturation. If too much hydrocortisone is administered ACTH will be suppressed and growth retardation will follow as a result of the excess quantity of glucocorticoid. In the salt-losing type of adrenal hyperplasia, growth retardation may occur if inadequate salt-retaining hormones are administered.

Pituitary Gigantism

Excessive production of growth hormones before fusion of the epiphyses will result in excessive linear growth. Eosinophil adenomas of the pituitary give rise to an increase in secretion of growth hormone. These tumours are usually small in childhood, and may not produce radiological changes in the pituitary fossa, or clinical signs of pressure on the optic chiasma. The growth velocity of the children is extremely rapid, and the feet and hands are markedly increased in size, with overgrowth of the soft tissues. The body proportions are normal, and bone maturation is compatible with chronological age. X-rays of the phalanges show cortical thickening, with tufting of the terminal phalanges. The diagnosis is established by demonstrating high levels of circulating growth hormone, which cannot be suppressed by the administration of glucose. In the normal child the administration of glucose will suppress growth hormone levels.

Surgical removal of the tumour is often a hazardous process, and the treatment of choice is probably irradiation. Yttrium implantation and cryosurgery have been used in an attempt to destroy the tumour.

Thyrotoxicosis

Accelerated growth occurs in hyperthyroidism. Children with this condition often experience a growth spurt at the time when they are losing weight. A child whose weight is falling off the percentiles at a time when his height is crossing the percentiles, should be suspected of having thyrotoxicosis. The diagnosis becomes clear from the history and examination.

MISCELLANEOUS CAUSES ASSOCIATED WITH TALL STATURE

Cerebral Gigantism

This is a condition of unknown aetiology. All cases reported have been sporadic. Excessive size of the infant is evident at birth. Growth is rapid, especially in the first 3 years of life, though final height may not be excessive. The hands and feet are large, and prognathism is present. Facial features are coarse. The health is good in childhood, but these children are usually dull mentally, and have poor concentration. Bone age is advanced and commensurate with height age. No chromosomal or metabolic disorders have been detected.

Marfan's Syndrome

This is a connective tissue disorder inherited as an autosomal dominant with wide variability in expression. Some cases occur sporadically. The children are tall, with long slim limbs, arachnodactyly, muscle hypotonia, and joint laxity, with scoliosis, kyphosis, and pectus excavatum or carinatum. Subluxation of the lens, due to a defect in the suspensory ligament, occurs. Aortic dilatation, sometimes associated with dissecting aneurysm or secondary aortic incompetence, is fairly common. The basic defect in connective tissue has not been determined, though there is an accumulation of mucopolysaccharide within the cells of the aorta.

Homocystinuria

Children with this condition are tall and slim, with long fingers, pectus excavatum or carinatum, and their characteristics resemble those seen in Marfan's syndrome. Most are mentally defective. Subluxation of the lens is common, occasionally associated with retinal detachment. Arterial and venous thromboses are also common. The hair tends to be fine, sparse, dry and light in colour. A malar flush is common with a tendency to patchy erythematous blotches elsewhere. Inheritance is as an autosomal recessive. These children have an excess of homocystine in their urine and plasma. Plasma methionine is also raised. A decreased cystathionine synthetase activity has been demonstrated in this condition.

A low protein intake and pharmacological doses of pyridoxine have been shown to decrease the levels of methionine and homocystinine in some of these patients. Whether or not this is beneficial to the patient remains to be demonstrated.

CONSTITUTIONAL TALL STATURE

There is a group of children who present with excessively tall stature, but who are normal in all other respects. Often they have one parent who is also excessively tall. This rarely presents a problem in boys. Girls who are taller than their contemporaries may become distressed by their excessive height, and seek help. The height that is regarded as excessive for a girl varies from community to community. In the U.K. a final adult height in excess of 178 cm (5 ft 10 in) would be considered socially undesirable for a girl. One of the problems in managing this group of children is the difficulty in predicting final adult height. The tables of Bayer and Bayley offer an approximate prediction of the height which they may attain according to their stage of bone maturation.

If the predicted height of a girl is greater than 178 cm, and certainly if it is greater than 183 cm (6 ft), it is desirable to attempt to produce acceleration in bone maturation and premature fusion of the epiphysis by the administration of oestrogen. In order for this form of therapy to be successful it should be started before completion of the adolescent growth spurt and menarche. Some workers have been doubtful as to the value of this form of therapy. The balance of evidence, however, is in favour of a beneficial effect in decreasing final height. Before treatment is commenced the problem must be discussed with the parents and the child. The oestrogen therapy may have to be given for a considerable period of time, until the epiphyses at the knees have fused. The oestrogen should be administered cyclically for 3 out of 4 weeks. Pigmentation, particularly of the nipples, and menorrhagia, may occur as side effects of this form of therapy.

REFERENCES

Greulich, W. W. and Pyle, S. I. (1959). *Radiographic Atlas of Skeletal Development of the Hand and Wrist.*, 2nd edition. Stanford: Stanford University Press.

5

Chronic Complications of Diabetes

Arnold Bloom

INTRODUCTION

Diabetes is a progressive disorder leading to degenerative changes in the vasculature, the eyes, the kidneys and the nervous system. These changes are referred to as complications of diabetes but they are better regarded as manifestations of a continuing metabolic disorder characterized by excessive glucose in the blood. Many questions remain unanswered. We do not know whether the elevated blood glucose in diabetes is the basic cause of the degenerative changes or whether it is merely a marker of other more significant disorders, perhaps of lipid metabolism. Certainly, the degree of elevation of blood glucose levels bears very little relation to the severity or progression of these complications. Nor have attempts to reduce blood sugar levels, either by insulin or by oral hypoglycaemic agents, been successful in preventing complications.

The relationship between the control of diabetes and the onset of complications is a controversial one. Even good control represents a deviation of blood sugar levels from normal since even the mildest of diabetics cannot maintain normoglycaemia throughout the day. Can it be assumed that it is this deviation which is responsible for the degenerative changes in diabetes? Numerous studies have been undertaken in an effort to establish whether or not the degree of hyperglycaemia is significant — whether good control is associated with a lower incidence of complications than poor control. Most of the findings are vitiated by the fact that the studies are retrospective and hence inadequately controlled. Furthermore, lack of precision in the definition of control makes comparison between studies invalid. Some rely on glucose output in the urine, some on blood sugar levels, and some on other factors. The implied or stated conclusion of those who find that good control is associated with a lower incidence of complications is that stricter care of the diabetic regime will lessen the risks of complications, but it is at least possible that the same factors which lead to poor control are also responsible for the degenerative changes. Hence, it cannot be assumed that poor control is necessarily the fault of the therapeutic regime or even that improving it will prevent or delay degenerative changes. If both complications and hyperglycaemia were caused by a common factor or by different independent factors, the reduction of hyperglycaemia would have no effect on the complications. Nevertheless, from a pragmatic viewpoint, until we are quite sure that complications are not adversely affected by the degree of hyperglycaemia, it remains our duty to advise patients to follow a regime designed to achieve as near normoglycaemia as feasible. It must be confessed that our present methods are singularly unsuccessful in the majority of insulin-requiring diabetics.

Until we know something of the aetiology of diabetes itself, it is not surprising that we are ignorant as to the nature of the degenerative changes. It is generally accepted that the earliest detectable structural change in diabetes is thickening of the capillary basement membrane, most actively studied by the electron microscope in the glomeruli and in the retinal vessels. Claims have been made that this basement membrane thickening has been seen in capillaries of subjects who are without hyperglycaemia but are genetically likely to develop diabetes (for example, the identical twin of a diabetic). Clearly, if this were substantiated it would be of fundamental importance; it would suggest that failure of insulin production and consequent hyperglycaemia may themselves be secondary, perhaps to structural changes in the microvasculature of the beta cells of the pancreas. However, these claims are disputed on the ground that more experience in the technique of electron microscopy is needed before the normal range of basement thickness can be delineated with confidence, and also because there is no certainty that even the identical twin of a diabetic will necessarily develop the ailment. In short, there is still no convincing evidence that basement membrane thickening ever occurs in diabetes before the blood sugars are elevated. Certainly the concept is gaining acceptance that the changes in the basement membrane may be a fundamental disorder in the pathogenesis of the changes in the diabetic kidney and to some extent the retina as well. The situation is less clear in neuropathy. Diabetic neuropathy could be due either to an impoverished blood supply to the nerves or to a more direct metabolic disorder of the nerve cells. The two hypotheses are not mutually exclusive, however.

VASCULAR DISEASE

Diabetics are prone to develop changes both in the large and small vessel. The term *arteriosclerosis* is usually taken to include both atherosclerosis and medial calcification, though these two components may occur as separate entities.

Atherosclerosis

This involves primarily the larger and medium-sized arteries and is characterized by fibrosis of the intima and the formation of sub-intimal fatty plaques. These plaques may calcify or they may ulcerate, providing an ideal surface for thrombus formation and consequent occlusion of the lumen. Although these pathological changes are not specific to diabetes, they occur at an earlier age in diabetics than in the population at large and tend to involve different vessels. Whereas changes in non-diabetics are most prominently seen in the aorta, the iliac vessels, the femorals and popliteals, in diabetes it is the tibials and popliteals that are commonly involved and the aorta and iliacs only rarely so.

Calcification of the Media (Monckeberg's Sclerosis)

This is liable to occur in long standing diabetes irrespective of age. It is commonly seen on x-ray in the pelvic and limb vessels, and sometimes in the digital vessels, but it does not appear to impair circulation or function.

Arteriolar Sclerosis

Intimal proliferation with hyaline changes are commonly seen in the arterioles in diabetes associated with hypertension, both efferent and afferent arterioles of the renal glomeruli being characteristically involved. Although these changes are not specific, they are more severe and extensive in diabetics than non-diabetics and many be seen even in the absence of hypertension.

Capillary Changes

Thickening of the basement membrane of the capillaries, particularly of the glomeruli and retinae but also in many other tissues, has been identified in diabetics by electron microscopy, the degree of thickening being more related to the duration of the diabetes than to any other ascertainable factor. Although thickening of the capillary basement membrane is characteristic of diabetes, similar changes can be seen in non-diabetic tissues — in hypertension or old age, for example — and variations in techniques may be responsible for some of the reported disparities. Nevertheless, thickening of capillary basement membrane may be regarded as the hallmark of long standing diabetes though whether or not these changes can actually precede discernible hyperglycaemia in subjects destined later to develop overt diabetes remains subject to controversy.

Clinical Manifestations

Peripheral vascular disease in the diabetic is usually associated with neuropathy and often with infection — a sinister triad likely to threaten the viability of the limb. The elderly diabetic is often divorced from his feet. Failing vision may make them difficult to see and loss of sensation may render them insensitive to trauma. Hence clear instructions must be spelt out to those at risk. Feet must be inspected each night and must be kept clean and warm, but never toasted near a hot fire. Toe nails should be cut transversely and, if eyesight is poor, preferably by somebody else. Socks and shoes should be loose and comfortable, and search made with the hand for sharp nails or rough protruberences. Symptoms of arterial insufficiency may be minimal. Intermittent claudication may appear gradually in both legs, sometimes more a feeling of heaviness than pain in the calves on walking, suggesting widespread peripheral arterial insufficiency; or it may appear more suddenly and unilaterally, denoting occlusion of a main artery. Pain may persist even at rest, and it may be difficult to distinguish on history alone from the pain of neuropathy. It must be stressed that in the presence of neuropathy quite severe tissue necrosis or even gangrene of the toes can occur in elderly diabetics with very little pain.

Examination of the legs for arterial insufficiency demands careful inspection of the skin, hair and nails. A dry skin with absence of hair on the dorsum of the feet and shins occurs both in ischaemia and neuropathy. Ischaemic feet are usually white but in severe ischaemia the skin may be dusky red, probably because of numerous small haemorrhages from fragile subcutaneous capillaries; they do not blanch on pressure. The venous filling time is a useful guide to the state of the collateral circulation. The legs are kept elevated until the dorsal foot veins are emptied and flat. The patient then sits with the legs dependent and the time is noted for the veins to fill. The end point is usually fairly definite and, if less than 20 sec, denotes a reasonably good collateral circulation.

The foot pulses are best palpated with the examiner seated by the bedside and the dorsalis pedis and posterior tibial vessels should be identified if present. The popliteal arteries can best be felt by using the tips of the fingers of both hands just lateral to the mid-line behind the knee with the knee in the semi-flexed position. The femoral pulses are normally easy to feel and can be assessed for strength and equality. The presence of a thrill should be noted and the stethoscope used to detect a bruit, since this denotes considerable narrowing of the lumen.

The use of an oscillometer offers further guidance as to the amplitude of the pulse at various levels in the thigh, calf and ankle but if surgery is contemplated, arteriography is invaluable. Using the transfemoral route, unequivocal information can be obtained as to the patency, size and regularity of the lumen of the vascular tree from the origin of the common iliac to the foot pulses. In diabetes, narrowing and occlusion of the popliteal and leg arteries are more common than involvement of the major vessels in the pelvis and thigh, a factor which militates against successful bypass surgery.

Treatment

Good control of the diabetic state is important since hyperglycaemia disposes of infection, particularly undesirable where there is ischaemia. This can often be achieved by simple dietary restriction in the elderly but, if not, tablets or insulin should be used. Prophylactic advice must be given, as already mentioned. Local areas of ischaemia or gangrene will often need rest and regular observation, making hospital care necessary in many cases. Where distal gangrene of the toes or foot has occurred, arteriography should be undertaken in most cases once the initial infection has been treated. Arterial reconstruction with techniques such as saphenous vein bypass grafts or thromboendarterectomy may so improve circulation to viable areas that amputation can be restricted to the local areas of damage without loss of the limb. Mid-leg amputations become necessary when gangrene extends from the toes to the metatarsal region without tendency to demarcate. Above-knee amputations should only be undertaken where there is extensive gangrene with infection of the foot and leg and where the circulation of the leg has been seriously impaired by a recent occlusion of the femoral or iliac arteries. A below-knee amputation offers a much better prospect of a pain-free stump and active rehabilitation with a prosthesis.

Treatment of intermittent claudication will depend on the severity of the symptoms and the opportunities for reconstructive surgery as suggested by the arteriograms. Where there is generalized narrowing and irregularity of the peripheral arterial tree, reconstruction is not feasible. Sympathectomy is occasionally warranted in such cases when the pain is severe and there is evidence of sympathetic activity in a skin capable of sweating. Vasodilating drugs are ineffective. Surprisingly, many cases of intermittent claudication show gradual symptomatic improvement, partly perhaps because of an improved collateral circulation and partly because exercise is gradually reduced by the patient to within the limits of tolerance.

Coronary Thrombosis

This has become the most common cause of death in the maturity onset diabetic. Although diabetes accelerates the development of coronary atherosclerosis, the pathological changes in the vessels are no different from those seen in non-diabetics. The relationship between diabetes and coronary atheroma has not been defined. Certainly, a high percentage of subjects suffering a myocardial infarct show an abnormal blood glucose response to oral glucose; similarly, in unselected adults, the more elevated the blood glucose levels in response to a glucose load, the greater the prevalence of coronary artery disease. Of course, diabetes is associated with abnormalities of lipid mobilization and metabolism and it may be that it is this hyperlipidaemia rather than hyperglycaemia which is implicated in the formation of atheroma.

DIABETIC NEPHROPATHY

The complex structure of the renal glomeruli has been actively investigated by both light and electron microscopy. The endothelial cells which line the capillaries are in direct contact with the lumen and blood. The epithelium lining Bowman's capsule is reflected over the capillaries of the glomerular tuft rather like the visceral layer of the peritoneum. Lying between these cellular continua is the basement membrane, probably composed of glycoprotein and sharply delineated microscopically by PAS staining. The basement membrane seems to be single structure and may well be the principal filter of the glomerulus. Since it has no pores, it cannot be a simple sieve. Some of the material from the blood (particularly protein) which passes through the basement membrane, may be recovered by the epithelial cells. Lying in the space between capillary loops is a special connective tissue matrix containing cells and known as the mesangium. The mesangium is prone to proliferate in response to various stimuli.

In 1936 Kimmelstiel and Wilson first described a glomerular lesion regarded as typifying diabetes. This lesion appears as a rounded, laminated, eosinophilic nodule in the periphery of the glomerulus but, although specific to diabetes, further experience has shown that this lesion is by no means common in the kidneys of diabetics with clinical renal disease. The pathology most commonly seen is diffuse glomerulo-sclerosis, and this includes hyaline thickening of the afferent and efferent arterioles of the glomerulus with thickened cellular capillary loops. On electron microscopy, two capillary lesions predominate. There is significant thickening of the basement membrane, sometimes folded and invaginated, and there is a variable increase of the mesangial tissue. It is not known whether the Kimmelstiel—Wilson nodule derives from excess basement membrane or mesangial material or from another source.

The nature of these lesions has given rise to much research and speculation. Diabetic glomeruli have insulin-binding capacity and can be shown to contain immunologically detectable insulin antibodies; this raises the possibility that the lesions are an immunological response to injected foreign insulin. This is unlikely wholly to be true since glomerulosclerosis occurs in diabetics who have never received insulin and in animals rendered diabetic experimentally and not maintained on insulin. It seems more likely that the glomerular changes are due to the metabolic disorder inherent in diabetes and, indeed, basement membrane thickening is widespread in the capillaries of many diabetic tissues apart from the glomeruli.

The clinical onset of diabetic nephropathy is insidious and is usually manifested by the appearance of intermittent proteinuria. The rate of deterioration is variable and may extend over many years. Proteinuria becomes more persistent and heavier; the ankles become oedematous and the blood pressure rises. Retinopathy is nearly always apparent and some degree of neuropathy as well. The patient may now enter a nephrotic phase with hypoalbuminaemia, prominent oedema and a rising blood urea. Paradoxically, at this stage, the insulin requirements may fall considerably, partly because there is a decreased intake of carbohydrate and partly because the damaged kidneys are inefficient in excreting insulin; hence less insulin is needed to achieve normo-glycaemia. Ultimately, renal failure and uraemia ensue.

Treatment of Nephropathy

Treatment is symptomatic. In the nephrotic stage, despite their mildly diabetogenic effect, thiazide diuretics should be used to relieve oedema. With deteriorating renal function and retention of urea, dietary protein should be restricted from 30 to 50 g per day and adequate nutrition maintained by increased carbohydrate. Hypertension may need to be controlled with agents such as methyldopa, particularly where there is evidence of left ventricular (LV) failure. Chronic haemodialysis and renal transplantation have been undertaken in diabetic subjects but all too often concomitant retinopathy and widespread arteriosclerosis militate against long-term programmes of this sort. In some cases pancreatico-duodenal allotransplantation has been performed in addition to renal transplantation in the hope that this would delay further vascular disease; it is too early to say whether this formidable procedure is likely to be of lasting benefit.

Pyelonephritis

Pyelonephritis is commoner in diabetics than non-diabetics and is a frequent concomitant of diabetic nephropathy, adversely affecting the prognosis. Acute pyelonephritis is most often due to a coliform infection, is commoner in women than men, and may be induced by pregnancy, bladder neck obstruction, or catheterization. It occurs more readily when the diabetes is poorly controlled and it should always be suspected in any unexplained febrile illness. Chronic pyelonephritis is more insidious and although it may follow repeated attacks of clinical acute pyelonephritis, it is found more often without antecedent symptoms. The diagnosis rests primarily on the demonstration of pyuria and a significant bacteria count on culture ($>10^5$/ml). The symptoms are vague and non-specific and may be attributed to the diabetes or, in the presence of proteinuria, to nephropathy. Malaise, headache and a low-grade fever often are present and should lead to careful examination of the urine. Intravenous pyelography may reveal a difference in size of the kidneys with variable narrowing of the corticles and blunting or dilatation of the calyces. Renal biopsy may confirm the diagnosis but a normal biopsy does not exclude it since the areas of involvement are not uniform and may be missed. Positive biopsy findings are characterized by interstitial fibrosis with mononuclear inflammatory cell exudate and tubular destruction.

The treatment of acute pyelonephritis will depend on the nature of the infecting organism and the use of appropriate chemotherapy. The diabetes must be rigidly controlled and it is usually advisable to change patients on oral therapy to insulin, at any rate during the period of infection. After the acute phase, it is wise to have further urine examinations to ensure that the infection has been overcome. Repeated attacks of acute pyelonephritis will demand prolonged chemotherapy with alternating courses of antibiotics and sulphonamides as indicated by culture and sensitivity tests. The treatment of chronic pyelonephritis is on similar lines but is complicated by the presence of a variable degree of renal function deficiency. The dose of potentially toxic agents must be adjusted in the light of possible cumulative effects.

Papillary Necrosis

Ischaemic necrosis of the renal papillae, and sometimes of the medulla as well, is prone to occur in diabetes, usually associated with pyelonephritis or with nephrotoxic drugs, particularly phenacetin. It may be unsuspected in life and seen at post-mortem as an infarct-like necrosis of the medullary pyramids. Clinically, papillary necrosis may present with loin pain, pyrexia, haematuria and the passage in the urine of renal material containing portions of renal papillae. The pathogenesis is unclear though infection and ischaemia are implicated.

NEUROPATHY

Involvement of the nervous system is common in diabetes and leads to widespread disorders, the main damage occurring in the nerve supply to the viscera and the limbs. Changes have been described in the anterior and posterior horn cell of the spinal cord but the most common and significant changes are seen in the peripheral nerves. On biopsy material from the sural nerve, for example, it can be seen that segments of axons have lost their myelin sheath and this patchy demyelination is associated with proliferation of the Schwann cells. These changes suggest a metabolic disturbance. Diffuse thickening of the vasa nervorum is also observed and this raises the alternative possibility that the neuropathy is ischaemic in origin.

From the clinical viewpoint, the longer the duration of the diabetes and the worse the control, the more likely is neuropathy to be present. This generalization has many exceptions. Occasionally severe peripheral neuropathy is the first indication that diabetes is present, though the diabetes is otherwise symptomless and evidence for the diagnosis only revealed by an abnormal glucose tolerance test. Nor is the response to therapy predictable. In most cases improvement of the diabetic state leads to an amelioration of neuropathic symptoms but not always. Sometimes neuropathic symptoms appear in well-controlled diabetes for no obvious reason and this is particularly true of the mononeuropathies. In the main, however, the incidence of neuropathy steadily increases with the duration of the diabetes. The relationship between the height and variability of blood glucose levels and the prevalence of neuropathy is much less certain, though most observers believe that a raised blood sugar disposes to the development of peripheral nerve disease. As has been mentioned, it remains possible that the factors responsible for the hyperglycaemia are also responsible for the deterioration of the nervous system.

Classification

With a disorder whose aetiology is ill-understood and whose manifestations are protean, some classification becomes necessary for ease of understanding. Nevertheless, the divisions are not absolute and many of the disorders may coexist. The manifestations can be discussed in three broad categories:

(1) *Somatic.* Somatic changes include peripheral neuropathy of the limbs, amyotrophy and mononeuropathies.

(2) *Visceral.* Visceral neuropathy includes involvement of the gastro-intestinal tract, the genito-urinary system and the eyes.

(3) *Other automatic disorders.* Other changes that occur can be seen to be due to further disturbances of the autonomic system.

SOMATIC CHANGES

Peripheral Neuropathy of the Limbs

The manifestation of peripheral neuropathy most commonly seen is sensory involvement of the legs. In the early stages of diabetes before control has been achieved, or in poorly controlled diabetes, pain and paraesthesia in the legs commonly occur, sometimes in association with lightning pains in the calves and numbness and tenderness in the feet. On examination, the reflexes may be normal or reduced and there may be a partial loss of sensation to cotton wool, pin-prick and vibration sense. The calf muscles are often tender. This type of neuropathy, sometimes described as hyperglycaemic, can be expected to improve with improvement of diabetic control. The picture changes in long-standing diabetes. Some degree of peripheral nerve involvement is usually present but more often the signs are more prominent than the symptoms. This chronic neuropathy appears unassociated with the degree of hyperglycaemia and is usually uninfluenced by changes in the diabetic regime. Inspection of the limbs may reveal muscle wasting, particularly of the small muscles of the hands and of the calves. Trophic changes are often seen in the feet and legs. The skin over the lower legs is pale and hairless and often pitted with small pigmented areas of

106

atrophy. The feet often have a marmorial appearance with shiny atrophic skin over claw-like toes. Deep painless ulcers may be observed on the soles of the feet. The knee and ankle jerks are either absent or severely reduced. There is usually some loss of sensation to all modalities: cotton wool, pin-prick, vibration sense, position sense and deep calf pain may all be impaired to a differing degree. Pain is variable not only between patients but in the same patient at different times. The pain is usually dull or boring but can become intolerably severe, giving the sufferer no respite day or night. Often the feet feel numb or heavy and paraesthesia can be troublesome with sensations of burning or formication. Often these symptoms, partly neuropathic and partly ischaemic, lead to a sense of general malaise and depression.

Amyotrophy

This is a term used to describe a variant of somatic neuropathy in which the intrusive changes are on the motor side, sensory changes being much less marked. The main features are wasting and weakness of the proximal muscles and particularly the thighs. Pain can become persistent and the weakness so profound that the patient is unable to stand up unaided. The wasting is often asymmetrical and sometimes associated with extensor plantar responses and fasciculation. CSF protein may be raised. Despite the painful and incapacitating nature of the illness, recovery is the rule and particularly so when control of the diabetes is improved. Although some aspects of the disorder suggest cord involvement, findings at post-mortem have been inconclusive.

Mononeuropathies

Diabetic mononeuropathy can occur at any time in the course of diabetes. It bears no relation to the duration or severity of the diabetes, making it likely that the lesion is vascular in origin. Cranial neuropathies most commonly affect the extra-ocular muscles, the third and sixth nerves being particularly susceptible. The ensuing palsy can be expected to recover in the large majority of cases though recurrence is not unusual. A true Argyll Robertson pupil is rare in diabetes but the pupils may be small and irregular and may react only poorly to light; when associated with a peripheral neuropathy the clinical picture closely resembles tabes and is sometimes called pseudo-tabes. Ocular palsies may sometimes be associated with pain due to involvement of one or more branches of the trigeminal nerve. Any major nerve trunk can be affected in diabetes. The femoral nerve or the sciatic nerve may be involved, giving rise to pain and weakness, but clinical examination and investigation will be necessary if other possible causes, such as pressure from a prolapsed intervertebral disc, for example, are to be excluded. Foot drop is not uncommon due to palsy of the peroneal nerve. The prognosis is good but the foot should be supported while recovery is taking place.

VISCERAL NEUROPATHY

The gastro-intestinal tract may be extensively involved in diabetic neuropathy. Various studies have demonstrated a disorder of oesophageal motility in diabetes characterized by a reduced resting pressure in the distal oesophageal sphincter and absent peristalsis on swallowing in the body of the oesophagus. These findings are probably due to involvement of the autonomic system and do not usually give rise to symptoms. Gastroparesis is very much more common and troublesome. There is delayed emptying of the stomach after a meal due to an enfeebled gastric contraction and a patulous pylorus. There may be an increase of gastric secretion. Episodes of vomiting are not uncommon in some long-standing diabetics; this is particularly troublesome where diabetic control is poor since it soon leads to keto-acidosis. Overfilling of a dilated stomach may initiate these episodes. It should be remembered that keto-acidosis itself may be associated with nausea and vomiting though this usually soon improves with appropriate therapy and hence is probably due to the metabolic disturbance. Dilatation of the stomach is often a prominent feature of diabetic coma and it may be difficult to decide whether vomiting led to keto-acidosis or whether keto-acidosis caused vomiting. This situation is made more difficult when abdominal pain is present, raising the possibility of a surgical lesions.

Diabetic Diarrhoea

This term is usually taken to mean an enteropathy assumed due to a disorder of the autonomic system. It should be remembered that diarrhoea may also occur in diabetics due to pancreatic insufficiency or to malabsorption from the small bowel.

Diabetic Enteropathy

This is often associated with other evidence of neuropathy and occurs most frequently in long-standing diabetes. The diarrhoea is usually intermittent and often occurs at night as well as during the daytime. During the acute stage as many as twenty loose stools may be passed during the day and faecal incontinence may occur at night. The diarrhoea may persist for several weeks or even months and is sometimes followed by constipation. Despite the distressing nature of the bowel disorder, the patients do not look ill, abdominal pain is infrequent, and the diabetic state is not noticeably disordered. Barium meal follow-through studies of the small bowel in these cases may reveal a disordered motility pattern with irregularity of the intestinal folds and variations of luminal calibre. Histological evidence of damage to the autonomic ganglion cells has not been forthcoming and the evidence that this enteropathy is due to a neuropathy is circumstantial and by exclusion. It has been found that a bout of diarrhoea due to diabetic enteropathy is often improved by a course of tetracycline, presumably acting on bacterial overgrowth.

Chronic Pancreatitis

Chronic pancreatitis can lead to diabetes and also to diarrhoea. Abdominal pain may be a prominent feature and pancreatic calcification may be seen on x-ray. Tests of exocrine pancreatic function (such as the Lundh test which measures the enzyme output into the duodenum after a fat load) will help to elucidate this cause.

Malabsorption

Malabsorption from the small bowel may be a cause of diarrhoea in diabetes sometimes associated with enteropathy and sometimes occurring independently of it. The stools are bulky, pale and foul smelling. They tend to float on water and can be demonstrated to carry a high fat content. The patient is put on a diet containing 100 g of fat per day and the stools collected over three days. The normal fat excretion is less than 6 g daily but is considerably in excess of this amount when malabsorption is present. The xylose absorption test, though more acceptable to the laboratory, is less reliable. A barium meal follow through may show dilatation of the small bowel with clumping of barium and thickened mucosal folds. Biopsy by the Crosby capsule may reveal blunting of the villi and cellular infiltration. Gluten sensitivity must be considered as a possible cause in the absence of other lesions and sometimes a gluten-free diet may prove effective. More often no cause can be found and steroids have been used to relieve symptoms, though this may entail an increase in the insulin dosage.

Bladder Dysfunction

Studies of bladder function in long-standing diabetics show that poor emptying of the bladder after micturition is relatively common but does not necessarily lead to symptoms in the early stages. After a time, urinary retention begins to occur and stasis of urine leads to infection. Ascending pyelonephritis may follow. Clinically, the patient may notice a poor urinary stream and infrequent micturition, though when infection ensues frequency, urgency and dribbling are likely to supervene. An asymptomatic enlargement of the bladder may be found on routine examination of the abdomen, suggesting a differential diagnosis of enlarged prostate in older men, and indeed the two conditions may coexist. Cystoscopy shows an increased bladder capacity and diminished bladder sensation. A micturating cystogram may reveal ureteral reflux. Treatment is difficult. Catheterization disposes to infection and should be avoided if possible. When necessary, a Foley's catheter can be used for about a week and the patient then encouraged to void the bladder at regular intervals, aided by manual abdominal pressure and para-sympathetic drugs. Where these manoeuvres are not successful, transurethral resection of the bladder neck can be performed to overcome the resistance of the internal sphincter.

Impotence

Impotence is not uncommon as one of the presenting symptoms of diabetes and can be regarded at this time as part of the constitutional weariness occasioned by the high blood sugar and other metabolic derangement. Recovery is the rule once the diabetes has been controlled. Impotence occurring in established diabetes is more likely to be associated with generalized neuropathy and is usually permanent. This loss of potency is probably due to involvement of the parasympathetic fibres responsible for maintaining an erection and is often associated with vesical disorders of similar aetiology. In most cases libido is unaffected and spermatogenesis is normal. Retrograde ejaculation is occasionally experienced in diabetic men. Although a normal orgasm occurs, incompetence of the internal vesical sphincter leads to retrograde ejaculation of the seminal fluid into the bladder. Treatment of neuropathic impotence is unsuccessful. As might be expected, testosterone or its analogues merely increase libido without improving potency.

OTHER AUTONOMIC NEUROPATHIC MANIFESTATIONS

Orthostatic hypotension is due to the failure of the normal reflex mechanism, probably mediated through pooling of the blood in the peripheral venous system on standing, and leading to constriction of the arterioles. Symptoms include giddiness and faintness on standing; less commonly syncope may occur. These effects are often attributed by the patient to hypoglycaemia. Care must be taken in diabetics when prescribing drugs which might intesify the tendency to postural hypotension — not only hypotensive drugs themselves but also, for example, diuretics, chlorpromazine, monoamine oxidase inhibitors and propranolol. Simple explanation to the patient of the dangers of getting up suddenly from the chair or out of bed or the bath is often enough to prevent trouble. When the symptoms are severe, fludrocortisone is usually successful, presumably by leading to salt and water retention. Care must be taken to avoid pulmonary oedema and an increase of insulin may become necessary.

Vasomotor Instability

This may also be manifested by postural tachycardia, by dependent oedema and by a failure of vasodilatation in the feet in response to a rise of body temperature. Valsalva's manoeuvre fails to produce the normal response in heart rate and blood pressure.

Since the sweat glands are innervated by the autonomic nervous system, changes in sweating pattern commonly occur in diabetic neuropathy. Anhidrosis may be found extensively on the face and trunk when the body is heated. Occasionally, free sweating at night occurs in neuropathic patients and may be attributed to a disordered nerve supply to the sweat glands.

Charcot's Joints

Diabetic neuropathic arthropathy is typified by the site of involvement, this being nearly always the inter-tarsal joints and less commonly the ankle joints or the tarso-metatarsal joints. Involvement in these areas is pathognomonic of diabetes and differentiates it from tabes which commonly affects the knees. The lesion starts in the cartilage with gradual destruction of the point surfaces, decalcification of the bone structure and disintegration with formation of loose bodies.

Trauma plays an important part since loss of sensation and absence of pain allow free movement despite the destructive changes. The foot becomes shorter and wider with a tendency to eversion and loss of the arch. Painless ulcers may form at pressure points but because the peripheral circulation is usually unimpaired, sepsis is uncommon. X-ray in the later stages will show disintegration of the tarsus, usually within a few years of onset. Although this deformity will necessitate the wearing of surgical boots and makes walking ungainly, the condition is painless and mobility is not materially affected.

Neuropathic Ulcers

These occur on pressure areas on the sole of the foot. They are usually circular in shape, punched out in appearance and painless, so that patients are often unaware of their presence. They may be initiated by protuberances or nails in the shoe, and elderly patients, divorced from their feet by failing eyesight and loss of sensation, must be warned of the hazards in this respect. They should be encouraged to make sure with their hands that the insides of their shoes are smooth and deliberately should inspect their feet as a regular habit. Once an ulcer has occurred, rest in bed may be advisable initially where there is sepsis to be overcome, but the disadvantages of prolonged immobilization in bed for elderly patients may make it preferable to get the patient on his feet before the ulcer has healed. A support in the shoe may help to relieve pressure from the ulcerated area.

RETINOPATHY

Diabetic retinopathy is probably the single most common cause of blindness in this country today and accounts for about 7 per cent of all new blind registrations. The prevalence of retinopathy in diabetes increases with the duration of the diabetes so that after ten years some 50 per cent of diabetics show retinopathic changes while in diabetics of twenty years standing 80 per cent are affected, though not necessarily to an extent that depresses visual acuity. Older patients are more likely to develop changes in the early years of diabetes than children or adolescents.

Although the evidence is based mainly on retrospective studies and often without adequate controls, consensus of informed opinion is that good control of the diabetes, particularly in the early years, reduces the incidence and progression of retinopathy. It remains possible that the factors which lead to the onset of diabetes may independently favour the development of retinopathy – an argument sometimes used to explain the many anomalies in correlation between good control and onset of complications. Against this hypothesis is the evidence in both experimental animals and in man that mechanical destruction of the pancreas can lead to retinopathic changes. Thus retinopathy has been reported in haemochromatosis, chronic pancreatitis and surgical pancreatectomy – evidence to suggest that diabetes itself leads to retinopathy and that there is not some other factor leading to both. From a practical viewpoint it is important to try and achieve as good a control of the diabetes as possible, as long as the probability exists that raised blood sugars contribute to the development of retinopathy.

From the clinical approach, a classification of the various elements of retinopathy has been suggested on a prognostic basis. Abnormalities of the veins, microaneurisms, haemorrhages and exudates are features of simple retinopathy and carry the better prognosis with only slow deterioration of visual acuity. Proliferative retinopathy includes new vessel formation, glial proliferation and vitreous detachment – changes associated with severe and progressive deterioration of vision.

Abnormalities of the retinal veins may precede other changes. The main veins appear irregularly dilated and tortuous, though the changes are seldom sufficiently characteristic to allow a confident prediction that other features will follow. Microaneurisms appear as small red dots or pin-points, sometimes in small groups and often near a main vein. It is important to realize that these are not permanent ophthalmological features but can be seen on one occasion and not the next. Photographs taken after an intravenous injection of fluorescein show that microaneurisms are usually much more prolific than is evident clinically, though some of the spots regarded as microaneurisms do not fill with fluorescein and can be presumed to be small haemorrhages. Various staining techniques have allowed microscopic examination of these lesions on necropsy material and have identified the microaneurisms as spherical saccular dilatations usually on the side of a capillary or arteriole and seldom on a venule. Using the electron microscope, it has been demonstrated that the basement membrane of retinal capillaries is significantly thickened in diabetes and it is thought that the microaneurisms may result as diverticula in this thickened membrane.

Haemorrhages are a characteristic feature of diabetic retinopathy. They may arise from rupture of microaneurisms and can be demonstrated to occur most frequently when associated with systemic capillary fragility. The haemorrhages are usually rounded blot-like areas situated in the deeper plexiform layer of the retina. These blot and blob haemorrhages do not as a rule interfere with vision, unless the macula is involved, and may gradually absorb over a few weeks. Flame-shaped haemorrhages are less frequent unless hypertension is present as well.

Exudates are most commonly seen in association with haemorrhages, though sometimes haemorrhages predominate and sometimes exudates. The exudates first are seen as small white flecks but these may coalesce and extend to form larger clear-cut white areas, often grouped in a circinate fashion round the macula. Further extension may produce large areas of yellow/white exudate involving a considerable proportion of the visible retina when viewed through the opthalmoscope. The nature of these exudates is unclear and they are probably misnamed in that there is no evidence that they result from vascular exudation. They lie in the outer plexiform layer of the retina and contain hyaline material rich in lipid, perhaps deposited in areas of neuronic degeneration from metabolic malnutrition. Soft exudates are less common than the hard exudates described. They are white or greyish in appearance, with blurred edges and are often seen in association with hypertension. They may be due to small vessel occlusion.

New vessel formation is mostly seen in younger diabetics after many years of diabetes and is seldom observed in the absence of other retinopathic changes. Fine new vessels may be seen at the disc itself extending into the vitreous or on the surface of the retina communicating between existing vessels. Numerous branching fan-like vessels may be seen — 'rete mirabile'. These new vessels may themselves show microaneurisms and are potentially dangerous because they are friable and liable to rupture. Haemorrhage may occur in the retina, in the vitreoretinal space with formation of subhyaloid haemorrhage, or in the vitreous itself. A subhyaloid haemorrhage lies in front of the retinal vessels and has a sharply defined border, particularly the upper border. Vision will be affected in a manner commensurate with the size and site of the haemorrhage. A large vitreous haemorrhage reduces vision down to light perception only and will obscure a view of the retina through the ophthalmoscope. Since new vessels may be attached to the posterior surface of the vitreous, vitreous detachment may cause bleeding in the retinovitreous space with further detachment of the vitreous. Gliosis may follow and formation of this connective tissue can now lead to retinal detachment.

Retinitis proliferans is a term used to denote the appearance of fibrous bands in the retina and is part of the process described. Vitreous haemorrhages, gliosis and retinal detachments are the end results of proliferative retinopathy and lead to blindness.

Retinopathy does not mean inevitable deterioration of vision since microaneurisms, haemorrhages and exudates can wax or wane over many years without causing serious deterioration of visual acuity. The presence of new vessel formation, gliosis or vitreous detachment carry a more serious prognosis for sight, and indeed for life-expectancy since these disorders are frequently associated with arteriopathy and renal disease.

TREATMENT

In the present state of ignorance as to the cause of diabetes and of retinopathy, treatment must be pragmatic. Good control of the diabetes, particularly in the early years after diagnosis, offers the best prophylaxis, and cases have been reported where considerable amelioration of retinopathic changes has occurred with better control of the diabetes. Unfortunately, once retinopathy is established a tightening of the regime is unlikely to be effective.

Since natural fluctuations occur in the severity of retinopathy, caution must be exercised in the assessment of claims for therapeutic success.

Corn Oil Diet and Clofibrate

In simple retinopathy the use of a corn oil diet and clofibrate to reduce serum cholesterol and lipids gradually leads to a striking reduction of exudative lesions. Unfortunately, a corresponding improvement in visual improvement is not apparent, and this suggests that the treatment does no more than remove lipids from retinal areas already irrevocably damaged through neuronal degeneration. Nevertheless, this treatment is free from obvious disadvantages and may possibly offer prophylactic advantage in preventing the formation of further exudates.

Pituitary Ablation

In 1953 Poulsen described a diabetic patient with severe retinopathy who suffered a post-partum pituitary necrosis; a striking improvement in the retinopathy followed. Therapeutic hypophysectomy has since been used for diabetic retinopathy though the rationale of the treatment is not understood. Various methods of pituitary ablation have been used including external irradiation, surgical hypophysectomy, transethmoidal cryosurgery and radioactive yttrium implantation. Selection of cases suitable for therapy is of first importance. There should be a reasonably good expectation of life and particularly no significant renal disorder. The blood urea should be less than 75 mg/100 ml. Exudates and gliosis are unimproved by ablating the pituitary and the patients most likely to benefit are those with new vessel formation and recent haemorrhages. In such cases, pituitary ablation leads to a significant improvement in the haemorrhages and a gradual diminution of new vessels with improved visual acuity. A controlled group of untreated patients showed no such improvement during a period of observation of over three years. Despite this potential visual improvement from pituitary ablation, the manoeuvre has formidable disadvantages. Insulin-sensitivity and consequent dangers of hypoglycaemia, impotence in the male and the need for steroid replacement therapy must be taken into consideration as well as the dangers of the particular manoeuvre adopted, carrying a post-operative mortality risk and morbidity from diabetes insipidus, for example. Nevertheless, until some surer technique is evolved to reduce the dreaded dangers of blindness, pituitary ablation will continue to be used in selected cases at special centres cognizant of the advantages and of the risks involved.

Photocoagulation

This technique is used to obliterate microaneurisms and new vessels by using polychromatic light from the xenon arc or by the ruby laser which delivers monochromatic red light. Both techniques are somewhat lacking in accuracy so that new vessels arising from the disc or near the macula cannot be treated for fear of damaging these vital areas. More recently the argon laser beam has been used. This emits light from the green part of the spectrum, well absorbed by haemoglobin and leading to generation of heat in the retinal and pre-retinal new vessels. This method is sufficiently precise to allow the surgeon to pick off vessels even when they are near the disc or macula, and, as it is a painless technique not requiring an anaesthetic, the treatment can be given in outpatients. The main objective of photocoagulation is to burn areas of retina with new vessels or microaneurisms and obliterate them by coagulation and necrosis. Clearly, the degree of success of this treatment will to a large part be proportionate to the experience and skill of the surgeon, but early reports suggest that this routine offers hope of delaying the ravages of haemorrhagic retinopathy.

Rubeosis Iridis

This condition of neovascularization of the iris is usually associated with advanced retinopathy and should be recognized as a possible precursor of glaucoma. The iris appears thickened and inflamed with many fine new vessels to be seen in the anterior surface of the iris just within

116

the pupillary margin. New vessels at the filtration angle and vitreous haemorrhages dispose to glaucoma; this is usually painful and, in view of the tendency of the iris to haemorrhage, difficult to treat surgically.

Cataract

A type of cataract specific to diabetes is sometimes seen in young diabetics where control is poor. The condition may be reversible in the early stage with improvement in therapy. Changes in the lens commonly begin under the posterior capsule and gradually extend to form a diffuse greyish opacity sometimes with linear streaks radiating from the centre. In older diabetics, cataracts are likely to form at an earlier age than the general population but they are otherwise no different. The indications for operation are basically the same as in non-diabetics but care must be taken to control the diabetes as meticulously as possible throughout the operative period. The presence of retinopathy may impair the success of cataract extraction but it is not in itself a contraindication to operation.

SKIN DISORDERS

Necrobiosis Lipoidica

Although occasionally lesions may appear on the arms, abdomen and thighs, far and away the most common site is the anterior aspect of the legs. The earliest lesions are small raised yellowish papules which gradually extend to form plaques of varying size, sometimes extending over the whole of the front of the shin but more usually the size of a hand. The plaques are usually reddish brown with an atrophic centre covered with a silvery scale. Histologically, necrobiotic changes can be seen in the collagen fibres with thickening of the capillaries and vascular occlusion. Deposits of lipid may be present towards the centre of the lesions. Local therapy is usually requested for cosmetic reasons and is successfully achieved by occlusive steroid applications.

Diabetic Dermopathy

This is a term sometimes used to describe small atrophic areas occurring especially on the front of the legs. The lesions are usually multiple and start as dull red raised papules, often with a scaly surface, and later leaving brown atrophic pitted scars. They remain discrete and cause no symptoms.

REFERENCES

Ellenberg, M. (1960). 'Diabetic neuropathy; a consideration of factors in onset'. *Ann. intern. Med.* **52**, 1067

Caird, F. I., Pirie, A. and Ramsell, T. G. (1969) *Diabetes and the eye.* Oxford: Blackwell Scientific Publications.

Siperstein, M. D. (Ed.) (1964). *Small blood Vessel Involvement in Diabetes Mellitus.* Washington: American Institute of Biological Sciences .

The Aetiology of Diabetes Mellitus and its Complications. (1964). *Ciba Fdn Colloq. Endocr.* London: Churchill

6

The Diagnosis of Common Colonic Disorders

Eric Beck

INTRODUCTION

Colonic symptoms are a major preoccupation of the layman whose introspection is stimulated by folk lore and the purgative industry. Numerous ills are attributed to the dreaded state of constipation. This background of superstition, fear and self medication often presents a formidable challenge to the clinician.

A common problem is the differentiation of functional colonic disorders from the organic. When the minority of patients presenting with colonic symptoms due to organic disease have been identified, they must be allotted to one of the disease categories. Unfortunately, diagnosis often ends here. If the patient has no organic disease a functional disorder is diagnosed by exclusion and is often thought not to merit further interest. Thus, at worst, the patient is told 'there is nothing wrong with you' — a statement which carries the implication that the symptoms of which he is all too aware are somehow not real. Alternatively, he may be reassured that he has not got the disease (often cancer) that he feared. Only rarely does the clinician make the effort to explain the causation of the symptoms and discuss their future management — that is to say take positive steps in diagnosis and treatment.

The accuracy in differential diagnosis of organic disease of the colon has inevitably progressed in recent years. However, the increasing clarity has often been obscured by confusing nomenclature and descriptive jargon. Although it is now well known that Crohn's disease affects the colon as well as ulcerative colitis, distinguishing between these two in certain cases can be very difficult and it is not helped by our ignorance of the causes of both. The increasingly recognized ischaemic

119

disease of the colon cannot always be correlated with an obvious interruption of blood supply. The detection of the presence of diverticula of the colon often raises the problem of whether they are an adequate cause of the patient's symptoms. These are some of the problems which will be discussed in this chapter.

COLONIC FUNCTION AND STRUCTURE

The function of the colon is to convert the liquid residue of small intestinal digestion and absorption into solid matter. Faeces are then discharged by defaecation which normally occurs with a frequency of between thrice daily and thrice weekly. Absorption and transit are thus closely interrelated. The fact that patients survive the operation of ileostomy to lead a near-normal life shows that the colon is a desirable rather than an essential organ.

Absorption of water and sodium is by an active transport mechanism and averages 500 ml and 70 mEq respectively daily, with a loss in the faeces of 100 ml and 5 mEq. Chloride is passively absorbed with sodium while a small amount of potassium (3 mEq) is secreted by the colon in addition to the equally small amount (5 mEq) entering it from the ileum. These are net figures representing the overall effect of bi-directional fluxes of water, sodium and potassium. Obviously, disease states will affect this function of colonic mucosa so that in total colitis the 'sodium pump' is damaged; this results in greater exsorption than insorption giving a net loss or secretion of sodium into the faeces. Conversely, hyperaldosteronism increases sodium absorption and, with it, water.

The colon contains a very large mixed population of bacteria with anaerobes, such as bacteroides, predominating. They metabolize unabsorbed products of digestion converting them to other substances which, at times, are of clinical significance. Carbohydrate, such as cellulose, starch, and unabsorbed sugars like lactose, when there is deficiency of lactose in the jejunal mucosa, or lactulose, used therapeutically, are all converted to lactic acid. This lowers the pH of the colonic contents despite the fact that the chyme entering from the ileum and the secretions of the colon are both alkaline. The more acidic the stools the greater the frequency of defaecation.

Amino acids such as tyrosine, phenylalanine, tryptophan and histidine, which are the end products of protein digestion, are converted by bacterial enzymes to products of putrefaction such as ammonia, phenol, cresol, skatole, indole and histamine. These are reabsorbed and, in a normal person, detoxicated in the liver by sulphation and glucuronation, to be excreted in the urine. In liver disease and portal hypertension this process is impaired and portosystemic encephalopathy ensues from their effect on the brain.

Unabsorbed triglycerides can be split into fatty acids by coliform bacteria thereby also contributing to diarrhoea. Carbon dioxide, hydrogen, hydrogen sulphide and other gases are also produced by bacterial metabolism.

The various absorptive mechanisms of the colon have a limited reserve capacity which means that if, as a result of disease of the small intenstine, too great a load is presented to the colon, diarrhoea inevitably follows. Thus, the maximum daily capacity for reabsorption of water is about 3 litres; moreover, unabsorbed substances may irritate the colon and inhibit absorption. An example of this is disease or resection of the terminal ileum where 95 per cent of bile salts are normally reabsorbed by a specific process; if this mechanism fails, cholerheic diarrhoea results from the action of bile salts on the colon.

Transit through the colon is dependent on the amount and nature of the chyme entering it, as discussed above, and movements within the colon. It has become apparent through modern pressure-recording techniques and cine-radiology that only infrequent powerful mass-movements of long segments of the colon associated with distal relaxation actually advance colon contents. Most colonic motor activity recorded is of segmental contraction waves, which, in spastic colon and diverticular disease, may reach considerable pressures. These may occur rhythmically over periods of minutes interspersed with longer periods of inactivity. The segments correlate with the pattern of haustration and are limited by rings of thickened muscle which are frequently in a state of contraction preventing the segmental movements from being propulsive. The paradox emerges that muscular activity of the colon largely slows transit and, conversely, that an atonic colon functions as a relatively open tube or drainpipe offering less resistance to flow. There are many factors which interact to influence motility of the colon. The nerve supply is particularly rich with the submucosal (Meissner's) plexus and the myenteric (Auerbach's) plexus which lies between the inner circular and outer longitudinal muscle layers. In addition, there is a periglandular and subserosal plexus. These networks of ganglia and nerve cells are responsible for the intrinsic activity of the gut and can be thought of as the final common pathway through which other influences mediate their effect. The response of the gut to stimulation at a particular point is to cause contraction with inhibition distally. The extrinsic nerve supply is both sympathetic and parasympathetic. Conflicting results obtained from stimulation experiments are probably due

121

to the different states of the intrinsic mechanisms. It is more likely that, physiologically, the autonomic innervation acts as a fine control over the local reflex and intrinsic muscular mechanisms. Many reflex arcs have been described or postulated to correlate activity in other parts of the gut with that in the colon. The best known, but least well experimentally based, is the gastro-colic reflex whereby increased colonic activity and defaecation is induced by eating or the sight or smell of food. It is possible that a hormonal rather than neural mechanism may be operative though present indications are that gastrin itself is not responsible. The compound 5-hydroxytryptamine, which is a powerful small-intestine stimulator, inhibits colonic motility, as does distension of neighbouring segments of colon; hydrogen ions stimulate. The role of the prostaglandins in normal colonic function has not yet been elucidated but they are likely to play an important part.

The blood supply to the colon has certain features peculiar to it. The superior mesenteric artery branches supply most of the jejunum, ileum, and the colon as far as two thirds along the transverse colon where the inferior mesenteric artery territory begins. The vessel branches are so arranged as to feed into a marginal artery which runs along the medial border of the colon and, at regular intervals, gives off short straight arteries which supply the microcirculation of the gut wall. This arrangement permits a rich anastomosis between the branches feeding the marginal artery, and is part of the usually efficient collateral circulation between coeliac, superior and inferior mesenteric arteries. Unfortunately, the marginal artery may be rather attenuated in the region of the splenic flexure — a fact which correlates with this being the most common site of ischaemic colitis. However, certain features of the microcirculation may also render the mucosa and gut wall vulnerable to ischaemic damage. The short arteries from the marginal artery form a submucosal plexus which gives off mucosal arteries, penetrating the muscularis mucosa, to form a superficial capillary plexus immediately below the mucosal lining cells. Arterial blood may bypass this superficial plexus by travelling instead through arteriovenous shunts; this is particularly likely to happen because the mucosal arteries are very sensitive to the constricting effects of circulating catecholamines. The normal pressure gradient between the arterial and venous system may also be reduced because of the absence of valves in the portal venous system and the relatively high pressure in the portal venous system. Unlike other organs of the body, there is little evidence of autoregulation in the visceral circulation. Mechanical pressures produced by muscular contraction, pressure within the lumen of the gut, and angulation of the gut, may all impede the microcirculation. These factors, no doubt, make necessary what otherwise appears to be a lavish blood supply.

122

IRRITABLE BOWEL SYNDROME (IBS)

As with many diseases of unknown aetiology, this syndrome has many synonyms. None can fully describe with precision the spectrum of symptoms arising from disordered function of the gut. Terms which include colitis (mucous colitis, muco-membranous colitis, spastic colitis) should not be used, as there is no evidence of inflammatory bowel disease; nervous diarrhoea and spastic colon describe the two main subgroups. Irritable colon syndrome has given way to irritable bowel syndrome (IBS) as it is realized that the disorder of function, attributed to muscular irritability of the bowel, may extend beyond the colon. The following two main clinical patterns occur.

Spastic Colon

This is characterized by alternating episodes of diarrhoea and constipation, the latter particularly being associated with abdominal pain. The most common site of the pain is in the left iliac fossa; frequently it is related to a tender palpable descending colon. It may be a continuous dull ache or discomfort building up at times into a sharper colicky pain prior to defaecation or after meals. There may be an associated sensation of fullness and distension which is not always relieved by passing wind. Not uncommonly, the pain is experienced in the right iliac fossa when the caecum may be palpable. Greater diagnostic difficulty occurs when the pain is situated in other sites along the course of the colon such as the right and left upper quadrants and the epigastrium. During the diarrhoeal phase the patient finds that she has to defaecate, often with urgency, immediately on rising in the morning, again after breakfast and often again during the morning. The stools are watery and may contain blobs of mucus. This is preceded and accompanied by borborygmi and flatus, the patient often being distressed by her inability to distinguish wind from water! She may then remain untroubled until the events are repeated next morning or each meal during the day may provoke further symptoms. However, sleep is not interrupted by these symptoms. After several such days a phase of constipation may supervene bringing with it abdominal pain as described and culminating in the passage of hard pellet or ribbon-like stools after which the pain is relieved. A period of normality may follow or the cycle repeats itself. Rectal bleeding is not a part of the syndrome but after a period of time there may be the complication of haemorrhoids which may bleed, adding to the diagnostic difficulty. The general health of the patient is good and weight loss does not occur. Mental stress is rightly emphasized as a precipitating factor and often the patient has noticed such an association. Frequently, a vicious circle is created by the patient's lacking such insight and then fear and anxiety are engendered by the symptoms which, in turn, reinforce them. The fear of cancer is often uppermost, perhaps as a result of friend or relative having recently died. The patient should always be encouraged to express her fears, without the risk of being ridiculed, so that they can be allayed.

There are no absolute diagnostic signs either on general examination or sigmoidoscopy. A helpful clue is provided if careful passage of the instrument reproduces the patient's pain, particularly when negotiating the recto-sigmoid junction. Excess mucus and mild hyperaemia are sometimes seen. The bowel may clamp down tightly on the sigmoidoscope and this may be exacerbated by air insufflation; indeed, pressure waves may be transmitted through what becomes a closed system into the inflating bulb.

This irritability of the colon with an excessive response of the smooth muscle can be more elegantly demonstrated by pressure recordings using either balloons or fluid-filled open tubes and transducers. Colonic motor activity in the basal state differs little between normals and spastic colon patients, however, in response to food or Prostigmin, or when psychologically stressful topics are discussed, much larger pressure waves than in normals are generated. A convincing demonstration may sometimes be obtained of pain coinciding with pressure waves and relief occurring with their abolition by intravenous propantheline. These essentially reasearch rather than routine diagnostic studies indicate that pain is caused by bowel distension from extra strong segmentation waves that are unable to overcome the pressure rings and result in a functional obstruction.

Other investigations such as blood count, stool culture and rectal biopsy are undertaken to exclude other diseases. This is also the main purpose of a barium enema examination; since this usually involves preparation with bowel stimulants and the instillation under pressure into an abnormally emptied bowel of an unphysiological suspension, it is not surprising that more is learnt of structure than function of the bowel. Nonetheless, the appearances may suggest the diagnosis if there is hypersegmentation of the colon with very prominent haustral markings and generalized narrowing of the lumen with even some segments completely shut down. These positive findings can often be better demonstrated by the more physiological technique of the oral cologram. 10 ml of micropaque are taken in sips with the evening meal and, by next morning, will have reached the colon and made the stools radio-opaque. A plain abdominal x-ray then shows the relationship of the colon to its contents when the appearances described above may be seen. In addition, whereas most of the descending colon in a normal person is usually empty of stool, in the patient with spastic colon

124

opacified stool may be seen in a chain of short, rounded segments which has been likened to the beads of a rosary. This technique will also allow measurement of transit time if serial films are taken until the stool reaches the rectum. It cannot be used to exclude other lesions of the colon which, if suspected, make a barium enema mandatory. Nor should this relatively physiological technique of stool opacification be confused with that of taking a late colonic film after a barium meal or follow-through examination since these procedures both present an unphysiological load to the colon and may, indeed, provoke diarrhoea or constipation.

Nervous Diarrhoea

This is usually painless and is either chronic or episodic, watery or semi-solid diarrhoea without weight loss. More often than in the spastic colon patients, there is a history of an abrupt onset dating back to a dysenteric illness. In the past this initial illness may have been experienced on military service in the Middle East or Asia when the continuing symptoms make it necessary to exclude persisting infection with shigella, salmonella or entamoeba species. Usually, the general well-being and long duration of symptoms make these unlikely and the absence of any features of malabsorption or steatorrhoea excludes tropical sprue. A common history nowadays is for a party of holiday-makers in Spain to be affected by a 'tummy bug' (usually unidentified) and for all but the patient to make a full recovery; from that time on diarrhoea persists, often being precipitated or exacerbated by dietary indiscretions or emotional disturbances that previously would have left her unscathed. The colonic smooth muscle appears to over-react to the multiplicity of stimuli which normally modify its action.

As mentioned above, manometric studies show that there is a low intraluminal pressure with a low resistance to flow resulting in accelerated transit in these patients with diarrhoea.

Aetiology of Irritable Bowel Syndrome (IBS)

The aetiology of IBS remains obscure even if there is increasing understanding of the mechanisms underlying it. It is certainly very prevalent, shows a female preponderance, and particularly affects the 20–60 age group. In the middle-aged it appears to overlap with diverticular disease with which it shares several features. The symptoms of uncomplicated diverticular disease and spastic colon are the same ones of alternating diarrhoea, constipation, left iliac fossa pain and tenderness. In both there is overactivity of muscle in the sigmoid colon. As yet no causal connection has been proved between the two conditions.

The colonic muscle hypersensitivity may be considered to be a hereditary predisposition which does not usually manifest itself until the end of the second decade. Perhaps this is because the provocative stimuli do not occur or have not been present for long enough until then. A positive family history is not uncommon. The importance of psychological factors has been stressed above and has resulted in the condition being cited as a classical psychosomatic disorder. However, this interpretation must encourage, rather than prevent, the physician and patient to identify the circumstances which precipitate the symptoms.

Diet, undoubtedly, is a factor. It may be the prime cause or, in the established case, certain foods may precipitate symptoms. It is hard to dissociate the diet of Western countries from all the other ills attributed to the stress of modern life. There is a striking difference between the low faecal residue when highly refined flour and carbohydrate is eaten and the high residue diet eaten by native Africans. This is mirrored by the small irritable colons of the younger population and high incidence of diverticulosis in the elderly of the West and the lack of reports of IBS and absence of diverticulosis in Africans. Instead, they are very prone to megacolon and its dangerous complication of volvulus.

True allergy to dietary factors is difficult to prove and probably rare but should not dissuade one from attending to this point in history taking. Rather than resorting to skin tests, it is probably better to try an exclusion diet if there is a suspected item such as milk.

Hypolactasia as a cause of IBS is not now thought to be of great importance. A high proportion of adults of Mediterranean or negro origin, and 5 per cent of the indigenous population, show a deficiency of lactase in the jejunal brush border. They are therefore unable to split the disaccharide lactose into its monosaccharide components of glucose and galactose. This can be shown by enzyme assay of a jejunal mucosal biopsy specimen or by the failure of blood glucose to rise after a 50 g load of lactose compared with a dose of 25 g glucose and 25 g galactose. The failure to absorb such a lactose load will often provoke diarrhoea and abdominal discomfort as colonic bacteria convert it to lactic acid which stimulates the bowel. However, the far smaller lactose intake in milk and its products under normal conditions rarely can be implicated, even if hypolactasia were demonstrated, in a patient with IBS.

The role of infection in aetiology has already been discussed. As so few of those exposed to the same infection go on to develop IBS, it is much more likely that it unmasks an underlying hypersensitivity. It is interesting that the hypersensitivity to cholinergic drugs demonstrated

126

by pressure studies in these patients can be shown to be still present when they are symptom free.

DIVERTICULA OF THE COLON

Diverticula of the colon are more properly termed pseudo-diverticula since they are formed by herniation of the mucosa through weaknesses in the circular muscle of the colon. They occur between the three bands of longitudinal muscle (taeniae) and are often better seen on barium enema than on inspection as they frequently track into the appendices epiploicae. Although they can occur throughout the colon, they are particularly common in the sigmoid region. At this site, they may give rise to the various symptoms discussed below, which tend to occur in younger patients. The combination of hypertonicity, increased irritability to various stimuli and eventual hypertrophy of colonic muscle gives rise to hypersegmentation of the bowel and the generation of excessive intra-luminal pressures. These factors are considered to be of aetiological significance as is the consistency of the stool which, in turn, is influenced by the roughage in the diet. The incidence of diverticula throughout the whole of the gut increases from the age of 40 onwards until, in the seventh decade, they are present, albeit asymptomatically, in about half the population of this country taking a Western diet. Attempts have been made to contrast the diverticula diffusely distributed throughout the colon (which have relatively short wide necks arising in a relatively thin-walled atrophied colon), with sigmoid diverticula, whose necks are long and narrow, as they penetrate the hypertrophied colonic muscular wall. It is by no means certain, however, that they differ fundamentally, the alternative view being that they represent opposite ends of the spectrum of colonic diverticula.

The terminology of disease states associated with colonic diverticula has been clarified in recent years *(Figure 6.1)*. Ninety per cent of patients with demonstrable diverticula are asymptomatic, and in these people the condition is described as *diverticulosis* and is often present throughout the colon. In those in whom the condition is confined to the sigmoid colon, and associated with muscle hypertrophy, there may be chronic or recurrent symptoms of alternating diarrhoea and constipation and cramp-like colicky pain, chiefly in the left lower quadrant, where tender colon may be palpated, resembling spastic colon. This was formerly called chronic diverticulitis. It is now realized that the diverticula are not inflamed at this stage but that symptoms are caused by muscular overactivity; the term *diverticular disease* is therefore preferable.

Acute inflammation of a sigmoid diverticulum is usually caused by an impacted faecolith and gives rise to *acute diverticulitis*. There may be a preceding history of diverticular disease or the patient may have had symptomless diverticulosis. Acute diverticulitis has been likened to left-sided appendicitis though a long sigmoid colon can loop over to

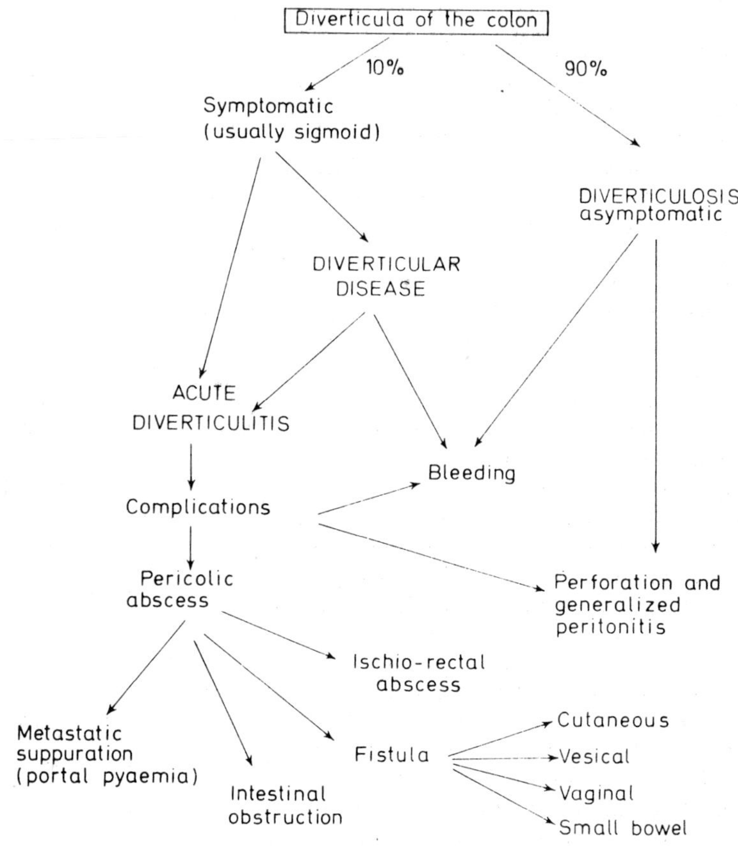

Figure 6.1. Disease states associated with diverticula of the colon

the right and appendicitis can be mimicked even more closely. There is usually an abrupt onset of lower abdominal pain later localizing to the left iliac fossa where tenderness and guarding occur and a mass may be palpable. There is accompanying fever, tachycardia, leucocytosis and constipation. On rectal examination, there is usually tenderness if the finger tip reaches the affected bowel. Vomiting may occur early as part of the malaise and does not necessarily imply colonic obstruction; it may sometimes be due to involvement of neighbouring small bowel. Likewise, irritation of the neighbouring bladder and vagina may give rise to frequency of micturition and vaginal discharge. In the majority of patients the acute diverticulitis, and associated pericolitis, settle spontaneously or with medical treatment.

Complications occur in a minority usually as a result of the formation of a pericolic abscess at the site of the inflamed diverticulum. By the time a pericolic abscess ruptures, it will generally have excited a marked local inflammatory response so that generalized peritonitis, fortunately, is rare; in fact, this may occur in a patient with previous symptomless diverticulosis where local defence mechanisms have not been alerted. The abscess may track through the pelvic peritoneum to form an ischio-rectal abscess, or it may become adherent to the anterior abdominal wall and form a cutaneous fistula. More often the abscess will rupture into an adjacent organ giving rise to internal fistulae with the bladder or vagina. This will give rise to the passage of wind, faeces and, sometimes, pus per urethram or per vaginam. Fistulae to the small bowel also occur and may give rise to malabsorption and steatorrhoea by introducing bacteria into the normally sterile small gut. Other fistulae to gall bladder and stomach have been reported.

Sigmoid colon obstruction may occur either in the acute stage from an inflammatory mass or from the distortion and fibrosis produced by repeated attacks. The differential diagnosis will then be from an obstructing sigmoid carcinoma and may prove to be very difficult. The recto-sigmoid junction frequently cannot be passed with a sigmoidoscope in such patients and barium enema may also show a block. This may be a situation in which fibre-optic colonoscopy could be of value but this method is not yet generally available. Hopes that detection of carcino-embryonic antigen (CEA) would provide a specific serological test for colonic cancer have not been realized as it is also found in patients with non-neoplastic disease of the colon. Further difficulty can arise from the presence of cancer and diverticulitis together. Similar age-groups are involved and the sigmoid is the most common site in the colon for both diverticulitis and cancer. Although dietary factors have been invoked as a link between the two conditions, there is no definite evidence that diverticulitis is a precancerous condition. Where doubt remains in this differential diagnosis, laparotomy must be undertaken. Portal pyaemia with metastatic suppuration is another complication; fortunately it is very rare.

Like perforation, profuse rectal bleeding may occur in previously asymptomatic patients, although usually it is small in amount. It tends to recur and, although it may be associated with sigmoid diverticula and their complications, the condition seems especially common in those with widespread diverticulosis. A problem then arises as to which of the many possible sites of bleeding is responsible. Again, the differential diagnosis can be difficult because carcinoma, ulcerative colitis, Crohn's disease and ischaemic colitis all have to be considered.

Barium enema examination remains the best method for diagnosis of colonic diverticula and their diseases and complications. The extent and distribution of diverticulosis will easily be seen. In the sigmoid type the muscular hypertrophy will give rise to narrowing and distortion of the lumen which is sometimes likened to a 'saw tooth' or an 'accordion' in appearance (*Figure 6.2*); pericolic abscess may superimpose a smooth

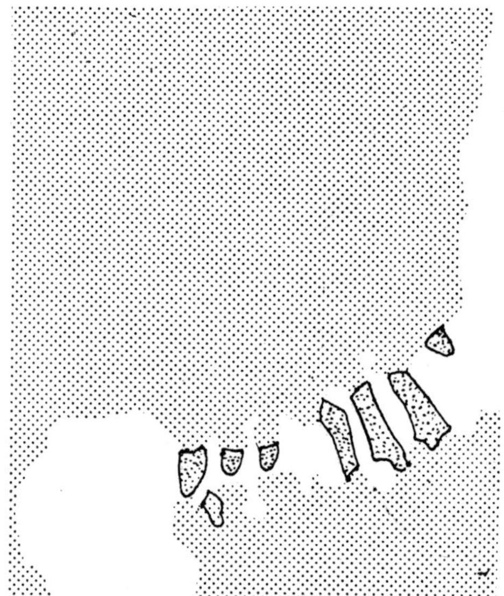

Figure 6.2. Barium enema in a patient with diverticular disease involving the sigmoid colon. Diverticula with circular muscular hypertrophy producing ridging

filling defect on the lumen. A fistula will be seen as a narrow track travelling beyond the bowel in continuity with its lumen; this may resemble the fissuring and fistula formation of Crohn's disease in which these lesions, however, are often multiple. Obstruction of the colon to barium enema has already been mentioned regarding its differentiation from carcinoma; sometimes relaxation of muscle, leading to improved definition, can be achieved with intravenous propantheline.

ISCHAEMIC DISEASE OF THE COLON
(ISCHAEMIC COLITIS)

In the past most forms of chronic bloody diarrhoea were attributed to ulcerative colitis. When unusual features were present such as severe pain or involvement of an isolated segment of colon with sparing of the rectum, the case was considered to be atypical and terms like segmental colitis were introduced. With the appreciation that Crohn's disease could involve the colon, some of the cases of atypical ulcerative colitis were indeed seen to be typical cases of Crohn's disease as discussed below. Other atypical cases of colitis are now recognized to be due to colonic ischaemia; since inflammation due to bacteria is a secondary rather than primary phenomenon, some would prefer the broader term of ischaemic disease of the colon to the more often used ischaemic colitis *(Figure 6.3)*.

The most severe form of ischaemic damage is that produced when full thickness necrosis and gangrene of the colon occur, resulting in large bowel obstruction, perforation and peritonitis. This is associated with shock. Even with early laparotomy the condition carries a high mortality. Fortunately, it only occurs in about one in ten patients with ischaemic disease of the colon. The patients are frequently elderly and known to have vascular diseases such as coronary heart disease, congestive cardiac failure, atrial fibrillation, with or without digoxin therapy, hypertension, intermittent claudication, or cerebrovascular disease. There is not usually evidence of preceding bowel disease. The history is short and abdominal pain of a few hours duration is the most constant feature. It is generalized and severe, not usually showing the transition from colicky to constant pain seen in small bowel infarction. Nausea, vomiting and diarrhoea are usually present but the stool may not contain fresh or altered blood; when present, however, it is a valuable clue. Examination reveals a very ill patient in a state of collapse, with subnormal temperature and showing the signs of generalized peritonitis without much distension. If sigmoidoscopy is performed, the mucosa usually appears normal as the rectum is rarely involved; if blood is present, it will be seen to be coming from above the reach of the sigmoidoscope. Investigations are rarely helpful, the blood count showing a neutrophil leucocytosis and haemoconcentration. Plain x-ray of the abdomen may show dilated loops of small and large bowel as in any form of obstruction. Blood cultures should always be taken prior to antibiotic therapy as clostridia from the lumen frequently invade the necrotic bowel. Central venous pressure monitoring is invaluable in the rapid correction of hypovolaemia required prior to laparotomy.

Most patients with ischaemic colitis present a less severe picture. Again there is a short history of abdominal pain usually localized to the lower half or left side of the abdomen. Diarrhoea soon follows and

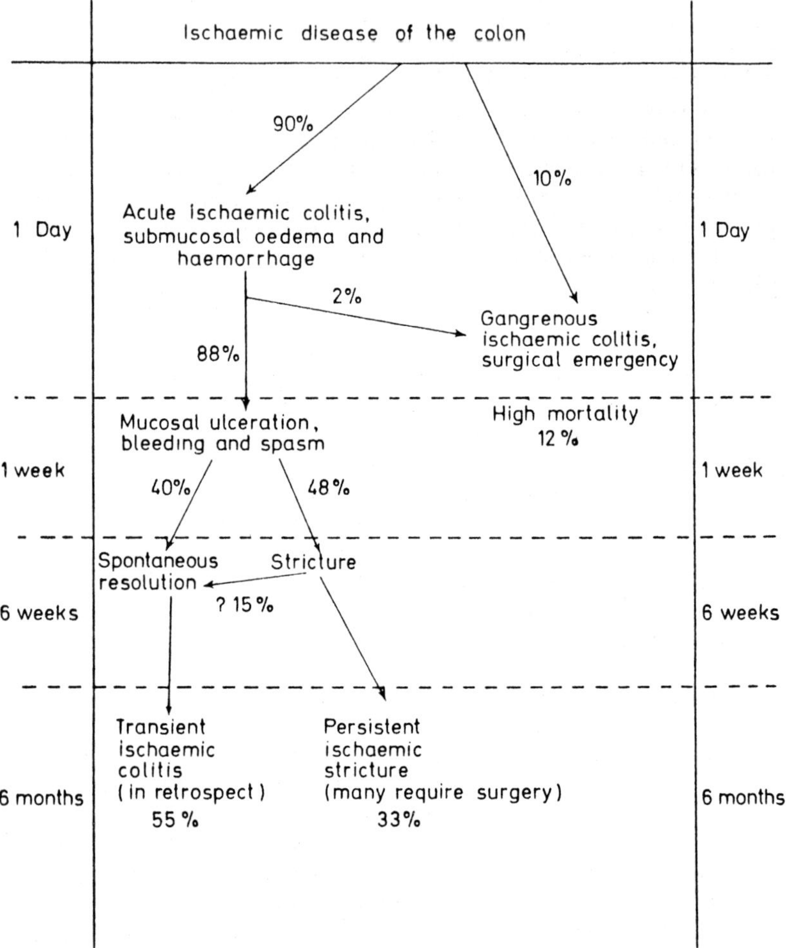

Figure 6.3. Disease states associated with ischaemic disease of the colon

contains fresh and altered blood, sometimes clots, mixed with stool. There may be nausea and vomiting. On examination, the patient is not shocked and has mild fever and tachycardia. There is left sided abdominal tenderness and guarding but a mass is not usually felt; bowel sounds are present and one should always listen for abdominal bruits as well. Sigmoidoscopy will confirm the presence of bleeding from higher up in the colon; on rare occasions, submucosal haemorrhage, sloughing and ulceration will extend to the rectum and can be visualized and biopsied. The most simple useful investigation is a plain abdominal x-ray. This may show a narrowed segment of colon often in the region of the splenic flexure. The lumen may show narrowing by irregular polypoid masses, when seen *en face,* or a scalloped appearance of indentation when seen in profile. These changes are more reliably seen on barium enema which should be performed at 48 hours. They have been described as 'thumb-printing' or pseudopolyposis (usually much larger than those seen in ulcerative colitis) and are due to submucosal oedema and haemorrhage *(Figure 6.4).* Within about 5 days the

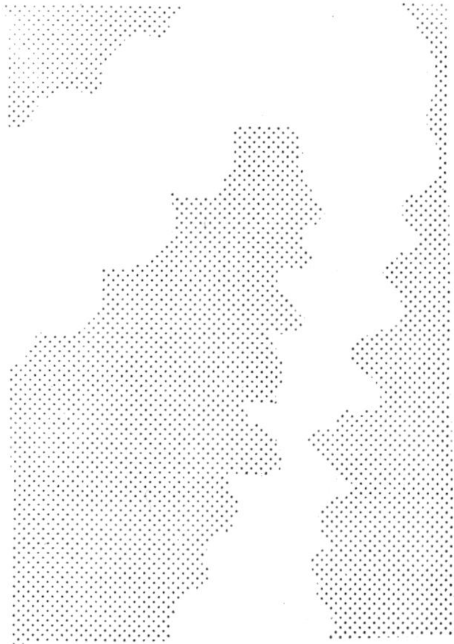

Figure 6.4. Barium enema at 48 hours in a patient with ischaemic colitis involving the descending colon. 'Thumb-printing' is due to submucosal oedema and haemorrhage

damaged mucosa sloughs off leaving an area of ulceration which may continue to bleed. The muscle layer is much more resistant to ischaemic damage but may show spasm. Very rarely at this stage the lesion extends to involve the full thickness of bowel transforming the situation to the previously described acute colon necrosis or gangrenous ischaemic colitis. If barium enema is not performed until seven days have elapsed pseudopolyposis may not be seen but instead there will be irregularity of bowel wall due to ulcers of varying size, some shallow and extensive and others narrow and fissuring. Secondary bacterial damage contributes to the clinical and radiological appearance. In nearly half the patients the bleeding and then the diarrhoea

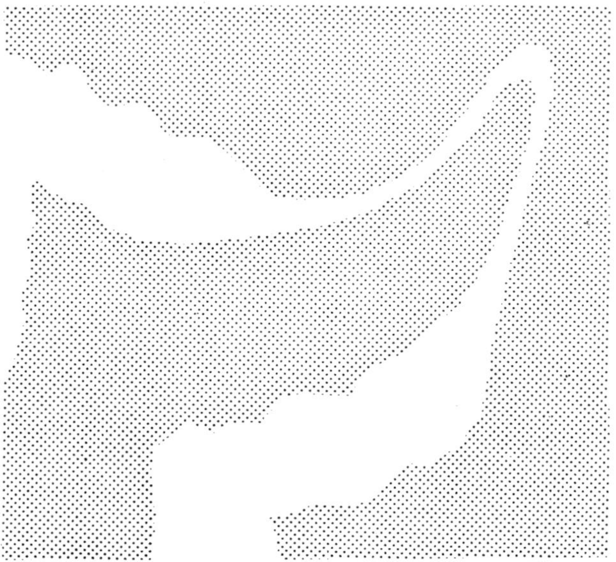

Figure 6.5. Barium enema at 8 weeks in a patient with ischaemic colitis. Long tubular stricture involving the splenic flexure showing marked funnelling

subside and, if barium enema is repeated at 6 weeks, there are no residual abnormalities. These patients are subject to the mildest ischaemia which damages the mucosa but spares the crypts from which the regenerative process is initiated. When the damage extends to the muscularis mucosa or circular muscle, the damaged muscle cannot regenerate but is replaced by fibrosis. Adjacent undamaged muscle, however, may undergo irregular hypertrophy. If this is regular and orderly a stricture will develop and be seen on the 6 week barium enema. This may be of considerable length (up to 25 cm) and tubular in appearance with a characteristic funnelling at its beginning *(Figure 6.5)*. If the pattern of damage and repair is more irregular, the appearance of sacculation is seen on the anti-mesenteric wall of the bowel. These broad bulges are quite different from narrow-necked diverticula *(Figure 6.6).* Bloody diarrhoea may persist if an ischaemic stricture is developing, and colicky pains of subacute obstruction may occur. Although such patients may require resection of their stricture, in others the symptoms are not severe enough to warrant it. If they are treated conservatively and the barium enema is repeated some months later, the signs of stricture may have totally disappeared. Although the acute lesions, and subsequent strictures, can affect any part of the large bowel from caecum to rectum, the distal, transverse, and proximal descending colon around the splenic flexure have been shown to be the most common site of involvement in all published series.

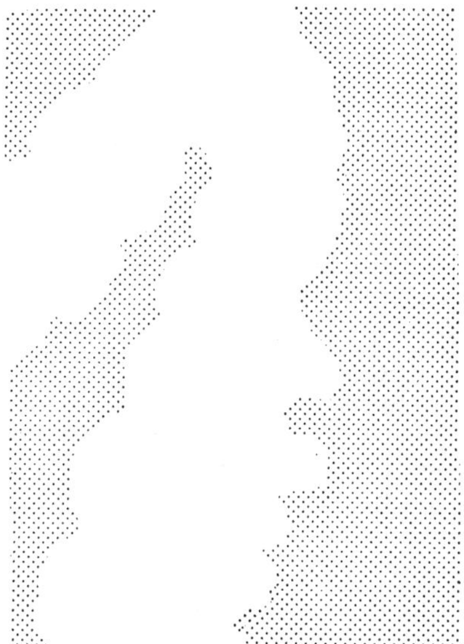

Figure 6.6. Same patient as in Figure 6.4. Barium enema at 10 days. Sacculation of anti-mesenteric border

At the time of initial presentation, diverticulitis, ulcerative colitis, Crohn's disease and carcinoma of the colon will enter into the differential diagnosis of acute ischaemic colitis. The gangrenous form is usually only distinguished from other causes of acute abdomen at laparotomy. In some patients the earlier stages may have gone unnoticed and they present with a stricture. Differentiation from carcinoma may be difficult and is often only resolved by laparotomy.

The precise aetiology and pathogenesis of ischaemic colitis often remains obscure in many patients. Occlusion of the inferior mesenteric artery at its origin by thrombosis, embolism, dissection, aneurysm or aortitis is found in a minority; even then there must be a failure of the collateral circulation from the superior mesenteric via the marginal artery or from the internal iliac via the middle haemorrhoidal artery. Sometimes there is small-vessel arteritis due, for example, to rheumatoid disease, polyarteritis nodosa, SLE, or diabetes. Venous thrombosis may rarely be the cause and has been postulated in those cases associated with the oestrogen contraceptive pill; mucosal oedema, giving rise to the thumb-printing appearance, may be much more prominent in these patients because of venous stasis. Not infrequently, laparotomy and angiography fail to reveal large vessel occlusion and even the vasa recta seem to have normal blood flow. The unique features of the microcirculation have already been discussed above and it is particularly in these 'non-occlusive' cases where impairment at this level is postulated. However, there is often a background of reduced cardiac output due to heart failure, hypovolaemia or recent blood loss or surgery. Secondary clostridial septicaemia and endotoxin shock contributes to the high mortality of gangrenous ischaemic colitis. It is also possible that a minor breach in the colonic mucosal defences allows pathogens normally present in the lumen of the colon to enter. The ensuing septicaemia and endotoxinaemia are known to promote intra-vascular coagulation. One of the histological features of 'non-occlusive' cases is the presence of platelet microthrombi in the capillaries and veins of the necrotic mucosa and submucosa and also in remote organs like the lungs and kidneys; this suggests that the gut is bearing the brunt of an intravascular coagulation syndrome. It is possible also that ill-understood conditions such as pseudo-membranous enterocolitis, acute nectrotizing enterocolitis and even clostridial and staphylococcal enterocolitis have a 'non-occlusive' ischaemic aetiology.

NON-SPECIFIC, INFLAMMATORY COLONIC DISEASE
(ULCERATIVE COLITIS AND CROHN'S DISEASE)

Although the aetiology of both conditions remains unknown, and despite many similarities, it is clinically useful to attempt to distinguish them because of differences in treatment and prognosis. Some would argue that the two diseases to be described below represent two ends of a spectrum and that there will always remain a group in the middle which is truly intermediate by clinical, radiological and pathological criteria. Others argue, from epidemiological data, that in the apparently bimodal incidence of all forms of Crohn's disease, the secondary rise in

136

the over 60 age-group can largely be accounted for by patients with colonic disease; they speculate that this may represent a third disease entity. Since ischaemic colitis and colonic Crohn's have become recognized, there have been doubts about the correct designation of many cases of ulcerative colitis beginning in the elderly in the past; this would tend to remove the second peak in the similar bimodal incidence curve for ulcerative colitis. By present criteria, ulcerative colitis would appear to be 8–10 times more common than Crohn's disease. However, the incidence of Crohn's disease seems to be increasing due either to more accurate diagnosis or to a true rise, or both. Genetically there is no clear-cut inheritance pattern but clustering within families is well recognized. Here there is overlap between ulcerative colitis, Crohn's disease and ankylosing spondylitis. Not only may ankylosing spondylitis occur in patients with ulcerative colitis or Crohn's disease but it occurs more commonly in their families. It is interesting that patients with Crohn's disease have a much stronger family history of ulcerative colitis than colitis patients have of Crohn's disease. No clear evidence as to the aetiology of either disease or to the differences between them yet exists to be of positive clinical value. Nonetheless, much promising reasearch is in progress which suggests that Crohn's disease may represent a continuing local reaction to a persisting antigen in the bowel wall of a person in whom there has been a change in natural tolerance. The antigen, which might be bacterial or a dietary constituent, would probably function as a hapten and might antigenically resemble normal tissue constituents thereby directing the body's immune response against them. Similar immunological phenomena have been found in ulcerative colitis where the patient's lymphocytes may be cytotoxic to colonic mucosa cells in tissue culture and antibodies to colonic mucosa cells and also to *Escherichia Coli* 014 are found.

The most common presenting symptom in ulcerative colitis is bloody diarrhoea, especially if the disease extends beyond the rectum. When it is confined to the rectum the stools may be formed or even constipated but, nonetheless, there may still be urgency passing blood and mucus. Severe abdominal pain rarely occurs but a mild discomfort associated with urgency and relieved by defaecation is not uncommon. In total colitis, malaise, anorexia, weight loss and mild fever may be present, whereas the patient who has proctitis only may be relatively well. Examination of the abdomen is usually unrewarding, though in a severe fulminating attack, toxic dilatation of the colon will be accompanied by increasing distension, loss of bowel sounds and disappearance of diarrhoea. The latter can be a dangerously misleading sign. Systemic signs of disease may be present. There may be clubbing of the fingers, skin lesions (such as pyoderma gangrenosum or erythema nodosum), aphthous ulceration, episcleritis and uveitis, asymmetrical, migratory arthritis affecting, particularly, large joints, sacro-iliitis and spondylitis, gall stones and liver disease. In long-standing complicated cases amyloidosis can occur. However, all of these signs have at some time occurred in both diseases and are not of great value in discriminating between ulcerative colitis and Crohn's disease. They do help, however, to distinguish these two diseases from ischaemic colitis, diverticulitis and other causes of chronic diarrhoea. Inspection of the perineum and anus may show excoriation in proportion to the diarrhoea. Sigmoidoscopy invariably shows evidence of inflammation which, in the case of proctitis, has a distinct upper border beyond which normal colonic mucosa is seen. There is uniform involvement of the affected area. The disease should be graded mild, moderate or severe, according to severity. Mild disease is signified if there is hyperaemia with contact bleeding when the surface is rubbed with a gauze swab. Moderate disease shows, in addition, granularity, petechial haemorrhages and purulent exudate. Severe disease is present when spontaneous bleeding occurs and gross ulceration is visible; pseudopolyposis is not common at this level of the bowel. Rectal biopsy shows the disease confined usually to the mucosa with hyperaemia and neutrophil infiltration, which may dilate the crypts to form crypt abscesses and, in more severe cases, ulceration of the surface. Radiological changes are seen if the disease is more than a proctitis. Barium enema is a safe procedure even in many severe cases if an instant enema technique, without bowel preparation, is used. If toxic dilatation is suspected then barium enema carries some risk of perforation and, instead, a plain abdominal x-ray should be taken. This will show a colon empty of faeces but, in the erect view, a few long fluid levels may be seen in distended segments usually of transverse colon; adjacent segments may be collapsed. Barium enema changes in total colitis show shortening (due to contraction of the taenia) and narrowing of the bowel with lack of haustration giving a featureless 'hose pipe' appearance. The margin of the bowel may have a fuzzy blurred appearance or the outline may be more ragged due to grosser ulceration which does not, however, go deep into the bowel wall. Pseudopolyposis is seen as multiple small filling defects *(Figure 6.7)*. The presence of a stricture, if the condition is ulcerative colitis and not Crohn's disease, suggests malignancy. This becomes a real hazard in patients with total colitis of ten years duration and few would allow their patients to retain their colons for this time. The disease is present in continuity and, if it involves the whole colon including the ileo-caecal valve, may spill back into the terminal ileum. Such incompetence of the ileo-caecal valve is then said to give rise to 'backwash ileitis'.

The contrasting features of colonic Crohn's disease begin with the history. Although diarrhoea may occur, bleeding is not usual. If the rectum is spared, as it may be in half the patients, urgency does not occur. Abdominal pain is a common presentation; when the right side of the colon is involved the lesion may be in continuity with terminal ileal disease and small intestinal colic may occur. As the disease process

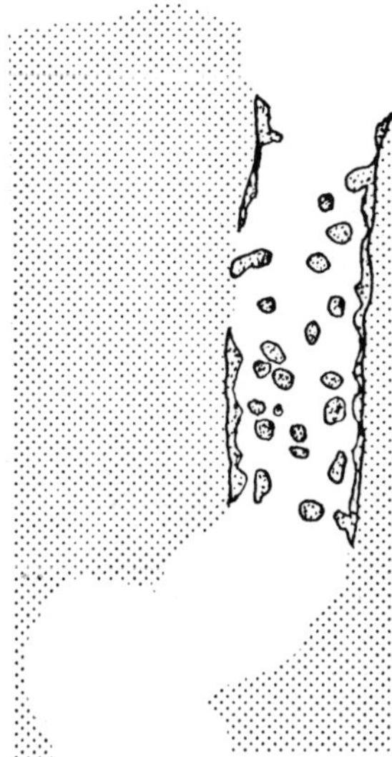

Figure 6.7. Barium enema showing descending colon in a patient with ulcerative colitis. Pseudopolyposis and shallow mucosal ulceration

involves the full thickness of the bowel wall, peritoneal irritation provides a second mechanism for pain production. Weight loss is much more prominent than in ulcerative colitis and is attributable partly to steatorrhoea and malabsorption from associated small intestinal disease. Vomiting is not uncommon. The similarity of systemic features in the two diseases has been indicated but sometimes characteristic mouth ulcers which show typical granulomas on biopsy are found. Abdominal signs of a right iliac fossa mass may be present or even signs of subacute obstruction in small or large bowel. Examination of the perineum is essential because four out of five patients with colonic Crohn's disease, and all those with rectal involvement, have an associated anal lesion. Multiple broad shallow apparently indolent and remarkably pain-free anal fissures are the most common finding. The peri-anal skin is often undermined and ulcerated and there are prominent oedematous skin tags. The peri-anal skin also often has a dusky cyanotic appearance.

Peri-anal or ischio-rectal abscesses occur which, on rupturing, give rise to fistulae which can be extensive. Two thirds of these lesions, if biopsied, will reveal characteristic granulomata of Crohn's disease, thus providing a readily accessible site for making a positive histological diagnosis. The anal lesions in about a quarter of patients may precede other symptoms and be the first manifestation of the disease. In the

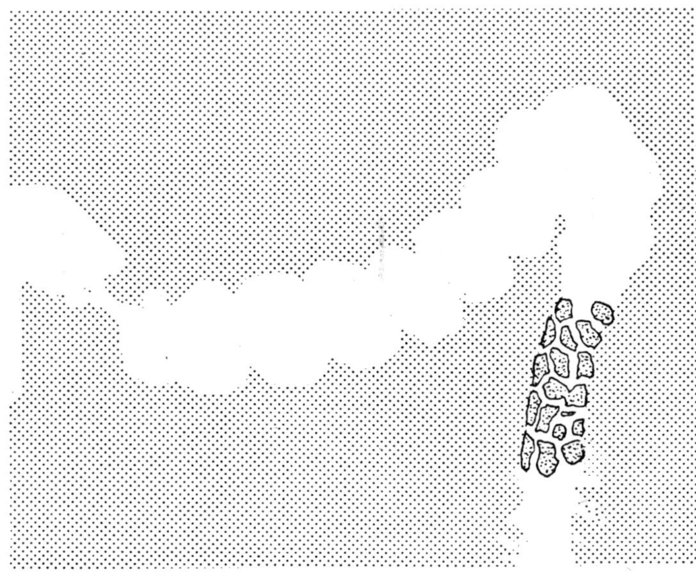

Figure 6.8. Barium enema showing transverse and descending colon in a patient with Crohn's disease. Stricture distal to hepatic flexure, normal remaining transverse colon 'cobblestone' appearance and fissuring 'rose-thorn' ulceration in descending colon

patients with rectal involvement on digital examination, nodularity of the rectum may be felt. On sigmoidoscopy this is shown to be due to swelling of the mucosa due to submucosal oedema. This gives a discontinuous cobblestone appearance due to linear ulcers limiting the areas of soggy mucosal swelling. Areas of inflammation may be seen but of great importance is the discontinuity of all these lesions with intervening areas of normal mucosa. A deep biopsy of an ulcer is the most likely source for the demonstration of a giant cell sarcoid-like granuloma; in addition, infiltration with lymphocytes and plasma cells of the submucosa and oedema gives rise to disproportionate inflammation in contrast to ulcerative colitis. The distribution of lesions seen on barium

TABLE 6.1

Differential Diagnosis of Ulcerative Colitis
and Crohn's disease of the Colon

	Ulcerative colitis	*Crohn's disease*
Symptoms		
Bleeding	Usual	Variable
Diarrhoea	Common	Common
Urgency	Common	Variable
Abdominal pain	Uncommon	Common
Weight loss	Variable	Common
Signs		
Abdominal mass	None	Common
Anal lesions	Uncommon and mild	Usual (80 per cent)
Internal fistulae	None	Occurs
Sigmoidoscopy		
Rectal involvement	95 per cent	50 per cent
Appearances	Continuous	Discontinuous
	Hyperaemia and bleeding	Oedema
	Granularity	Ulceration
Barium enema		
Distribution	Continuous	Discontinuous
Distal ileum	Backwash ileitis in total colitis	Commonly right ileo-colitis
Ulceration	Superficial	Fissuring
Strictures	Rare and malignant	Common and benign
Fistulae	None	Occur
Rectal biopsy		
Inflammation	Neutrophil	Lymphocyte
	Superficial	Disproportionately submucosal
Hyperaemia	Marked	Unremarkable
Oedema	Absent	Prominent; submucosal
Crypt abscesses	Common	Rare
Fissuring	Absent	Common
Pareth cell metaplasia	Common	Rare
Giant cell granulomata	Absent	Common

enema as well as their appearance differs from ulcerative colitis *(Figure 6.8)*. The lesions are frequently discontinuous with normal intervening bowel (skip lesions). The mucosal lesions seen on sigmoidoscopy appear radiologically as 'cobblestones' with deep fissuring ulcers seen *en face.* When seen in profile, these ulcers penetrate deep into the bowel wall giving a 'rose thorn' appearance. Such fissures may perforate the bowel; the bowel usually adheres to a neighbouring viscus which is then penetrated to form an internal fistula. These may occur with the ileum or other parts of the gut, bladder or vagina. Strictures are a common feature in Crohn's disease and take a variety of forms. The long narrow stricture described in the ileum as the 'string' sign may also occur in the colon. A 'purse string' stricture is due to eccentric contractions due to involvement of only part of the circumference of the bowel wall. Extrinsic pressure by an abscess, from a fistula, may also produce narrowing of the lumen. Other complications seen in ulcerative colitis are much rarer in Crohn's colitis; acute toxic dilatation leading to perforation, and also carcinoma have been reported. It is suggested that as ulcerative colitis primarily affects the surface of the bowel, which is therefore constantly regenerating, cancer is more common than in the full thickness non-ulcerating inflammation of Crohn's disease. A barium follow-through should always be performed to look for coexisting small bowel involvement.

The differential diagnosis of ulcerative colitis and Crohn's disease is summarized in Table 6.1.

REFERENCES

Brooke, B. N. (Ed) (1972). 'Crohn's disease' In *Clinics in Gastro-enterology,* Vol 1, No. 2. London: W. B. Saunders and Co.

Kyle, J. (1972). *Crohn's Disease.* London: Heinemann.

Marston, A. (Ed) (1972). 'Vascular disorders of the alimentary tract.' In *Clinics in Gastroenterology,* Vol 1, No 3. London: W. B. Saunders and Co.

Morson, B. C. (Ed) (1969). 'Diseases of the colon, rectum and anus' In *Tutorials in Postgraduate Medicine.* London: Heinemann.

Williams, L. F. (1971). 'Vascular insufficiency of the intestines'. In Progress in Gastroenterology, *Gastroenterology,* **61,** 757.

7

Renal Glomerular Disease

B. I. Hoffbrand

INTRODUCTION

For over a century following Richard Bright's classic work, the study of glomerulonephritis consisted largely of attempts, such as those of Longcope and Ellis, to correlate clinical, laboratory and autopsy observations. With the introduction of percutaneous renal biopsy in the early 1950's it became possible to obtain renal histology in a large number of non-fatal cases. This showed how poorly clinical and microscopic estimates of glomerular damage were related in many cases. Inevitably, the range of histological changes in living tissues proved greater than that seen in post-mortem material. Serial biopsies also provided information about the natural history of the renal disease.

There are a number of reasons for current interest in glomerular disease. One is the appreciation that in a majority of patients needing renal transplantation, or chronic haemodialysis, the original disease is glomerulonephritis. The potential value of prevention or effective treatment is self-evident. Other reasons are the advances that have been made in the study of renal biopsies. Electron microscopy and immunofluorescent techniques have proved of value in two ways. In the first place they have clearly shown that immunological reactions play a part in the pathogenesis of many cases of glomerulonephritis. This, in turn, has led to much work on the mechanisms of tissue-damaging processes which is of great relevance to considerations of treatment. In the second place immunofluorescent studies in particular are leading to far more precise classification of glomerulonephritis with the recognition of characteristic patterns of fluorescent staining. It is becoming increasingly possible to pick out groups of patients who we can more or less confidently believe, are suffering from the same disease. This means that we can look, with far greater hope of success, for environmental and genetic factors of aetiological importance.

No classification of renal glomerular disease made in ignorance of the aetiology can be fully acceptable. As indicated in Table 7.1, the

TABLE 7.1

Renal Glomerular Disease

Group	*Specific disorders*
1 — Primary	Glomerulonephritis Minimal change Membranous Proliferative
2 — Secondary. Glomerular disease as part of systemic disease due to drugs, toxins, etc. (*see* Table 7.2)	Diabetes mellitus Amyloidosis Systemic lupus erythematosus (SLE) Henoch-Schönlein purpura (HSP) Polyarteritis nodosa Subacute bacterial endocarditis (SBE) Goodpasture's syndrome Haemolytic–uraemic syndrome Quartan malaria nephropathy
3 — Hereditary and metabolic	Hereditary nephritis Fabry's disease
4 — Glomerular disease as part of disease of renal circulation, tubules, interstitium and urinary tract	Hypertension, renal artery and renal vein occlusion Acute tubular necrosis Chronic pyelonephritis Nephropathy due to analgesics, hypercalcaemia and hyperuricaemia Urinary tract obstruction Multiple myeloma Renal calculous, tuberculous and polycystic disease, etc. Interstitial nephritis due to drugs, irradiation, etc.

term glomerulonephritis is reserved on the whole for primary (group 1) glomerular disease, be it due to known aetiological agents, as with post-streptococcal glomerulonephritis, or not. However, the renal lesions of many diseases in Group 2 (Table 7.1) are also often described as glomerulonephritis — for example, in systemic lupus erythematosus (SLE) and in Goodpasture's Syndrome. The use of the term is purely conventional and it is applied to disease with a non-inflammatory histological picture, such as membranous glomerulonephritis, and even to glomeruli with no significant histological abnormality at all — for example, minimal change glomerulonephritis. The term 'nephritis' tends to be used clinically where histological confirmation of glomerulonephritis is lacking or where more widespread inflammatory changes are recognized; examples are interstitial nephritis and hereditary nephritis. The term 'glomerulitis' describes histological appearances confined to the glomerulus while 'nephropathy' adds up to nothing more specific than 'kidney disease'. Unhappily, nephrology is not celebrated for the precision of its semantics and these terms get used interchangeably. Group 3 diseases, such as the hereditary nephritides and Fabry's disease, are of relatively minor importance numerically but of great interest as pointers to mechanisms of tissue damage other than immunological ones.

Group 4 diseases will not be discussed in detail in this chapter. They are included as a reminder that the integrity of the renal glomerulus is dependent on the wellbeing of the rest of the nephron and of its supporting anatomy. It is imperative in the differential diagnosis of suspected glomerular disease to consider these and many other conditions that affect the glomerulus as part of more widespread renal involvement. It is apparent that this list includes common disorders for which treatment directed to limiting nephron loss is highly effective. This cannot, unhappily, be said at present for the majority of the conditions in Groups 1—3.

NORMAL GLOMERULAR STRUCTURE

The afferent arteriole enters the parietal layer of Bowman's capsule and divides eventually into 20 or more capillary loops, which recombine into the efferent arteriole *(Figure 7.1)*. The tuft of the capillary loops is subdivided into *lobules* which are not very apparent in the normal glomerulus. The lobular structure is accentuated in many glomerular diseases. The capillary walls are composed of three layers; *endothelial cells,* continuous with the arteriolar endothelium; the *glomerular basement membrane (GBM)*; and the *epithelial cells* of the visceral layer of Bowman's capsule. These epithelial cells have long foot processes or *podocytes* which rest on the basement membrane. The podocytes coalesce in any condition where there is a heavy glomerular leak of protein. The space between the capillaries of the tufts is occupied by a supporting structure, the *mesangium*. This consists of *mesangial cells* (closely resembling structurally the endothelium cell), and a contiguous *matrix* of GBM-like material. The mesangial cells are believed to be

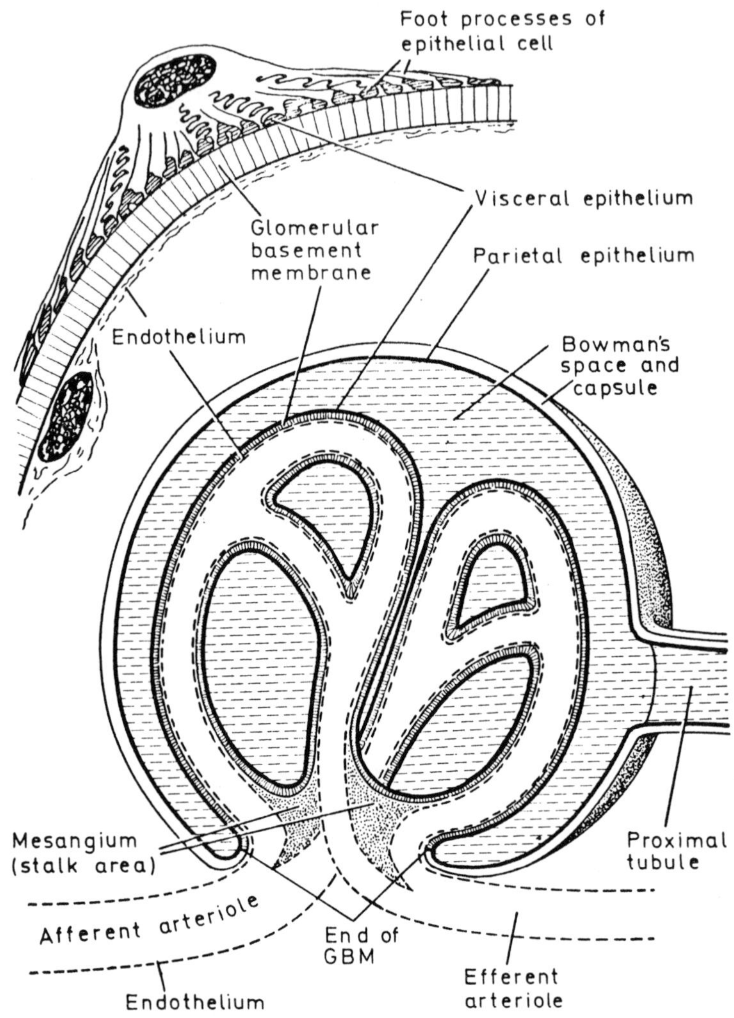

Figure 7.1. A simplified view of the normal renal glomerulus. The details of the stalk area in particular are still controversial

important in scavenging and repair both in health and in disease. In the latter, they may interfere with normal function by laying down connective tissue elements such as GBM-like material or collagen, or by excessive proliferation.

PATHOGENESIS OF GLOMERULAR DAMAGE IN GLOMERULONEPHRITIS

Two immunological mechanisms can produce glomerulonephritis:

(1)   Deposition of circulating antigen–antibody complexes formed in antigen excess.
(2)   Anti-GBM antibodies.

Complement activation occurs with both mechanisms and can generate chemotactic factors attracting polymorphs and vasoactive substances increasing vascular permeability. It can also probably initiate coagulation. These reactions have, of course, great tissue-damaging potential. The importance of complement activation in experimental glomerulonephritis is better documented for the anti-GBM antibody variety (Masugi nephritis).

Glomerulonephritis due to Antigen–Antibody Complexes

Here the antigen is not glomerular, the kidney suffering because it filters off circulating (synonyms: immune; soluble; toxic) complexes from the circulation. The classical example is serum sickness. The hallmarks of this situation are the presence of discrete, granular deposits of immunoglobulin and complement on or in the GBM; these are seen as dense deposits on electron microscopy (lumps, bumps, humps). In SLE and chronic quartan malaria glomerular disease, the antigens have, in a number of cases, been identified as DNA and malarial substances respectively. There is some evidence of streptococcal antigen in the classical immune complex 'humps' of acute post-streptococcal glomerulonephritis (acute PSGN). However, in the majority of cases with evidence of immune complex glomerulonephritis the antigen has not been identified. One working hypothesis, based on several animal models, is that the antigens are viral or self-antigens modified by viruses. The other factor likely to prove important in immune complex production is a genetic tendency of the host to produce antibody inadequate in quality or quantity to produce the innocuous insoluble complexes that are removed from the circulation by the reticulo-endothelial system.

As the vast majority of cases of immunologically mediated glomerulonephritis is of the immune complex type, there must be important biological differences in complexes to produce the known range of histological and immunofluorescent pictures. Complex size is one such factor of proven significance experimentally.

147

Glomerulonephritis due to Anti-GBM Antibodies

The most clear-cut example of this mechanism is provided by Goodpasture's syndrome, the characteristic immunofluorescent pattern being a linear deposition of immunoglobulin and complement on the GBM. The circulating antibodies have been isolated in anephric patients prior to transplantation, where total removal of GBM allows the serum titre to rise to easily detectable amounts. Linear staining has been described in some cases of rapidly progressive glomerulonephritis and occasionally in other types, but it is generally rare, being found in 2 per cent or less of cases of glomerulonephritis.

The following points should be stressed:

(1)   Complexes can be deposited in areas of glomerular damage due to other, non-immunological causes so that their detection in a biopsy is not proof of their aetiological importance.

(2)   Immunofluorescent deposits often consist of complement only or immunoglobulin only and may not correlate with areas of histological abnormality.

(3)   Immunofluorescent deposits may or may not be detectable in histologically identical cases.

(4)   There is an alternative pathway of complement activation at the $C'3$ level which need not involve antigen—antibody interaction. It can be appreciated that so-called 'immune complex disease' may often be more complex that immune! Experience to date does, however, suggest that the immunofluorescent pattern is specific for each individual and may be the first sign of recurrence of glomerulonephritis in a transplanted kidney. Although the fluorescence technique is itself immunological, one should regard the findings as indicating changes in tissue proteins, which themselves may or may not be of immunological importance. The mechanisms of glomerular damage in other forms of glomerular disease will be discussed with the specific conditions.

CLINICAL FEATURES OF GLOMERULAR DISEASE

In spite of the many pathological processes that can involve the renal glomerulus, there are a limited number of manifestations of glomerular disease. These fall into two general patterns, the nephritic and the nephrotic, in addition to acute and chronic renal failure. Nephritic features are haematuria, hypertension and oedema due to salt and water retention, nephrotic ones being heavy proteinuria, and oedema with a low serum albumin. Glomerular disease may present as purely nephritic (acute PSGN, for example) or purely nephrotic, (for example, minimal change glomerulonephritis). As a very general rule, patients who show prominent features of both types prove to have disease with a less favourable prognosis. The presence of variable amounts of acute and/or chronic renal failure also affects the balance of diagnostic possibilities. The specific diseases mentioned below will be dealt with more fully in a later section (*see* Table 7.1 and page 161).

Symptomless Proteinuria

Normal urine contains up to 100–150 mg/24h. Orthostatic and functional proteinurias, after exercise and with fever, for example, may give considerably greater amounts than this and are often associated with increased numbers of urinary cells and casts. The urinary abnormalities here are, of course, intermittent with characteristic relationships to posture, exercise, etc. Protein excretion of over 1–2 g/24h, if persistent, is very suggestive of glomerular disease although, even here, the amounts may increase with the patient erect or after exercise. Common diseases affecting the kidney such as chronic pyelonephritis, non-accelerated (benign) hypertension, obstructive nephropathy, calculous and polycystic disease, may reach advanced stages with no or very little proteinuria. In glomerular disease, proteinuria tends to decrease in amount as the glomerular filtration rate falls to low levels.

Nephrotic Syndrome (Massive Proteinuria, Hypoalbuminaemia, Oedema)

Symptomatic proteinuria (that is, oedema) occurs with daily excretion rates of about 5 g or 3.5 g/1.73 m^2 body surface area. These are the figures generally used in conventional definitions of nephrotic syndrome. However, hypoalbuminaemia and oedema can occur with greater or lesser degrees of proteinuria, the degree being dependent on a variety of other factors. A high protein diet and heavy physical activity tend to maintain serum albumin levels. The presence or absence of oedema should not affect the differential diagnosis. An occasional patient presents complaining of frothy urine, a symptom that can be elicited more frequently on direct questioning, to help date the onset of heavy proteinuria. The hypoalbuminaemia is related primarily to the degree of urinary protein loss, but other factors operate. These are poor dietary protein intake, impaired albumin synthesis, increased renal degradation of albumin and, possibly, an intestinal albumin leak. The typical electrophoretic protein strip shows increased $\alpha2$ and β globulins and low γ globulin, as well as a low albumin. Oedema in the nephrotic syndrome, as in the acute nephritic syndrome, is commonly periorbital, on waking. The site is attributed to the absence of orthopnoea. The

149

presence and severity of oedema are only roughly related to serum albumin concentration, the relationship being even less marked in children. Oedema can occur with serum albumin levels over 3 g/100 ml and may be absent at concentrations well under 2 g/100 ml. Anasarca with pleural and peritoneal effusions as well as dependent oedema, occurs only at levels under (usually well under) 3 g/100 ml. Oedema may be intermittent, irrespective of changes in glomerular pathology or treatment. Dietary intake of protein and salt are important in this respect.

TABLE 7.2

Causes of the Nephrotic Syndrome

Congenital	
Circulatory	Renal vein thrombosis IVC obstruction Congestive cardiac failure Sickle cell disease Chyluria
Drugs and toxins	Troxidone and paramethadione Probenecid Penicillamine Gold and other heavy metals Organic and inorganic mercury
Allergens	Pollen Bee stings Poison ivy
Infections	Quartan malaria Syphilis (secondary and congenital)
Malignancy	Multiple myeloma Cancer Lymphoma

This table excludes those causes of the nephrotic syndrome discussed elsewhere in this chapter (*see* Table 7.1, groups 1–3, and related text).

There are a large number of associated physiological and metabolic abnormalities in the nephrotic syndrome. The best recognized is hyperlipidaemia with elevation of serum cholesterol, triglyceride and low density lipoprotein levels. The serum cholesterol and albumin concentrations usually show a close inverse correlation, the cholesterol returning to normal as the albumin rises in remission. The cause of the lipid abnormality is unknown. Greater clinical importance is attached to the fact that patients with the nephrotic syndrome tend to have low blood volumes and generalized protein depletion. Hypovolaemia can be severe enough to give severe pre-renal uraemia and even frank acute tubular necrosis although other factors, for example, tubular protein cast obstruction, may contribute. Overvigorous treatment with diuretics can precipitate this complication. Protein malnutrition may be the reason why nephrotics seem especially prone to the catabolic side-effects of corticosteroid therapy affecting bone, muscle and skin. A tendency to infection (partly due to secondary hypogammaglobulinaemia), and vascular thrombosis, are other important features of the nephrotic syndrome. Renal glycosuria can occur occasionally with other features of proximal tubular dysfunction such as amino-aciduria. This may be part of the primary disease or secondary to the tubular protein load. Diabetic glomerular disease should not be mis-diagnosed in these circumstances.

The associations, proven and alleged, of the nephrotic syndrome are legion. Table 7.2 gives the more important ones from a clinical and aetiological viewpoint not dealt with elsewhere in this chapter.

Haematuria

This may range from the microscopic to the massive. A frequent complaint is one of recurrent haematuria occurring with, or just a day or two after, some non-specific upper respiratory tract infection, sore throat (usually not streptococcal) mild febrile illness, or after exercise. Although renal histology in such cases may range from entirely normal to diffuse proliferative glomerulonephritis, this story is characteristic of two conditions: focal glomerulonephritis, now known to have a high incidence of diffuse mesangial IgA deposition; and hereditary nephritis. Loin pain is common and clot colic can recur.

In view of the enormous number of renal and extra-renal conditions that can give haematuria, the importance of microscopy of the sediment of freshly passed specimens of urine cannot be overstressed. The finding of red cell casts, however few the number, is diagnostic of renal bleeding and usually excludes the need for urological investigation of the lower urinary tract.

Acute Nephritic Syndrome

The classical picture of acute PSGN consists of haematuria, oliguria, oedema, hypertension, proteinuria, circulatory congestion and azotaemia. These develop 1–3 weeks after a streptococcal sore throat or skin infection and are assocated with some malaise and backache. Although the cardiovascular state may include cardiomegaly, pulmonary congestion, a gallop rhythm and raised JVP, these changes are probably due entirely to salt and water retention and not to myocardial failure. For example the cardiac output is not reduced and increased normally on exercise. The hypertension, which is usually only modest, is almost certainly due to the same cause. Hypertensive encephalopathy can occur nonetheless. The most feared complication is the development of severe oliguric renal failure (*see* below).

In practice, acute PSGN, more often than not, does not live up to the full textbook description. A variety of other conditions can present as 'acute nephritis', a term that should not be used synonymously with acute PSGN. A vague onset, heavy proteinuria in the early stages, extreme oliguria, and the absence of hypertension, should all rouse suspicions that one is not dealing with acute PSGN. There may be evidence of chronic renal disease such as signs of long standing hypertension or anaemia or evidence of a systemic disease, all of which would point to other diagnoses. A previous history of renal disease, a short latent period after the start of any predisposing infection and clinical and laboratory evidence of chronic renal disease help in the diagnosis of acute exacerbations of chronic glomerulonephritis. In membranoproliferative glomerulonephritis the serum complement often remains low whereas in acute PSGN it returns to normal in 4–6 weeks. In rapidly progressive glomerulonephritis the serum complement is normal throughout and hypertension is uncommon. Focal glomerulonephritis may occasionally be associated with nephritic features other than haematuria but these again develop with, or only a day or two after, the sore throat. Henoch Schönlein purpura (HSP), SLE, Goodpasture's syndrome, polyarteritis nodosa, Wegener's granulomatosis and scleroderma are well recognized causes of 'acute nephritis'. Although the glomerulonephritis of subacute bacterial endocarditis (SBE) can present with uraemia and microscopic haematuria, hypertension and noncardiac oedema are rare. Membranous glomerulonephritis with a nephrotic syndrome can mimic 'acute nephritis' as microscopic haematuria is common and oliguria with severe uraemia can occur. Of non-glomerular diseases, acute pyelonephritis and malignant hypertension are the two most likely to be confused with an 'acute nephritic syndrome'.

Acute Renal Failure

The clinical picture here merges into that of the acute nephritic syndrome with oliguria and azotaemia more prominent and hypertension and haematuria less so. The patient may well be thought to have acute tubular necrosis (ATN) even in the absence of any obvious precipitating cause. The differential diagnosis of acute renal failure is enormous. Glomerular disease covered by Groups 1–3 (Table 7.1) is not a common cause. Pointers to glomerulonephritis as a cause of acute renal failure are:

(1)   Recent and past history – for example, sore throat, proteinuria.

(2)   Absolute anuria, which is uncommon in ATN although a feature of bilateral cortical necrosis. Urinary tract obstruction needs particularly careful exclusion in these circumstances.

(3)   Such urine as there is may contain many red cells and red cell casts which are rare in ATN where granular and hyaline casts are frequently found. Heavy proteinuria is also suggestive of glomerular disease.

(4)   With glomerulonephritis, urine osmolality tends to be well above that of serum but its sodium concentration is low (10–20 mEq/1). In ATN the reverse is more characteristic; urine osmolality is close to that of plasma and urinary sodium high, usually above 40 mEq/1. Undue reliance should not, however, be placed on the biochemical results.

All the glomerular diseases considered under the acute nephritic syndrome, can present as acute renal failure, including acute PSGN. The most characteristic though fortunately rare 'disease' to present in this way is rapidly progressive glomerulonephritis. The glomerular disease of the haemolytic–uraemic syndrome and thrombotic thrombocytopenic purpura (TPP) can best be described under this heading. Acute renal failure sometimes can be the most prominent feature of the nephrotic syndrome, as discussed above.

Chronic Renal Failure

Uraemia, with its many manifestations, is the unhappy outcome of many forms of progressive glomerular disease. The almost invariable development of hypertension in most forms of proliferative glomerulonephritis hastens glomerular destruction. Although patients presenting *de novo* with uraemia due to glomerular disease may give a history of one of the other clinical patterns already discussed, the majority do not. The histology, when obtainable, is often complicated by secondary pyelonephritis and arteriolar nephrosclerosis – so called 'endstage kidney'. The few immunofluorescent studies to date on such material have not proved very informative. The relationship of advanced chronic glomerulonephritis to acute PSGN and the other glomerulonephritides remains uncertain. It is likely that a majority are chronic from the start.

153

Hypertension

A raised blood pressure is a particularly prominent feature of the acute nephritic syndrome and of renal failure, especially chronic. When it is the initial finding, pointers to a glomerular cause are the presence of other features of renal disease, historical, clinical or laboratory. It must be remembered that hypertension itself causes glomerular damage with proteinuria at all stages. In accelerated (malignant) hypertension, proteinuria can be massive, haematuria is common, and renal failure (which can be acute oliguric), occurs all too frequently. The hen and egg situation sometimes cannot be resolved. However, a history of hypertension preceding proteinuria or vice versa is helpful. When non-accelerated hypertension is due to chronic glomerulonephritis, one nearly always finds proteinuria much heavier than expected for the degree of hypertension. The absence of proteinuria in a concentrated specimen of urine (SG >1020) makes glomerulonephritis an extremely unlikely cause of hypertension.

Occasionally, acute PSGN can present with hypertension and heart failure and only insignificant urinary abnormalities.

INVESTIGATIONS IN GLOMERULAR DISEASE

Investigations will depend on the particular features of the individual case. They should be directed especially at excluding the reversible causes of glomerular damage such as urinary tract obstruction. The sparing of nephrons comes second only to the saving of life in the priorities of managing a renal problem.

Urine Microscopy

The finding of excess red, white and epithelial cells in the urinary sediment has little value in the localization of disease within the urinary tract. However, abnormal amounts of casts (red cell, white cell, granular and mixed) indicate renal disease. Hyaline casts can occur in any concentrated urine and are of no significance. Red cell casts are very suggestive of active glomerulonephritis; white cell casts are found typically in pyelonephritis but occur in glomerulonephritis, especially with acute inflammatory (exudative) changes. The characteristic cast of chronic renal failure is broad. Fat droplets are frequently seen in the nephrotic syndrome. More than one *fresh* specimen should be examined. Casts do not form well in alkaline urine due to the solubility at high pH of Tamm—Horsfall mucoprotein, which is responsible for the matrix of urinary casts.

Protein Excretion

(1) *Twenty-four hour urinary protein* excretion. This should be measured by a modern laboratory technique. This estimation is of value in diagnosis, and in following the course of the disease and its response to therapy.

(2) *Differential protein clearances.* There is a relationship between the renal histology and the 'leakiness' of the glomerulus to macromolecules. As a general rule the less damage the glomerulus shows histologically, the less protein of high molecular weight, such as β lipoprotein or IgG, appears in the urine. In the nephrotic syndrome due to minimal change glomerulonephritis, the proteinuria consists almost entirely of albumin, transferrin and other relatively small-sized protein molecules. In membranous and proliferative glomerulonephritis appreciable amounts of high molecular weight proteins are excreted. An index of 'leakiness' is given by comparing the clearance of a high molecular weight protein with that of transferrin or albumin — for example, measuring clearance of IgG/clearance of transferrin. A low value would indicate a highly selective differential protein clearance and a high value a poorly selective one.

Unfortunately, there is a wide range of degrees of selectivity within any single histological group, the values overlapping with those found in other groups. Consequently, these measurements are not sufficiently discriminating to be of much help in diagnosis. Proliferative glomerulonephritis and secondary glomerular disease, such as advanced amyloid can show highly selective proteinuria. The most useful application of differential protein clearances is in children with the nephrotic syndrome. Here, over 90 per cent or so of cases are due to minimal change disease. A child with the nephrotic syndrome without nephritic features and with highly selective proteinuria can be safely treated as having minimal change lesions. On the other hand, poorly selective proteinuria is strongly suggestive of some other pathology and indicates the need for renal biopsy. Moderately selective proteinuria is found with both minimal change and other pathology. The selectivity of proteinuria is of no help in indicating which patient with steroid sensitive nephrotic syndrome will relapse.

Endogenous Creatinine Clearance

With all its drawbacks this remains the most useful measurement in clinical practice for assessing and following glomerular function. High creatinine clearance values are found frequently in the nephrotic syndrome, due to high glomerular filtration rates and other factors. The serum creatinine level provides a good general guide to progress. Although the blood urea level is related roughly to many of the clinical features of chronic renal failure, it is too dependent on protein metabolism, determined by dietary intake and many other factors, to reflect glomerular function closely.

Renal Radiology

This is important for two reasons:

(1) To exclude a structural abnormality of the kidneys and urinary tract.

(2) To assess the size of the kidneys for prognosis and with renal biopsy in mind.

When there is no renal failure, all that is needed is a good quality IVP. The major problems arise when the patient is in renal failure, acute or chronic. Plain abdominal x-ray and high dose IVP, with or without nephrotomography, may provide the necessary information. However, angiography, isotopic renography, and cystoscopy with ureteric catheterization, may be needed, depending on the clinical situation. If the patient has abnormal kidneys due to glomerular disease, instrument-ation of the urinary tract could be especially dangerous in introducing infection. Nonetheless, if urinary tract obstruction remains a possibil-ity, this hazard must be accepted.

There are no characteristic radiological features of glomerulo-nephritis. In acute glomerulonephritis and the nephrotic syndrome the kidneys may be large and later return to normal size. In chronic glomerulonephritis the kidneys are typically small, smooth, and symmetrical but secondary pyelonephritis and arteriolar nephrosclerosis may produce irregular scarring.

Serum Complement

Both total haemolytic complement and its major component quantitatively $C'3$ (synonym: $\beta_1 C$ globulin) are low in acute PSGN, SLE with renal involvement, membrano-proliferative glomerulo-nephritis, and in the glomerulonephritis of SBE and chronically infected ventriculo-atrial shunts ('shunt nephritis'). A normal serum complement early in a case of acute glomerulonephritis makes a post-streptococcal origin unlikely and is therefore a valuable aid in making this important differential diagnosis. The serum patterns of comple-ment components differ in various conditions, low levels of $C'1q$ and $C'4$ being characteristic of SLE with nephritis. The alternative pathway of

$C'3$ activation, involving properdin and bypassing the early components $C'1$, $C'4$ and $C'2$, is now being actively studied in renal disease. Abnormalities are being reported both in serum levels and glomerular deposition. In the majority of cases of glomerulonephritis with complement deposited in the glomeruli, serum levels are normal or elevated. $C'3$ levels in the nephrotic syndrome from any cause may be elevated. This is probably a non-specific serum protein response. $C'3$ is also elevated with infection, tissue injury, etc., so that raised complement levels are of little diagnostic help.

Renal Biopsy

An adequate percutaneous renal biopsy will provide a definitive histological diagnosis on which to base immediate treatment and future management.

Unless there are strong contra-indications a biopsy should be performed in every adult case of the nephrotic syndrome. This will permit the proper use of steroid and immunosuppressive drugs by picking out minimal change glomerulonephritis (for which disease these drugs are of real value), from proliferative and membranous disease in which such value as the drugs have, may be outweighed by their side-effects. In any group of patients with the nephrotic syndrome renal biopsy may show some totally unexpected findings. A high incidence of renal amyloid, unsuspected clinically, has been found in some reported series.

In some circumstances — for example, oliguric renal failure and recurrent haematuria — a tissue diagnosis of glomerulonephritis will spare the patient unnecessary and potentially hazardous investigations as well as helping with treatment and in assessing prognosis. In view of the relative rarity of acute PSGN in this country most adult patients with an acute nephritic syndrome should have a renal biopsy at some stage of their illness.

One common clinical problem is the symptom-free patient with mild persistent proteinuria. The yield of significant histological abnormalities with a daily protein excretion under 2 g is not large. If other investigations prove normal the case for carrying out a renal biopsy may not be strong. The prognostic value of a biopsy and the reassurance that normal histology provides must then be weighed against the risks of biopsy which in experienced hands are probably smaller than those of liver biopsy. It should be added that unexpected non-glomerular lesions, such as chronic pyelonephritis and myeloma, may also be revealed. Even in known secondary glomerular disease, the management of a case may depend on accurate histological assessment. Thus, in diabetes mellitus, hypertension, pyelonephritis and diabetic renal disease could all be contributing to renal failure to varying extents. Moreover, the presence of diabetes is not proof against glomerulonephritis. In SLE, the detailed renal histology is important in planning combined steroid–immunosuppressive treatment.

There may be problems in visualizing the kidneys and in controlling advanced uraemia and severe hypertension before attempting biopsy. Small kidneys are a contra-indication to biopsy as the risks are much greater and the information obtained less helpful. Unexpected bleeding tendencies can occur in the nephrotic syndrome due to low levels of certain coagulation factors. There are many other contra-indications to renal biopsy but as a general rule the patient with known, or strongly suspected, glomerular disease should have the very real benefits of an accurate histological diagnosis whenever possible.

PRIMARY GLOMERULAR DISEASE

Glomerulonephritis has been subdivided into three major histological groups: minimal change; membranous; and proliferative. These groups are *not* different stages of any one pathological process. Although the histological appearances of all three groups are found in association with recognized aetiological factors, in the vast majority of cases the origin of the condition is unknown. The idiopathic minimal change and membranous cases often run fairly consistent clinical courses and have enough features in common to be described as 'diseases'. It should be appreciated, however, that several different causes could be responsible for one final picture.

Proliferative glomerulonephritis is patently a heterogeneous group of diseases, having in common only an excess of cells in the glomerulus, be they mesangial, endothelial, epithelial or inflammatory, in varying proportions. The subdivision used here (*see* page 161) is an attempt at an up-to-date consensus of the experience of leading nephrology units. Two points are immediately apparent. In the first place these putative diseases are described variably on aetiological, clinical, histological and immunological grounds. It is not surprising that the subdivisions as described are by no means clear-cut but run into one another. Ostensibly synonymous terms are freely used in the literature, but it is often difficult to be certain that any two authors are using them in identical fashion. The 'synonyms' given here are more or less approximations and 'best fits'. Ellis's classification is now obsolete and should not be used. His 'type 2 nephritis' includes most types of primary glomerular disease with the nephrotic syndrome. Subacute glomerulonephritis also is a particularly confusing term. The second point to be appreciated is that a majority of cases of proliferative glomerulonephritis cannot be classified more specifically at present. These are mainly those presenting a more chronic clinical picture. Proliferative glomerulonephritis accounts for all cases of the acute nephritic syndrome, about 40 per cent of adult and 10 per cent or fewer of childhood nephrotics, and for a majority of cases of primary glomerular disease presenting with chronic renal failure, haematuria or symptomless proteinuria.

MINIMAL CHANGE GLOMERULONEPHRITIS
(SYNONYMS: LIPOID NEPHROSIS; IDIOPATHIC NEPHROTIC SYNDROME)

Here light microscopy of the glomerulus is normal or shows only slight focal hypercellularity and/or increase in mesangial matrix. The tubules show fat droplets in the cytoplasm (hence 'lipoid nephrosis') and on electron microscopy there is fusion of the epithelial foot processes. These changes, it should be stressed, are non-specific and reversible, being seen with heavy glomerular protein leaks from any cause. Immunofluorescent studies show no abnormal deposits. Reports of IgE deposition have not been confirmed.

This is the major cause of the nephrotic syndrome in children in this country, and it is responsible for 90 per cent or more of cases. It is found in about one quarter of adult cases. The onset may be insidious or fairly acute and is often preceded by a non-specific upper respiratory tract illness. There are only occasional and then usually transient nephritic features such as hypertension or haematuria. The blood urea may be elevated but this is due to prerenal causes or tubular obstruction, as discussed earlier. Spontaneous remission and relapse is common, relapses becoming less frequent with the passage of time. Corticosteroids or ACTH induce a remission in 95–100 per cent of children, the figure for adults being less well documented but probably somewhat less favourable.

Although there are ever-present dangers to minimal change nephrotic patients (notably injudicious treatment, acute renal failure, overwhelming infection and vascular occlusion), the development of progressive renal failure is rare. When it occurs the recently recognized condition of *focal glomerulosclerosis* should be suspected. Here there is a localized increase in mesangial matrix which affects the glomeruli segmentally at first but progresses to complete glomerular obliteration. IgM and β lipoprotein have been found in the lesions. Nephritic features and poorly selective proteinuria occur. The condition is probably in no way related to minimal change disease, confusion arising because patchy lesions of focal glomerulosclerosis may not be picked up by an initial renal biopsy.

The relationship of idiopathic minimal change glomerulonephritis to the normal glomerulus on light microscopy, seen in the nephrotic syndrome due to pollen sensitivity, certain drugs, a distant cancer and other causes, is unclear.

MEMBRANOUS GLOMERULONEPHRITIS
(SYNONYM: EPIMEMBRANOUS)

On light microscopy there is a uniform thickening of the capillary wall affecting each and every glomerulus diffusely. Electron microscopy shows that this is largely due to electron dense lumps distributed profusely on the epithelial side of the GBM (hence the word *epi*membranous). These are surrounded by spiky projections of basement membrane which often show up well on silver methenamine preparations. There is no increase in cellularity. Immunofluorescent preparations show a characteristic appearance of profuse discrete deposits of IgG in the lumps with only small amounts of complement or none at all.

Clinically, these patients present with the nephrotic syndrome or symptomless proteinuria. There is a much higher incidence of nephritic features than in minimal lesion disease. Membranous glomerulonephritis is rare in children but is widely held to be responsible for about 30 per cent of cases of the nephrotic syndrome in adults though some authorities put the figure much lower than this. The course of the disease is variable but generally progresses to terminal renal failure due to progressive obliteration of the capillaries and cellular elements. There is some suggestive anecdotal evidence that a number of patients with this condition respond to steroids. As the responses are usually slow, and spontaneous remission is said to occur, the significance of these reports is uncertain.

The majority of patients have no known cause, but similar or identical histological findings have been described in association with:

(1) Renal vein thrombosis
(2) Cancer and lymphoma
(3) SLE
(4) Chronic active hepatitis.

The immuno-pathology, as well as these associations, suggests that membranous glomerulonephritis is an immune complex disease. The most intriguing and best documented association is with renal vein

160

thrombosis. It is unclear whether renal vein thrombosis can predispose to immune complex deposition or whether membranous glomerulonephritis gives rise to a special tendency to local venous thrombosis. The latter may be more likely as bilateral glomerular changes have been seen with unilateral venous thrombosis.

PROLIFERATIVE GLOMERULONEPHRITIS

A separate section will be devoted to each of the following subdivisions of proliferative glomerulonephritis:

(1)   Acute post-streptococcal glomerulonephritis (acute PSGN)
(2)   Mesangial sclerosis
(3)   Rapidly progressive glomerulonephritis
(4)   Membrano-proliferative glomerulonephritis
(5)   Focal glomerulonephritis
(6)   Chronic glomerulonephritis and unspecified cases of proliferative glomerulonephritis

Acute Post-streptococcal Glomerulonephritis (Acute PSGN)
(Synonyms: Diffuse Exudative Glomerulonephritis; Acute Ellis Type 1)

This is a less common disease than of old. It remains predominantly a disease of children and young adults but occurs at any age. Males are affected more commonly than females. It follows infection with a Group A β haemolytic streptococcus, most frequently type 12, but also types 4, 1, 49 and others. In this country the most frequent site of infection is the pharynx but skin infections (impetigo) are responsible for probably a majority of cases in warmer countries as well as for some recent well-documented epidemics — for example, Red Lake, Trinidad (*see* chapter 11, page 257). The clinical features of the classical acute nephritic syndrome have been presented above.

The histological appearance at the height of the disease is characteristic, showing proliferation of endothelial and mesangial cells together with exudation (oedema and infiltration of polymorphs and macrophages). The electron microscope shows prominent discrete 'humps' on the epithelial side of the GBM. These can sometimes be seen easily on light microscopy and they last about 6 weeks. Immunofluorescence shows that they contain IgG and large amounts of C′3. Diffuse mesangial deposits are also found. These changes affect all glomeruli and are associated with variable amounts of capillary thrombosis and necrosis, Bowman's space haemorrhage, and tubular and interstitial abnormalities. Epithelial cell proliferation with capsule formation is unusual.

The relationship of this disease to the preceding infection and the histological and immunofluorescent appearances, with a low serum complement over the same period of time, is good evidence of immune complex deposition. However, streptococcal antigen has been found in the humps only sporadically and other immunological mechanisms have been invoked. These include the presence of a shared antigen between the kidney and the streptococcus, and renal antigens altered by streptococcal products initiating auto-immune reactions. Why some streptococci are nephritogenic remains a mystery.

The diagnosis of acute PSGN is usually straightforward – once it has been considered. Previous antibiotic treatment makes isolation of streptococci and a significant antistreptolysin-O titre (ASO) less likely. The differential diagnostic features of other types of glomerular disease presenting as acute nephritis have been discussed. It should be appreciated that β haemolytic streptococcal infections can apparently precipitate acute relapses in chronic glomerulonephritis and episodes of haematuria in focal glomerulonephritis. There may well be evidence of a recent streptococcal infection in other conditions so that such evidence does not constitute proof of the nature of the glomerular condition. The illness varies widely in severity, hypertension and oedema being absent in less severe cases. In the majority, signs and symptoms subside within one to two weeks, a diuresis occurring even in the absence of oedema. Nowadays, probably well under 5–10 per cent of the figure quoted of old, die in the acute stage. There is no evidence that steroids or immunosuppressive drugs are of value.

The most serious complication is anuric renal failure. A small percentage merge from the acute illness into a progressively down-hill 'subacute' phase. An unknown number enter a latent 'persistent' stage with continuing urinary abnormalities and later progression to renal failure. The vast majority, 95 per cent or more, of children recover completely. The percentage in adults is certainly smaller but inadequate numbers of cases, biopsy proven in the acute phase, have been followed for precise figures to be given. Proteinuria usually clears within 2 years but it can disappear after longer periods. One outstanding problem is how often a previous unrecognized attack of acute PSGN leads to chronic glomerulonephritis.

Mesangial Sclerosis (Synonym: PSGN)

Following recovery from acute PSGN, histological abnormalities in the mesangium may persist for a variable period of time. There is an increase in mesangial cells and matrix which contains fibrils.

These changes may accentuate the normal lobular structure of the glomerulus. Identical appearances may be found in patients, both children and adults, presenting with proteinuria, a nephrotic syndrome, or haematuria but without any clinical or laboratory evidence of a recent streptococcal infection. A relationship to acute PSGN is likely but not proven. The ultimate prognosis in such cases appears good, although steroid treatment is of no apparent benefit.

Rapidly Progressive Glomerulonephritis
(Synonyms: Glomerulonephritis with Epithelial Crescents,
Rapidly Progressive Ellis Type 1, Subacute Glomerulonephritis)

Although this condition (fortunately a rare one) may follow proven acute PSGN, the majority of cases do not. A history of recent infection is, however, frequently obtained.

The histological picture is one of acute glomerulonephritis with endothelial and mesangial cell proliferation but the most striking feature is epithelial cell proliferation to form large crescents that tend to compress and obliterate the glomerular capillaries. The crescents are interspersed with fibrin which provides the theoretical basis for anti-coagulation therapy in this condition. Crescents form in other types of proliferative glomerulonephritis and in polyarteritis and malignant hypertension suggesting that ischaemia plays a part in their aetiology. They are, however, never as large or widespread as in rapidly progressive glomerulonephritis. Immunofluorescent studies have shown a variety of deposits. A few cases have a diffuse linear pattern of IgG on basement membrane (anti-GBM antibody).

The disorder can occur at any age although it is found especially in young adults of both sexes. The onset may be an acute nephritic syndrome with oliguria prominent, frank acute renal failure, or a nephrotic syndrome, with nephritic features. In almost all instances renal failure progresses and death occurs within weeks or months. Occasionally remissions occur. A normal blood pressure is the rule and the serum complement is not reduced at an early stage as in acute PSGN. However, renal biopsy is needed for a firm diagnosis. Although intensive steroid and immunosuppressive treatment will probably be used, it is of uncertain value. Identical light microscopic appearances are seen in Goodpasture's Syndrome (where anti-GBM immunofluorescent staining is characteristically found) and rare cases of Henoch Schönlein purpura (HSP). These histological findings are associated with a similar clinical course.

Membrano-proliferative Glomerulonephritis
(Synonyms: Lobular, Hypocomplementaemic, Mixed
Nephritic—Nephrotic, Mesangio-capillary)

This is a characteristic form of proliferative glomerulonephritis show-ing the usual mesangial, endothelial and variable epithelial proliferation with two, more specific, histological features:

(1)   Widening of the GBM due to deposition of mesangial matrix on the endothelial surface with intervening mesangial cytoplasm giving the basement membrane a 'split' appearance.

(2)   A prominent accentuation of the lobulation of the glomeruli. In addition, many patients have a more or less persistently low serum $C'3$.

Clinically, there is a mixed nephritic and nephrotic picture — hence the various synonyms. Some authorities describe lobular and membrano-proliferative glomerulonephritis as separate entities.

The condition occurs at any age but especially in older children and young adults. The general outlook is poor although in some patients the disease does not progress for long periods. Steroid therapy is generally considered unhelpful.

Major interest has centred on the low serum complement levels which are not invariable or consistently found in a single patient during the course of this illness. Although the characteristic immunofluores-cent finding is $C'3$ deposition on the GBM, this is not the cause of the hypo-complementaemia which persists after bilateral nephrectomy. There is evidence of reduced complement synthesis and of increased catabolism, possibly related to a circulating 'toxic' factor. It will be appreciated that, clinically, histologically and immunologically, this condition bears no resemblance to membranous glomerulonephritis.

Focal Glomerulonephritis

This term has been a source of confusion as it has been used in two ways:

(1)   *Pathologically*, to describe histological changes involving a proportion only of glomeruli and then often just one or two lobules of the affected tufts ('segmental', 'local'). These changes can occur in a variety of conditions, the major ones being: (a) Henoch Schönlein purpura (HSP); (b) SLE; (c) subacute bacterial endocarditis (SBE); (d) polyarteritis nodosa; (e) Goodpasture's syndrome; (f) hereditary nephritis; and (g) idiopathic focal glomerulonephritis.

(2)   *Clinically*, to refer to patients with attacks of haematuria often

recurrent, occurring out of the blue, following exercise or, most characteristically, at the height of or just a day or two after a non-specific respiratory infection. A considerable proportion of these patients *do* show focal glomerulonephritis histologically but in others renal biopsy may be normal to light microscopy. Some show a diffuse proliferative glomerulonephritis or one of the more specific varieties described previously. Moreover, focal glomerulonephritis can be found on biopsy in patients presenting with other features of glomerular disease such as symptom-free proteinuria, nephrotic syndrome, persistent microscopic haematuria, or an acute nephritic syndrome. The use of the term in the clinical sense should be abandoned.

The details of the histological picture are not diagnostic. There is variable proliferation of endothelial cells and mesangial cells and matrix with rather less epithelial involvement. There may be adhesions locally across Bowman's capsule and associated areas of necrosis and sclerosis. Such changes are the ones most usually seen in HSP glomerular disease, SLE, subacute bacterial endocarditis (SBE) and the 'microscopic' variety of polyarteritis nodosa. They are also seen at an early stage in Goodpasture's syndrome and hereditary nephritis. In idiopathic focal glomerulonephritis (which forms a large proportion of most series of proliferative glomerulonephritis), the most frequent clinical picture is that described above, of recurrent haematuria. There are occasionally other nephritic features such as transient oedema and hypertension. There is usually no evidence of a streptococcal infection and the serum complement remains normal. The patients are predominantly male children and young adults. Loin pain and fever are frequent in the attacks which may also be associated with erythematous rashes and arthralgia. The prognosis, even with multiple attacks, is usually excellent. Steroids are again not thought to influence the disease process. The finding of heavy proteinuria would suggest a more diffuse glomerulonephritis but the only certain way of making the diagnosis is by renal biopsy. Immunofluorescent examination is especially helpful. Idiopathic focal glomerulonephritis is characterized by diffuse mesangial deposits of predominantly IgA with lesser amounts of IgG and $C'3$. It is of great interest that these deposits occur in glomeruli normal to light microscopy and in normal segments of affected glomeruli. A substantial proportion of cases, however, have other patterns of immunofluorescent staining or none at all.

There is a considerable overlap between idiopathic focal glomerulonephritis and HSP glomerulonephritis. On the one hand, some of the clinical features described above are found in HSP. On the other hand, the glomerular disease of HSP can present years after the acute illness with identical clinical histological and immunological findings to those found in idiopathic focal glomerulonephritis. As some reported series of the latter have also included cases with a family history of haematuria there may also be some overlap with hereditary nephritis.

Chronic Glomerulonephritis

This heterogeneous group forms a large proportion of cases of proliferative glomerulonephritis. Histologically, there is a variety of proliferative changes progressing at different rates in different glomeruli to shrinkage and hyalinization with GBM-like substance and collagen. There is interstitial fibrosis and infiltration and tubular atrophy and dilatation. Hypertensive and pyelonephritic changes may become dominant. Immunofluorescence may show staining but is generally not very helpful. There is usually no history of previous acute PSGN. It is doubtful whether many cases arise from subclinical attacks, because of reported series of acute PSGN only the more severe cases fail to heal completely.

The patients are of any age and there is a preponderance of males. The clinical presentation is with any of the clinical features of glomerular disease. Persistent proteinuria and casts are a prominent feature. In practice, the major differential diagnostic problems are hypertensive renal disease and chronic pyelonephritis. The prognosis is very variable but generally the disease tends to progress.

SECONDARY GLOMERULAR DISEASE

DIABETES MELLITUS

The major glomerular abnormality in diabetes is an excess of mesangial matrix and the chemically closely-related GBM itself. Electron microscopy has been especially valuable here in precise anatomical localization of the pathological process in its early stages.

The mesangial matrix is laid down initially in the stalk area of the lobules between the capillary loops — hence the term 'intercapillary glomerulosclerosis'. The basement membrane is thickened at an early stage. The diffuse mesangial excess and the basement membrane thickening are contiguous and are referred to as 'diffuse' intercapillary glomerulosclerosis. The 'nodular' variety consists of nodules of excess mesangial matrix lying more peripherally in the lobules. It was these latter lesions, described by Kimmelstiel and Wilson in 1936, which were the first specific features of diabetic glomerular disease to be recognized. Controversy concerns the inter-relationship of the two types of diffuse lesion and the nodules. A majority of observers now believe that the diffuse mesangial lesion precedes the GBM thickening and that the nodule is an expression of more severe 'diffuse' pathology. Exceptions to this time sequence of events certainly do occur.

Other lesions are seen, notably hyaline degeneration of the afferent and efferent arterioles and similarly staining hyaline nodules around the capillary loops and Bowman's Capsule (hyaline caps, capsular drops, etc.).

The clinical features of diabetic glomerulosclerosis are proteinuria, initially intermittent but later persistent and heavy, with progressive renal failure and hypertension. A nephrotic syndrome occurs in about one third of these patients.

The first signs tend to develop in juvenile diabetics after 10 years and are almost invariable after 20 years. Renal biopsy has shown changes of diabetic glomerulosclerosis, however, at the time of first presentation and even in pre-diabetics. There is a close association between glomerular disease and diabetic retinopathy. The severity of the clinical disease correlates best with the extent of the 'diffuse' lesions. The Kimmelstiel—Wilson nodules are *not* especially associated with the nephrotic syndrome and the use of their names in this context is incorrect. Advanced histological disease, including nodules, can be found without any *clinical* evidence of glomerular involvement. The progress of the disease is also highly unpredictable but heavy proteinuria usually heralds death in uraemia within 3 years or so.

The aetiology of the glomerular lesion is unknown but may be metabolic as it is found in diabetes secondary to non-genetically determined diseases such as pancreatitis. Normal GBM and mesangial matrix contains a good deal of carbohydrate as mucopolysaccharide and glycoprotein which may be relevant to the high incidence of glomerular involvement in diabetes.

Good diabetic control is sound practice but probably has no influence on the development of glomerular disease, which appears to be determined by the duration of the diabetes more than any other factor. Insulin requirements may drop as renal failure progresses; this contrasts with the equally unexplained carbohydrate intolerance and insulin resistance in non-diabetic patients with uraemia.

Diabetics are also rather more prone than non-diabetics to papillary necrosis and chronic pyelonephritis. The former is very rare and the latter highly controversial though probably true for women, at least. Renal changes due to hypertension and vascular disease are, of course, not uncommon in diabetics (*see* Chapter 5, pages 102—105).

AMYLOIDOSIS

There is no generally agreed way of classifying the clinical conditions in which amyloid tissue is found. The chemical and ultrastructural features (amyloid fibrils) are the same in them all. A modification of the old clinical basis of classifying amyloidosis is probably the soundest.

(1) *Primary*, localized or generalized

(2) *Hereditary*, such as familial Mediterranean fever and the neurological syndrome

(3) *Secondary* to chronic inflammation, infectious, as in tuberculosis and osteomyelitis, or non-infectious, as in rheumatoid arthritis and ulcerative colitis

(4) *Associated with malignancy*, notably multiple myeloma, but also cancer and lymphoma.

The kidney can be involved in all forms of generalized amyloidosis. Although looked upon as being particularly common in the secondary varieties, the incidence is probably no less in many of the other types. Renal amyloid is common in multiple myeloma, accounts for most deaths due to familial Mediterranean fever, and has been found in no fewer than 10 per cent of adults with the nephrotic syndrome considered, prior to renal biopsy, to have primary glomerular disease.

Amyloid accumulates in the mesangium and on both sides of the GBM but it is also found around the tubules, in the interstitium and in blood vessels. Special stains can help but metachromatic staining is very variable. Electron microscopy, if needed, will show the amyloid fibrils and make an unequivocal diagnosis. Rectal biopsy can provide a likely answer, liver biopsy may be more dangerous in amyloidosis due to a high incidence of haemorrhage, while the Congo Red test is obsolete. The only certain way of making a diagnosis of renal amyloid is by kidney biopsy.

Proteinuria may be the first finding, particularly if the patient is already under observation. Renal amyloid commonly presents with a nephrotic syndrome but may present with renal insufficiency or renal vein thrombosis (acute onset of a nephrotic syndrome or rapidly developing uraemia). Nephrogenic diabetes insipidus due to medullary deposits has been recorded. The kidneys may be enlarged and hypertension is not frequently seen, at least until there is advanced renal failure. In familial Mediterranean fever, proteinuria develops about 10 years before terminal uraemia. The nephrotic syndrome is usually followed by death in 3 years or so.

In secondary amyloidosis the progress of the renal disease can be halted if there is a curable cause such as tuberculosis or chronic osteomyelitis; otherwise treatment is symptomatic. Corticosteroids are contraindicated and immunosuppressive drugs are of no value.

SYSTEMIC LUPUS ERYTHEMATOSUS (SLE)

Glomerular involvement occurs in over 50 per cent of cases of SLE. It is especially important in younger patients, being a major cause of death. In the middle-aged and elderly, glomerular involvement is less common, while in drug-induced SLE it is almost unknown.

Three histological pictures are described:

(1)   Focal proliferative (lupus glomerulitis)
(2)   Diffuse proliferative, often with epithelial crescents and marked interstitial changes (lupus glomerulonephritis)
(3)   Diffuse membranous

These subdivisions are by no means mutually exclusive and their relationship to one another is uncertain. Changes from (2) to (3) have been described following azathioprine treatment. Only the rare finding of haematoxylin bodies is specific for SLE although other changes are suggestive. Necrotizing lesions, fibrinoid necrosis and patchy basement membrane thickening ('wire loops') are frequently seen. Electron microscopy shows that GBM thickening is frequent and that usually there are deposits within and on the endothelial and epithelial sides of the basement membrane as well as in the mesangium. Immunofluorescent studies show granular deposits of immunoglobins, especially IgG, and complement ($C'3$ and $C'1q$). There is good evidence that the glomerular disease is due to immune complexes consisting of DNA and anti-DNA antibody. Positive serum anti-DNA antibody tests are fairly specific for active SLE.

The clinical manifestations of renal SLE range from symptomless proteinuria and haematuria to rapidly advancing uraemia with acute nephritic features, the nephrotic syndrome, or both. Hypertension is a relatively late feature. A low serum cholesterol in the nephrotic phase is not now thought to be of prognostic significance. The urine microscopy may show nephritic, nephrotic and chronic renal failure features at the same time ('telescoped sediment').

The most severe glomerular disease is due to lupus glomerulonephritis, the other variants taking a more benign course. Renal biopsy is important in assessing the detailed histology, as the glomerulonephritis in particular should, in general, be treated energetically. High dose steroid therapy has been shown to be of value in this condition although at some cost in terms of side-effects. There is much evidence, albeit uncontrolled, that azathioprine, in combination with modest doses of steroids, can be extremely effective in improving histological appearances as well as giving remissions in the nephrotic syndrome. Renal function may remain steady and proteinuria diminish. Cyclophosphamide may prove preferable here, as appears to be the case in minimal change glomerulonephritis. The treatment of advanced renal failure along these lines is generally unrewarding. Serum complement levels are low with active glomerular disease and may rise with effective therapy.

HENOCH-SCHÖNLEIN PURPURA
(SYNONYMS: ANAPHYLACTOID, ALLERGIC PURPURA)

This condition, with its characteristic rash, polyarthralgia and abdominal symptoms, is mainly a disease of early childhood although it can occur at any age. Glomerular disease can be present with normal urine and as most hospital series show a preponderance of the more severe cases, the exact incidence of glomerular involvement, usually quoted at about 50 per cent, is unknown. In a majority, the evidence of renal disease consists of haematuria, microscopic or macroscopic, with a modest amount of proteinuria. This almost always clears completely although short relapses can occur in the early stages, with further episodes of purpura, joint or abdominal pain.

A far smaller number of patients develop an acute nephritic syndrome, a nephrotic syndrome or, most seriously of all, a combination of the two. The renal disease may then prove fatal within weeks or months, remit incompletely with persistent proteinuria and renal insufficiency, or heal apparently completely. On the whole, the more severe the extra-renal manifestations, the more severe the renal disease. Older children and adults tend to have the worst illnesses.

There is little evidence, even anecdotal, that steroids and immunosuppressive drugs are of any value. In view of the excellent prognosis of patients with evidence of only mild renal involvement these agents should not be used in the majority of cases. A careful trial in patients with the more severe illnesses is probably justified.

The renal biopsy findings reflect the clinical evidence of renal disease. In the mildest cases the changes are those of focal glomerulonephritis. The most severe cases with rapidly developing advanced renal failure show the histological picture of rapidly progressive glomerulonephritis with extensive epithelial crescents. Electron microscopy shows electron dense deposits around the GBM, mainly in a subendothelial position. Immunofluorescence shows diffuse mesangial and granular capillary wall deposits of immunoglobulins, mainly IgA but also IgG, $C'3$ and fibrinogen. The abnormalities are seen in histologically normal glomeruli and segments. These findings resemble those in idiopathic focal glomerulonephritis.

The nature of HSP is uncertain although it is believed that the cutaneous vasculitis, as well as the glomerulonephritis, is due to immune complex deposition. Although a history of a preceding respiratory illness is commonly obtained and may be streptococcal, the nature of the antigen(s) involved is unknown. Serum complement levels remain normal.

POLYARTERITIS NODOSA

Renal involvement (urinary abnormalities and azotaemia) occur in about 80 per cent of cases. Macroscopic haematuria, and loin pain due to renal infarcts occur in about 10 per cent. There are two, often coexisting, renal lesions:

(1)   Renal polyarteritis affecting medium and small-sized arteries as in other organs. Glomeruli are affected due to ischaemia and frank renal infarcts occur.

(2)   Proliferative glomerulonephritis ('microscopic' renal polyarteritis). This is less common. There are widespread focal changes with necrosis prominent. Some glomeruli show fibrosis ('healing') and others may appear normal Sometimes the histology is indistinguishable from that seen in rapidly progressive glomerulonephritis described previously. The clinical picture may also be similar — an acute nephritic syndrome with progressive renal failure and a normal blood pressure. Remissions and relapses are more common and hypertension develops if the patient survives the acute phase. High-dose steroid treatment can be life-saving and a precise diagnosis is important.

Systemic features such as abdominal pain, fever, broncho-pulmonary disease, mononeuritis multiplex, leucocytosis and eosinophilia may make the diagnosis obvious but occasionally the renal disease predominates. A nephrotic syndrome can sometimes occur. The renal disease in Wegeners granulomatosis is similar to that in polyarteritis with more necrotizing lesions.

SUBACUTE BACTERIAL ENDOCARDITIS (SBE)

Focal 'embolic' glomerulonephritis probably occurs frequently and accounts for the high incidence of microscopic haematuria in SBE. A diffuse proliferative glomerulonephritis, indistinguishable histologically, immunologically and on electron microscopy, from acute PSGN, is less common. It is this condition that accounts for severe renal impairment seen only occasionally in SBE nowadays but which occurred in 10 per cent or so of cases in the pre-antibiotic era. Hypertension and an acute nephritic syndrome are rare.

Both forms of glomerular disease, which can coexist, are believed to be due to immune complex deposition. Micro-embolism of fibrin may account for some of the focal changes and renal infarcts can occur. All organisms including fungi, and infections on the right side of the heart can lead to glomerulonephritis. The serum complement is low and rises with effective treatment which prevents progression of the renal disease. The presence of rheumatoid factor also provides evidence of chronic immunization in SBE. The danger of making a diagnosis of connective tissue disease in culture negative SBE needs no emphasis.

GOODPASTURE'S SYNDROME

This rare condition is of great interest because the immunological process involved has been convincingly shown to be mediated by an antibody against GBM which appears to share antigenic determinants with alveolar basement membrane antigens. The antigen–antibody combination activates complement. Although no age is exempt, the typical patient is a young man. The presenting symptom is usually haemoptysis which often follows an upper respiratory or 'flu-like' illness. The patient may be breathless and anaemic. The chest x-ray may show transient shadows due to lung haemorrhage. Haematuria and proteinuria may be present initially or develop shortly afterwards. Renal biopsy at this stage shows a focal glomerulonephritis.

Although haemoptysis often continues and may be profuse, advancing renal impairment becomes the dominant clinical feature. The histology is now that of rapidly progressive glomerulonephritis, immunofluorescent studies showing smooth linear deposition of IgG and $C'3$ on the GBM. The disease usually proves fatal within weeks or a month or two, but not invariably. Steroids alone do not appear helpful but in combination with azathioprine or cyclophosphamide they are worth trying. Renal replacement is needed, nevertheless, in the majority of cases. It is encouraging that after bilateral nephrectomy and haemodialysis for at least one year, circulating anti-GBM antibodies disappear, following which transplantation may be successful.

HAEMOLYTIC–URAEMIC SYNDROME AND THROMBOTIC THROMBOCYTOPENIC PURPURA

The main features of these conditions are micro-angiopathic haemolytic anaemia, thrombocytopenic purpura, intracranial neurological involvement and glomerular disease. The former is described mainly in children (predominantly around one year of age) and usually follows a non-specific gastro-intestinal or respiratory illness. The latter occurs in adults with a higher incidence in women. However, there is a good deal of overlap in the clinical pictures and the histopathology is indistinguishable. The major findings are subendothelial deposits of fibrin and amorphous thrombi in the terminal arterioles of many organs including the sternal marrow, biopsy of which helps in making the diagnosis. The kidneys show similar arteriolar changes with varying degrees of proliferative glomerulonephritis. Cortical necrosis is seen, especially in children. In adults there is usually a fatal course of a few months with occasional remissions. Twenty per cent of adult cases are found to have features of SLE. The neurological features tend to be the most prominent in adults but anuric renal failure occurs. Surviving children may recover completely or have renal impairment with hypertension prominent.

It is widely believed that the pathogenesis of this condition(s) is disseminated intravascular coagulation (DIC) with consumption of coagulation factors including platelets, excess fibrinogen turnover, and secondary red cell damage and breakdown. This forms the theoretical basis for heparin therapy which is as yet of unproven value. An experimental model (probably a poor one) is the Schwartzmann reaction in the rabbit (DIC and cortical necrosis following 2 injections of endotoxin 24 hrs apart). Firm evidence of DIC is found in some cases of post-partum renal failure and in association with renal failure following frank gram negative septicaemia. There is also evidence of similar mechanisms contributing to the renal lesions of malignant hypertension, polyarteritis nodosa, toxaemia of pregnancy, renal transplant rejection and many cases of proliferative glomerulonephritis, especially the rapidly progressive variety. Anticoagulation with heparin or warfarin and dipyridamole which inhibits platelet aggregation, have been used in all these situations.

QUARTAN MALARIA NEPHROPATHY

An aetiological relationship has been firmly established between glomerular disease presenting with the nephrotic syndrome and chronic quartan *(Plasmodium malariae)* malaria. It is probably the most common world-wide cause of the nephrotic syndrome. There is good evidence that immune complex deposition is involved. Granular staining for IgG, IgM and C′3 is found in the capillary wall while malarial antigen has been detected in a number of cases. In Nigerian children a specific glomerular lesion has been recently described. This consists of minute lacunae containing inclusions of unknown composition, lying in a thickened GBM. Capillary obliteration due to the GBM-thickening and mesangial sclerosis is, at first, segmental but later involves the entire glomerulus. Secondary tubular atrophy and interstitial cellular infiltration occur. Descriptions from Uganda stress proliferative changes.

Response to anti-malarial treatment, steroids, cyclophosphamide and azathioprine is uncertain. The patients with less advanced histological changes and those with highly selective proteinuria tend to have a better prognosis.

HEREDITARY AND METABOLIC GLOMERULAR DISEASE

There are many hereditary forms of renal disease. Polycystic disease is by far the most common to present with such 'glomerular' symptoms as haematuria, hypertension and chronic renal failure. As it is a disease that affects the entire renal parenchyma it will not be considered further.

HEREDITARY NEPHRITIS (ALPORT'S SYNDROME)

Although uncommon, this condition is not rare, and it is being recognized with increasing frequency. Its salient features are recurrent haematuria, nerve deafness and progressive renal failure, all more severe in males than females. Many patients also have ocular abnormalities such as cataracts, nystagmus, spherophakia, anterior lenticonus and myopia.

The earliest symptoms are often recurrent haematuria or, especially in females, recurrent attacks of frank acute pyelonephritis. Men tend to die of renal failure in their 30's or 40's but women rarely develop advanced uraemia and the nephrotic syndrome is rare in both sexes. Families with osseous abnormalities and others without deafness or eye disorders have been described The inheritance in many families is dominant but this does not explain the findings in others.

The histology reported varies from a picture of focal or chronic glomerulonephritis to chronic pyelonephritis with, often, features of all three. The most characteristic finding is lipid-containing foam cells in the interstitium. They are not specific for hereditary nephritis but are never found as commonly in other conditions. Their significance is unknown.

FABRY'S DISEASE
(SYNONYMS: GLYCOLIPID LIPOIDOSIS, ANGIOKERATOMA CORPORIS DIFFUSUM)

This is a very rare disorder but an example of glomerular disease due to an enzyme defect. There is a deficiency of ceramide trihexosidase which is involved in the breakdown of sphingolipid. Gaucher's disease results from a failure in breakdown at a later step. Ceramide trihexoside accumulates in many tissues giving foam cells. The glomerular epithelial cells are especially involved.

Clinically, in childhood and young adults, there are attacks of severe bizarre pains in the limbs with fever and oedema. Later, an angiomatous rash develops on the hips, buttocks, genitalia and arms. Proteinuria may be present already but progressive renal failure develops. Again, males are involved far more severely. The condition can be recognized in both sexes by a characteristic corneal dystrophy seen on slit lamp microscopy. The urine may contain foam cells.

MANAGEMENT OF RENAL GLOMERULAR DISEASE

There are two ends in view — those of limiting glomerular damage and correcting any functional disturbance (providing symptomatic treatment). On the whole we can do little about the first but we do have the means to provide reasonable symptomatic treatment.

Indications have been given already (under each of the headings for individual glomerular diseases) of which diseases respond to treatment directed at the pathogenic mechanisms and which do not. The symptomatic treatment of renal failure (acute and chronic) is an enormous subject and, as it is by no means a specifically glomerular disorder, it will not be discussed here. The nephrotic syndrome, on the other hand, is, with the notable but rare exception of chyluria, always due to a glomerular leak of protein.

NEPHROTIC SYNDROME

In children in this country the nephrotic syndrome is almost always due to primary glomerular disease. In adults about 20 per cent of cases are due to secondary glomerular disease but among these the remediable causes are relatively rare. It is important to exclude drugs, toxins and allergens. Desensitization has proved curative in seasonal nephrotic syndrome due to pollen sensitivity. Secondary syphilis can give a nephrotic syndrome probably by an immune complex mechanism. In contrast to quartan malaria nephropathy, 'removing' the antigen by treating the infection appears to be curative. The diagnosis of renal vein thrombosis is usually made too late to permit thrombectomy or anticoagulation. Nonetheless it is wise to give anticoagulants as pulmonary embolism can occur. The possibility of a distant cancer or lymphoma should be considered.

Symptomatic Treatment of the Nephrotic Syndrome

Bed Rest

This may induce a diuresis but should never be prolonged in view of its catabolic effects and the increased tendency to venous thrombosis.

Diuretics

Frusemide and ethacrynic acid, sometimes in large doses, may be needed with or without spironolactone. Less powerful thiazide diuretics may be adequate initially or for maintenance. Added potassium is usually needed if the patient is not uraemic, probably because of the frequency of secondary hyperaldosteronism (steroids, if used, also increase the tendency to hypokaliaemia sharply). A diuresis of more than 1–2 kg loss of body weight per day should be avoided. Excess fluid loss can precipitate severe hypovolaemia, shock, acute renal failure and venous thrombosis.

Diet

The patient should have a high protein diet (1.5–2.0 g/kg per day). Preferably, this should be combined with a reduced sodium intake but this proves difficult without resorting to unpalatable formula foods. Ion exchange resins such as Katonium may be needed but the added K^+ can be a hazard if the patient is uraemic.

Plasma Expansion

Plasma expansion with a salt free albumin infusion can provoke a diuresis if the oedema is otherwise refractory. A large dose of frusemide should be given with the infusion which can also be used if severe hypovolaemia develops.

Antibiotics

These should be held at the ready and used early, with bacterio-logical control. Prophylactic use is not recommended. Cholesterol-lowering agents such as clofibrate have been advocated in view of the evidence of an increased tendency to atherosclerosis and arterial throm-bosis. Usually the serum lipids return to normal if a remission occurs.

Corticosteroids and Cyclophosphamide

These agents are effective in inducing remission in nephrotic synd-rome due to minimal change glomerulonephritis. Their mechanism of action is totally unknown — hence their consideration under symp-tomatic treatment.

In minimal change disease, steroid treatment is justified unless the patient quickly improves spontaneously with loss of proteinuria. High doses of prednisolone will induce a remission in the vast majority of children and in a high percentage (about 80 per cent) of adults. The dose can be reduced but if there is no response after 8 weeks treatment, steroids should be discontinued. A variable number (about 50 per cent) relapse on stopping or tailing off the steroids which should be attempted in every case that responds initially. If the dose of steroids needed to keep the patient in remission is likely to give side-effects, a short course of cyclophosphamide in doses that need not induce leuco-penia may induce a prolonged remission or permit lower doses of steroids to be used. However, cyclophosphamide can produce prolonged impairment of ovum and sperm production and should not be used without this consideration in young patients. Patients on cyclophos-phamide have also had dangerous or fatal viral illnesses such as measles.

Cyclophosphamide is not as useful in the rare steroid-resistant as opposed to the common steroid-dependent case of minimal change nephrotic syndrome. In resistant cases the diagnosis should be recon-sidered, particularly with focal glomerulosclerosis in mind. These drugs have little or no place in the treatment of the nephrotic syndrome due to membranous and proliferative glomerulonephritis.

HYPERTENSION

It is generally accepted that hypertension in glomerular disease needs energetic and early treatment designed to limit hypertensive renal damage. Drugs that maintain renal blood flow, such as alpha-methyldopa and hydrallazine, are popular although there is no documented evidence that they are superior to other agents.

In chronic renal failure and the acute nephritic syndrome, hypertension should be controlled by correcting salt and water excess before resorting to drugs. Hypertensive encephalopathy in acute PSGN can occur at relatively mild degrees of diastolic hypertension.

THE AVOIDANCE OF URINARY INFECTIONS

One must be careful not to make difficult situations worse by risking urinary tract infections with unnecessary bladder catheterization. Patients with glomerular disease get superadded urinary tract infections nonetheless. Urine cultures should be carried out regularly and any infections found should be treated.

REFERENCES

Black, D. A. K. (1972). *Renal Disease.*, 3rd edition. Oxford: Blackwell Scientific Publications.

Cameron, J. S. (1970). 'Glomerulonephritis: current practice' and 'Nephrotic syndrome' *Br. Med. J.* **4**, 285 and 350

Strauss, M. B. and Welt, L. G. (1971). *Diseases of the Kidney.*, 2nd edition., Boston: Little, Brown.

8

Adverse Reactions to Drugs and Diseases of the Chest

P. D. B. Davies

However drugs are administered to a patient they may be returned to the lungs by the venous system and so it should come as no surprise that drug-induced pulmonary reactions are really quite common. They have followed the administration of drugs by the most unlikely routes. For example, oil-embolism has followed myelography using a radio-opaque iodized oil, and pulmonary eosinophilia has followed the application of a sulphonamide-containing cream to the vagina. It follows, then, that whenever a clinician sees a patient with an unusual pulmonary reaction who is, or has been, taking a drug either for treatment or for an investigation, he should consider the possibility of a drug-induced disorder. To try to decide the matter he should ask himself three questions:

(1)   Could a drug (or drugs) be responsible for the disorder?
(2)   If so, which drug (or drugs) is responsible for the disorder?
(3)   What is the mechanism responsible for the disorder?

The first question is decided by careful history-taking with the possibility of a drug-induced reaction in mind. Sometimes the possibility is suggested by the finding of some associated reaction. It might be a clinical finding, such as the development of a rash or fever, or a pathological finding, such as eosinophilia in the peripheral blood. Sometimes the possibility is suggested by observing the effect of withdrawal of all drugs.

The second question makes demands upon the clinician's knowledge of the likely reactions produced by individual drugs. Sometimes a suspicion may be confirmed by the use of special tests such as those involving the release of histamine from sensitized tissues, lymphocyte transformation, or the detection of specific antibodies. If it is considered safe to do so, the diagnosis may be confirmed by a provocation challenge. It is important to bear in mind that the finding of a reaction to one drug in no way excludes the possibility of a reaction to another. This is commonly seen, for example, in the treatment of pulmonary tuberculosis with streptomycin and PAS; about half the patients who develop rash and fever while taking these two drugs will be shown by provocation challenge to be sensitive to both of them.

The third question is really a research question. Nevertheless, in ordinary clinical practice a very important pathogenetic distinction can be made by asking a further series of three questions.

(4)   Is it a toxic reaction? That is to say, is it explicable by the normal pharmacological activity of the drug?

(5)   Is it an idiosyncratic reaction? That is to say, is it a consequence of a genetically determined biochemical abnormality?

(6)   Is it an allergic reaction? That is to say, is it a manifestation of hypersensitivity produced by immunological mechanisms?

It should be remembered that drugs may cause reactions by more than one means. For example, again in the case of streptomycin, toxic reactions in the form of labyrinthine disturbance, leading to ataxia nystagmus and giddiness, are common, and so are allergic reactions of which the most common are rash and fever. Moreover, one drug may produce the same reaction by more than one means. For example, sulphonamides may induce anaemia as a result of an idiosyncratic reaction in a patient deficient in glucose-6-phosphate dehydrogenase or as the result of allergy, by immunological mechanisms.

TOXIC REACTIONS

Toxic reactions may be of three types (Table 8.1).

Direct Effects

Overdosage

A good example of the production of toxic effects by overdosage was the increase in incidence of reactions to digoxin which followed a change in the method of its manufacture. This led to greater absorption of the drug from the intestine and so to higher blood levels than before. Digitalis also illustrates well immediate and cumulative overdosage and absolute and relative overdosage. It has been shown that about 10 per cent of patients given digitalis alone develop toxic reactions to it, whereas about 25 per cent of patients do so if given digoxin together with diuretic; the result of the depletion of potassium induced by many oral diuretics. This is an example of drug interactions potentiating pharmacological response which can also be brought about by enzyme inhibition, by displacement from protein binding or by competing for renal excretion.

TABLE 8.1

Toxic Reactions

Direct effects	
Overdosage	Immediate or cumulative; absolute or relative
Intolerance	Quantitative increase due to lowered threshold to action of a drug
Indirect effects	
Side effects	Undesirable but unavoidable actions of a drug
Secondary effects	Undesirable but not inevitable actions of a drug

Intolerance

Intolerance simply means that some patients seem to develop toxic reactions to drugs much more readily than others. The classical example is quinine. The basis of intolerance is certainly in some cases, and probably in all, an inherited abnormality of biochemical function. This differs from idiosyncrasy in that the reaction produced is merely a quantitative increase in the normal response to the drug and not the development of a completely new type of reaction as in idiosyncrasy, for example, porphyria precipitated by barbiturates. A good example is the intolerance that certain patients show to isoniazid. There is an inherited variation in the speed of inactivation of isoniazid and patients who inactivate the drug slowly develop toxic effects more frequently than those who inactivate it rapidly. Again, the prolonged apnoea which may follow the use of suxamethonium compounds is due to a genetically determined abnormality of the enzyme pseudo-cholinesterase.

Side Effects

These are the undesirable but unavoidable actions of a drug and they can be well illustrated by the use of corticosteroids. These drugs inevitably (though variably) induce the features of Cushing's syndrome and so obesity, hypertension, glycosuria and osteoporosis may all be the consequence of the use of corticosteroids in large doses over long periods.

Secondary Effects

Secondary effects, the indirect and not inevitable actions of a drug, can also be well illustrated by the use of corticosteroids. Opportunistic lung infections and reactivation of quiescent tuberculous lesions may complicate corticosteroid treatment. Another complication, less well authenticated, is the development of spontaneous pneumothorax in patients having corticosteroid drugs as part of the treatment of pulmonary tuberculosis and possibly other lung diseases too. Though this association is not fully proven, it is certain that when a spontaneous pneumothorax develops in a patient taking corticosteroid drugs it may be difficult to close the broncho-pleural fistula. Perhaps this is because zinc is essential to the healing of wounds and one of the effects of corticosteroids is to deplete the body of zinc.

ALLERGIC REACTIONS

Allergic reactions, unlike toxic effects, are not dose-dependent. They can be reproduced by minute quantities of the allergen. Nevertheless, massive exposure may serve to induce hypersensitivity. For example, if patients in renal failure are given streptomycin, they may have exceedingly high levels of the drug in the blood and then develop not only toxic but allergic reactions. The main mechanisms whereby allergic reactions may cause tissue damage are classified in Table 8.2.

It is important to realize that the appearance of antibodies does not necessarily lead to tissue damage or clinical signs of allergy; nor may it necessarily be associated with a favourable immune response.

An example of this is the severe atypical measles with pneumonia which may result from exposure to measles after immunization with a killed (inactivated) vaccine. In atypical measles the rash is unlike that of ordinary measles in its site of origin (feet instead of hairline), its progression (towards the head instead of away from it), its distribution (densest in the lower limbs and creases), and its character (a mixture of papular, petechial, vesicular and urticarial components). This is associated with high fever and symptoms and signs of involvement of viscera. The lungs are often involved. There is lobar or segmental pneumonia with enlarged hilar lymph nodes and pleural effusion; the chest x-ray may remain abnormal long, even years, after all other evidence of the disease has cleared. The explanation seems to be that although there is an adequate serum antibody response to the killed vaccine there is a failure to develop secretory IgA antibody. The result is that after infection by natural measles there may be replication of the virus in the respiratory tract and an accelerated serum antibody response leading to the formation of tissue-damaging immune complexes.

TABLE 8.2

Allergic reactions

Type 1	Immediate anaphylactic-type hypersensitivity mediated by reaginic antibodies (IgE)
Type 2	Hypersensitivity directed against tissue or cellular antigens: auto-allergy
Type 3	Intermediate Arthus-type sensitivity mediated by precipitating antibodies (IgG)
Type 4	Delayed tuberculin-type hypersensitivity mediated by lymphoid cells without circulating antibodies

Penicillin provides another good example of the difficulties of associating the finding of antibodies to a drug with the development of disease and the production of tissue damage. It is probably true that all patients given penicillin develop antibodies and in fact many patients already have antibodies as a result of the ingestion of penicillin in foodstuffs. Despite this, reactions are by no means the rule and severe reactions are quite rare. Another difficulty is that hypersensitivity may be induced by a metabolite of the complex penicillin such as penicilloic acid. Again, penicillins may polymerize and then, as polymers, more readily combine with proteins to form haptens. It has been shown, too, that hypersensitivity reactions to penicillin are sometimes induced by the presence of contaminants within the commercial preparations; this is the basis of the use of the compound Purapen from which the contaminants have been excluded. A further difficulty is that all penicillins contain the basic nucleus, the beta-lactam ring 6-amino-penicillanic acid, and although cross-sensitivity between the different compounds is the rule, there is a higher incidence of adverse reactions to ampicillin than to other penicillins. In fact, hypersensitivity reactions are no more common with ampicillin than with other penicillins, but 90 per cent of patients with glandular fever or lymphatic leukaemia, given ampicillin, develop an erythematous maculo-papular rash over the extensor aspects of limbs and trunk. Mucous membranes may be affected; there may be itching and malaise. This does not seem to be an allergic reaction. It has a short incubation period of 5–8 days, it is not associated with other anaphylactic reactions, and it does not recur if ampicillin is given after recovery, either as a test dose or for treatment of other diseases. It is not suppressed by steroids. No reaginic antibodies have been demonstrated and lymphocyte transformation is negative. The explanation is quite unknown.

There is, then, a theoretical basis for an analysis of the pathogenesis of adverse reactions to drugs within the respiratory tract, and some drug-induced pulmonary reactions have been fully analysed. Perhaps the best examples are the reactions which may complicate the use of pituitary snuff as replacement therapy for patients with diabetes insipidus. Some patients may develop rhinitis, some may develop asthma, and others may develop extrinsic allergic alveolitis in which there is sustained dyspnoea with cough, widespread crepitations, and extensive mottling in the chest x-ray, together with a restrictive impedance to ventilation and impairment of the capacity for gas transfer.

Pituitary snuff can, then, evoke reactions at all levels in the respiratory tract and it does so by more than one immunological mechanism. The rhinitis and asthma are largely a manifestation of type 1 hypersensitivity (*see* table 8.1), mediated by reaginic IgE antibodies. This has been conclusively demonstrated by Prausnitz–Kustner passive transfer test and by immediate whealing reactions to skin tests, though in some cases there may be a late component to the asthmatic reaction which may represent type 3 hypersensitivity. On the other hand, extrinsic allergic alveolitis is an example of type 3 hypersensitivity mediated by precipitating IgG antibodies. This has been demonstrated by the finding of precipitating antibodies to the antigens and by a late Arthus-type oedematous response to intradermal testing.

An interesting and important finding during the analysis of this reaction was that the antibodies evoked by the taking of pituitary snuff will not only react as expected with porcine and bovine pituitary tissue antigens but will also react with human pituitary antigens. This raises the possibility that, in certain circumstances, the taking of drugs might lead to the development of auto-antibodies and so to the development of auto-immune disease.

On the other hand, it must be realized that the basis of many, if not most, drug reactions is poorly understood. An example of this are the respiratory reactions evoked by the use of iodides: acute reactions, iodism and polyarteritis nodosa.

Many patients, given iodine-containing contrast-media intravenously for radiological purposes, develop some paraesthesiae of the skin; some develop transient hypotension, and a few may develop severe, even fatal, circulatory collapse. In some ways this reaction resembles ana-phylaxis but it can occur in patients who have never before been given the compound; skin tests are negative and antibodies have not been demonstrated. It is therefore postulated that these iodine-containing compounds have some direct angiotoxic action leading to the release of histamine.

Iodism may complicate the use of any iodine-containing compound. The respiratory tract may be involved throughout its length with upper respiratory symptoms and signs, tracheobronchitis, asthma or pneu-monia. The skin and alimentary tract may also be involved. The reaction may be immediate or delayed; it may be of every degree of severity (it may even cause death), and every degree of chronicity. Although the incidence of iodism seems to be related to the dose, some patients react much more unfavourably than others. Moreover, the reaction is so capricious that symptoms resulting from small doses may disappear if the dose is doubled.

There are a number of case reports in which polyarteritis followed the use of iodides and the development of iodism but the pathogenesis is quite uncertain because the evidence for the association is purely circumstantial.

EPIDEMIOLOGICAL STUDIES LINKING THE TAKING OF A DRUG WITH THE DEVELOPMENT OF A DISEASE

The majority of drug-induced pulmonary reactions have to be described simply syndrome by syndrome and only here and there can a likely pathogenetic mechanism be put forward. We shall consider first three situations in which the evidence linking the taking of a drug with the development of a disease came from epidemiological studies, though in each case, of course, it was a clinical observation which first prompted an epidemiological survey.

Trhomboembolism and the Contraceptive Pill

The first suggestion that these compounds might be associated with the development of venous thrombosis and pulmonary embolism came from a general practitioner, Dr. Jordan, of Bungay in Suffolk, who in 1961 treated a 40-year old district nurse for endometriosis with a contraceptive pill (Enavid). After a few weeks she developed an episode of severe vomiting which was followed by bilateral pulmonary embolism. Thereafter, the Royal College of General Practitioners showed superficial thrombo-phlebitis to be 3 times as common in women taking a contraceptive pill as in controls, and the Medical Research Council and the Committee on Safety of Drugs showed that deep vein thrombosis, pulmonary embolism and cerebral thrombosis were between 4 and 8 times as common as in controls. The Committee on Safety of Drugs then established that the vital element in the development of these reactions was the oestrogen content of the combined contraceptive pill. They compared the incidence of these adverse reactions in pills of different oestrogen content. If the pill containing 50 μg of oestrogen is used as the baseline, pills containing 75 μg carry a risk 1.2 times as great, 100 μg 1.6 times as great, and 150 μg 2.4 times as great. Further work has shown quite conclusively that these contraceptives specifically influence the factors responsible for the development of intravascular thrombosis, their most constant effects being to increase clotting factors VII and X, and to enhance platelet adhesiveness and aggregation. To counteract this tendency new contraceptive pills have now been developed which contain only a progestogen. It has been shown that pills of this type may reverse the accelerated clotting patterns in women who have been taking combined preparations and will produce no change in clotting factors in women who have not previously taken oral contraceptives.

The diagnosis of pulmonary embolism in a woman taking a contraceptive pill, can be extremely difficult. There are three reasons for this:

(1) Pulmonary embolism does not invariably or even usually produce pulmonary infarction. In a healthy young woman with a normal pulmonary venous pressure and systemic arterial pressure it may well, in fact, not do so. The presence of even a massive pulmonary embolism is perfectly compatible with normal chest x-ray appearances. Increase in size of a pulmonary artery due to the presence of a thrombus within it and marked reduction of vascular markings distal to an embolus, are uncommon radiological signs. Lung scanning using radioactive macro-aggregates has many limitations especially in patients with underlying disease, particularly airway obstruction. Pulmonary angiography, a major procedure, may be needed.

(2)   The pulmonary circulation has an enormous reserve. Over half the total cross-section of the pulmonary arteries must be obstructed before there is any change of pressure and over two thirds before the rise of pressure causes cardiac embarrassment. The majority of pulmonary emboli therefore cause no cardiac (or pulmonary) disturbance. Cardiac catheterization may be needed to demonstrate pulmonary hypertension (a 'float' catheter is both simple and safe).

(3)   There may be no clinical evidence of peripheral venous thrombosis. Venography, ultrasound and radioactive fibrinogen may all have to be used to demonstrate the presence of a thrombus.

All women taking a combined contraceptive pill require full investigation if they complain of dyspynoea (the most common symptom) either sustained where there is pulmonary hypertension due to multiple pulmonary emboli, or paroxysmal, with or without wheeze and prolongation of expiration.

Primary Pulmonary Hypertension and Aminorex

In 1967 a physician working in a cardiac clinic in Switzerland noticed that over 15 per cent of his cardiac catheter studies in that year had shown evidence of so-called primary pulmonary hypertension. The more usual figure for a normal year was less than 1 per cent. When this finding was investigated he found that 55 out of his 70 patients had been taking aminorex, a drug with a structure resembling amphetamine for treatment of obesity. The drug had only been released for sale in Switzerland, Austria and Germany; a survey showed that more than 10 per cent of those who had taken more than 300 tablets developed pulmonary hypertension which progressed rapidly and did not remit when the drug was stopped. When the drug was withdrawn from sale, the 'epidemic' of pulmonary hypertension ceased. The histology of the condition resembled spontaneous primary pulmonary hypertension, quite different from both thrombo-embolic disease and the reactive hypertension induced by hypoxia in grossly obese patients (the Pickwick syndrome). In this country practitioners have been invited since 1970 to report to the Committee on Safety of Medicines, any cases of pulmonary hypertension associated with the use of appetite suppressants, including amphetamine, but no further clinical reports have been made and what is more it has proved impossible to reproduce the disease in animals.

Death from Asthma and Pressurized Aerosols

In 1965, Dr. Martin Greenberg, a chest physician working in Cambridge, reported sudden death in 8 young patients suffering from asthma all of whom had been using pressurized sympathomimetic aerosols. Surveys showed that between 1961, when these aerosols came on the market, and 1966 there had been a severe increase in the mortality from asthma. In the age group 10–14 the mortality had increased 7 times; in the 15–34 age-group, the mortality had increased 3 times. The Medical Research Council investigated 184 deaths from asthma; such pressurized aerosols had been used in 84 per cent of them. In 1967 a warning was therefore issued to doctors about the overuse of these compounds and in 1968 they were available to the general public in the U.K. on prescription only. Animal investigation suggested that the basis of the catastrophe was cardiac arrhythmia, including ventricular fibrillation, brought about by the effects of the sympatho-mimetic agent, usually isoprenaline, on a hypoxic myocardium. With the understanding of the cause of the condition there came a drop in sales and sympatho -mimetic agents with a more selective action on the beta-receptors in the bronchial tree than on the heart were developed (orciprenaline, salbutamol, terbutaline). The mortality from asthma then fell to the previous figures. Nevertheless, at this stage, some facts remained unexplained, the most important being that this epidemic of deaths from asthma was reported in the U.K., in New Zealand, Australia and Eire, but not in the U.S.A., Canada or the Netherlands, though pressurized sympatho-mimetic-containing aerosols had been used in those countries. At first, attention was directed to the possible adverse effects of the propellant and indeed a number of deaths were reported in drug addicts in the U.S.A. who used an aerosol containing only the propellant (this was sold for the cooling of drinking glasses). The drug addicts filled plastic bags with the contents of the aerosol and then inhaled it. The effects were apparently pleasurable but in some cases disastrous. On investigation it was found that the propellants used with the benign sounding names of Arcton and Freon were in fact fluorinated hydrocarbons with a structure not unlike chloroform and halothane which occasionally cause fatal cardiac arrest during anaesthesia. However, further investigation showed that the amount of these compounds absorbed after the inhalation of pressurized aerosols for the relief of bronchial asthma was too small to have any significant effect upon the myocardium. Finally, a further investigation showed that the link between deaths in asthma and use of pressurized aerosols was to be explained by the use of the high dose preparation containing 0.4 mg per dose of isoprenaline. Sales of this powerful compound represented 30 per cent of the total in the U.K. at the relevant time. It is now realized that these big-dose aerosols were released for sale in the countries which suffered epidemics of sudden deaths from asthma and were not licensed for sale in the U.S.A. and in Canada. In the Netherlands they were only introduced late and sales were low. Thus, this serious and dangerous drug-induced pulmonary reaction has finally been fully explained.

ASTHMA

Drugs may cause asthma in a variety of ways, most straightforwardly by simple irritation. The increase of cough, wheeze and dyspnoea which some patients notice after the inhalation of disodium cromoglycate (Intal), is the reason for the use of the compound Intal-co in which a small dose of isoprenaline is incorporated to counteract the irritative effect. Cromoglycate can be a considerable irritative agent. Some patients have developed chronic laryngitis after using the compound for a considerable time. Moreover, when the drug has been withdrawn it has taken several weeks or months before the chronic laryngitis has remitted.

Drugs may cause asthma by a direct pharmacological action. An example of this is the increase of airways obstruction which asthmatic patients may suffer if they use a beta-blocking agent for the treatment of a cardiac condition. Fortunately, successively more selective agents have been developed so that, in succession, pronethalol, propranolol and practolol have shown fewer and less serious actions upon the bronchial tree, while preserving their activity upon the heart.

Most commonly, of course, drugs may cause asthma by means of the development of an allergic reaction. In some cases the drug may cause asthma without inducing any other manifestation of hypersensitivity, but in some other cases asthma may merely be one part of a generalized reaction. The reaction may be immediate, it may be mediated by reaginic IgE antibodies, and may or may not be associated with the general picture of anaphylactic shock. In other cases the reaction may be late, a manifestation of type 3 hypersensitivity, mediated by precipitating IgG antibodies, and may then occur either in isolation or as part of a serum sickness syndrome.

Piperazine provides an interesting example of a drug which can induce allergic asthma. Workers manufacturing tranquillizers derived from piperazine have become hypersensitive to it as the result of inhaling minute quantities. This is an example of 'late' or 'intermission' asthma probably dependent on a type 3 response, but specific IgG antibody has not yet been identified. Piperazine itself is, of course, a useful drug for the treatment of round and thread worms.

Asthma is a common feature of cases of hypersensitivity angiitis, and allergic granulomatous angiitis, which may complicate the use of drugs such as sulphonamides.

In some cases the cause of a drug-induced asthma is quite unknown. Aspirin asthma usually occurs in late onset asthma, in non-atopic subjects many of whom have nasal polypi. The asthmatic reaction comes on about half an hour to two hours after taking the drug. The attack may be severe, even fatal; death has followed the taking of one tablet, 300 mg. It is important to remember that aspirin is an ingredient of many proprietary compounds, for example, Beecham's powders and Alka-seltzer. The asthmatic reaction may be accompanied by profuse watery rhinorrhoea and flushing of the skin of the head, neck and extremities and this may be followed by nausea, vomiting, colic and diarrhoea. The patients do not exhibit skin sensitivity to aspirin and there is no cross-sensitivity with other salicylates so that the basis of it is unlikely to be allergic. Some other drugs structurally dissimilar to aspirin can induce the same reaction. These compounds, of which indomethacin is an example, are all peripherally-acting analgesics (with the exception of tartrazine, a colouring agent used in foods and drugs). Most probably the mechanism of this reaction is connected with the prostaglandin content of the lung. Prostaglandins of the E series are bronchodilator and of the F series bronchoconstrictor. Analgesics can differentially affect the synthesis of both types and asthmatics may show atypical responses to them.

PULMONARY EOSINOPHILIA

Pulmonary eosinophilia is an unsatisfactory term which was coined in order to described those conditions in which lung shadows seen in a chest x-ray are associated with an excess of eosinophils in the peripheral blood. Even this unsatisfactory criterion is not always satisfied in that patients who have similar clinical and radiological conditions may have no excess of eosinophils in the peripheral blood and yet histological examination of the lung may show a true eosinophilic pneumonitis. Many drugs have been incriminated in this syndrome. The most common is nitrofurantoin with, perhaps, para-aminosalicylic acid (PAS) the next most common as well as penicillin, mephenesin, sulphonamides, imipramine, streptomycin, isoniazid, furazolidone, aspirin and methotrexate.

Typically, pulmonary eosinophilia is a clinical syndrome of sudden onset, often with fever. The striking symptom is usually dyspnoea and the most conspicuous physical sign widespread crepitations audible over the lungs. Most patients have no wheeze or prolongation of expiration but on rare occasions there may be signs of airway obstruction and a few patients have rhinitis as well. The cough may be productive of mucoid sputum though haemoptysis is not a feature. The chest x-ray usually shows patchy shadowing which may be very extensive and there may be pleural effusion. There is often an eosinophilia of the peripheral blood though this is not invariable.

Lung function tests show impairment of ventilatory capacity both restrictive and, less commonly, obstructive together with reduction of transfer factor.

In some cases in which the diagnosis is made only after repeated episodes the interval between the use of the drug and the development of the reaction becomes progressively shorter. Sometimes the condition persists for weeks or months after the withdrawal of the drug and disappears only when steroids are used. This prolonged syndrome may lead to progressive pulmonary fibrosis; it seems to be particularly likely to occur with nitrofurantoin and methotrexate.

In the acute cases, the alveoli are packed with histiocytes and sheets of eosinophils in a protein-rich oedema with a mild perivasculitis. In the rare chronic cases there is interstitial pulmonary fibrosis. The allergic basis of the condition has not yet been worked out but the specificity of the reaction has been confirmed by provocation challenge and by lymphocyte transformation.

POLYARTERITIS

Polyarteritis nodosa is the best understood of a group of conditions which have in common a necrotizing vasculitis. The variants which may be associated with the use of drugs, hypersensitivity angiitis, and allergic granulomatous angiitis, are distinct from classical polyarteritis nodosa in that smaller vessels are involved, veins as well as arteries. The lesions often contain eosinophils and there may be granuloma formation with giant cells. In this group of drug-induced polyarteritis the lungs are much more often affected than in classical polyarteritis nodosa. A common presentation is asthma, transient shadows in the chest x-ray and a considerable increase of eosinophils in the peripheral blood. There may be destructive granulomatous lesions in both the upper and lower respiratory tract. The course is usually more relentless than that of classical idiopathic polyarteritis nodosa in which spontaneous remissions are a common feature. Remission sometimes follows withdrawal of the drug and sometimes follows the use of corticosteroids or cytotoxic agents.

The drugs which have been most frequently incriminated include sulphonomides, penicillin, phenothiazines, thiouracils, hydantoins, gold salts and iodides. However, the evidence linking the use of the drug with the development of the disease is purely circumstantial. Symptoms and signs which prompted the use of the drug may themselves have been the first manifestation of idiopathic polyarteritis. Nevertheless, in some cases, the repeated use of the drug has been shown to be clearly linked with exacerbation of the disease. The resemblance between serum sickness and Arthus-type lesions, resulting from experimental hyper-immunization in animals and the lesions of polyarteritis in man, has suggested that this disease might be a manifestation of type 3 hypersensitivity.

BUSULPHAN LUNG

This was originally described as hexamethonium lung. The ganglion-blocking hypotensive agents, hexamethonium, pentolinium and mecamylamine, which are known to have caused the condition, are now little used, whereas busulphan is much used in the treatment of chronic granulocytic leukaemia. Other cytotoxic drugs such as cyclophospha-mide, bleomycin, and, perhaps, vincristine, may also cause the condition, and it has been attributed to amitryptyline.

In the acute stage there is a picture resembling pulmonary oedema, though the absence of orthopnoea or other evidence of left ventricular (LV) failure is an important clue to the diagnosis. In the chronic stage the picture is that of diffuse pulmonary fibrosis, with progressive dyspnoea associated with the presence of widespread crepitations (clubbing is not a feature). In the acute stages, the radiological picture also is that of pulmonary oedema, with 'bat's-wing' shadows. In the chronic stages there is widespread nodular or patchy shadowing throughout the lung fields. In the extremely chronic cases there may be a picture resembling honeycomb lung. Lung function studies show a restrictive impedance to ventilation and impairment of gas transfer and hypoxia.

The histological picture is of an alveolar fibrinous oedema in which fibrous tissue is laid down. The pathogenesis in the cases associated with the use of hypertensive drugs is thought to be a combination of LV failure and vasodilatation induced by the drugs. In the case of busulphan, electron microscopy has demonstrated abnormalities of type 2 alveolar lining cells — a local manifestation of a widespread abnormality of cells throughout the body. These cells produce the surfactant lipoprotein which normally lines the alveolar walls and it is thought that the intra-alveolar oedema follows disturbance of surfactant activity.

An interesting feature is that although the condition may remit if the drug is withdrawn, it may be found possible later to use the drug again without inducing a recurrence of the condition. Certainly, though a small number of fatal cases have been described, knowledge of this complication should not inhibit the use of busulphan in the treatment of chronic granulocytic leukaemia for which it is a most useful drug.

SYSTEMIC LUPUS ERYTHEMATOSUS (SLE)

Many drugs may cause the appearance of antinuclear antibodies, antinuclear factor, anti-DNA antibodies and LE cell factor, and some drugs produce the full clinical syndrome of the disease. Curiously, there seems to be an almost inverse relationship between the capacity of a drug to induce the appearance of antibodies and the capacity of the same drug to induce the development of the full clinical syndrome. About 30–40 per cent of all patients who take procainamide for 6 or more months, develop antinuclear antibodies but only 1–2 per cent of those who develop antibodies have any symptoms or signs of the disease. Hydrallazine, on the other hand, comparatively infrequently leads to the appearance of antibodies. Less than 2 per cent of those who took the drug for 6 months developed antibodies, whereas 15 per cent of patients developed symptoms and signs of the disease. It is for this reason that the drug has fallen into disfavour. No drug induces both antibodies and disease in more than a small proportion of patients but it is probably true that about 20 per cent of all patients admitted to hospital with SLE have a disease which is clearly drug-induced.

The incrimination of the drug as the agent responsible for the disease is as difficult as in the case of polyarteritis. It is well known that patients with SLE are remarkably sensitive to drugs and frequently develop adverse reactions to them. Of course, the symptoms or signs for which the drug was prescribed may have been the first sign of the disease. Moreover, patients with drug-induced disease often have features in common with those who spontaneously develop the condition. Females predominate and there are often strong past and family histories of rheumatic disorders. The disease associated with procainamide seems to be exceptional; it is more common in men than women, the lungs are particularly frequently involved and the kidneys never involved. Antibodies to single strand (denatured) DNA are found but not to double strand (native) DNA as in the idiopathic disorder and there is no deficiency of complement.

Among the drugs thought to have caused the syndrome are penicillin, tetracycline, gold, phenylbutazone, griseofulvin, hydrallazine, isoniazid, carbamazepine (Tegretol), phenytoin, mephenytoin (Mesantoin), streptomycin, procainamide, sulphonamides (various), para-aminosalicylic acid, thiouracils, trimethadione (Tridione), guanoxan (Envacar), methsuximide and methyldopa.

As with polyarteritis, the appearance of lesions experimentally produced in animals resembling the lesions of SLE, suggests the possibility that the disease is a manifestation of type 3 hypersensitivity.

The role of antinuclear antibodies is difficult to determine. They are not known to be capable of entering healthy cells. On the whole it seems that they are a manifestation of the disease rather than the pathogenetic agent. On the other hand, the auto-antibodies directed against red cells are undoubtedly destructive *in vivo;* they are responsible for the haemolytic anaemia which is a common feature of the disease.

The respiratory system is commonly involved in patients with SLE. Three main patterns are seen:

(1)   Pleurisy, often with effusion, usually bilateral, and frequently with pericarditis, severe illness and fever; after corticosteroids recovery is usually rapid.

(2)   Recurrent febrile attacks with cough, dyspnoea, pleurisy and severe illness, which can clinically resemble pneumonia, pulmonary oedema or pulmonary infarction; after corticosteroids recovery is usually rapid.

(3)   Dyspnoea with tachypnoea and reduced chest expansion with progressive elevation of the diaphragm, which moves poorly on screening. Respiratory function tests show the lungs to be small and stiff with a reduced capacity for gas transfer. This syndrome is the result of widespread alveolar atelectasis without airway obstruction or external compression. The dyspnoea usually improves with corticosteroids, but the vital capacity improves less dramatically and the diaphragms do not return to their normal position or motility.

LIPOID PNEUMONIA AND OIL EMBOLISM

The inhalation of oily material can lead to the development of lipoid pneumonia and the introduction of oils into the circulation may cause oil embolization.

Iodized vegetable oils, used for bronchography, may cause lipoid pneumonia. The oil lies in pools enclosed by fibrous tissue with focal collections of endothelial cells, lymphocytes and giant cells; associated with this is a severe endarteritis obliterans. Eventually, these changes lead to complete destruction of normal lung and its total replacement by fibrous tissue in which are found a few residual epithelium-lined alveoli and bronchiolectatic air passages, surrounded and infiltrated by hyperplastic lymphoid nodules. These changes may produce a diffuse interstitial fibrosis or a localized mass easily mistaken for a carcinoma.

Similar changes may follow the aspiration of liquid paraffin, used either in oily nose drops (a use now abandoned) or as a lubricant for surgical manoeuvres within the oesophagus. Oil-containing medicines or foods can also cause lipoid pneumonia in patients who have dysphagia as the result of regurgitation or 'spill-over'. Animal fats are more irritating than mineral oils and vegetable oils less irritating. If lipoid pneumonia is suspected, fat globules should be looked for in the sputum.

Black fat is a tobacco to which mineral oil and vaseline are added to moisten and flavour it. Patients who smoke this tobacco develop diffuse lipoid pneumonia due to inhalation of the oils.

Iodized oils are also used for lymphangiography. The material is returned via the thoracic duct to the great veins at the base of the neck and so oil embolization is inevitable. The condition is usually symptomless but there may be dyspnoea and cough productive of sputum which is sometimes blood-stained. Deaths have been reported in patients with pre-existing lung disease, with impaired lung function. The chest x-ray may show a fine stippling which lasts several days. Fat droplets can sometimes be demonstrated in the sputum within 2 to 4 hours. Respiratory function tests may show a fall in the transfer factor; more rarely, reduction of arterial oxygen tension. The effects usually disappear within 48 hours. Animal studies and lung biopsies in humans show, at first, a mechanical phase of oil emboli causing capillary obstruction. Within 24 hours the oil is discharged into the interstitial tissue and alveoli. This leads to a chemical phase, produced by hydrolysis of the oil, releasing fatty acids which damage the capillaries and alveolar cells and cause haemorrhage and consolidation.

Lymphangiography is safe in patients without pulmonary disease if not more than 0.25 ml/kg body weight is used. It should not be carried out in a patient with diffuse pulmonary disease.

OXYGEN-INDUCED LUNG DISEASE

Patients, particularly new-born babies, treated with oxygen and assisted ventilation may develop progressive dyspnoea, rales may be heard over the lungs, shadows may appear in the chest x-ray, and hypoxaemia may develop. It may be found impossible to 'wean' some of these patients from the ventilator and eventually some may die. Though it is difficult to distinguish the effects of the basic underlying disease, such as the respiratory distress syndrome, from the effects of long-continued positive pressure ventilation, especially where a positive end expiratory pressure is deliberately employed to prevent atelectasis, there can be no doubt that oxygen itself can cause a severe, even fatal, fibroplasia of the lung.

Volunteers breathing 100 per cent oxygen develop, within a few hours, cough and a feeling of substernal distress. This is associated with

195

a decrease of vital capacity and reduction of lung compliance. The effects are progressive and no one has been able to continue the experiment for more than 100 hours. More prolonged exposure to 40 per cent oxygen has the same effect. These changes depend on the partial pressure of oxygen inhaled and the duration of inhalation. They do not directly depend on the concentration. During the early flights, American astronauts breathed pure oxygen but at a third of an atmosphere. A disastrous fire led to a change to oxygen—helium mixtures. Russian cosmonauts breathe compressed air.

When high concentrations of oxygen have been administered for some time abnormal alveolar lining-cells and hyaline membrane appear. It is possible that this is associated with the disappearance of surfactant and an increase of surface tension, leading to atelectasis and oedema. The histological picture is one of a generalized pulmonary change, involving mucosal, alveolar and vascular tissues, superimposed upon simple atelectasis. Macroscopically, the lungs appear heavy 'beefy' and oedematous. Microscopically, there are two phases that merge. First, there is an exudative phase, associated with the clinical and radiological appearance of pulmonary oedema; there are pulmonary congestion, alveolar oedema, intra-alveolar haemorrhage and a fibrinous exudate with the formation of a prominent hyaline membrane, without an associated inflammatory component. Later there are proliferative changes associated with the clinical and radiological appearances of diffuse pulmonary fibrosis. There are marked alveolar and interlobular septal oedema with fibroblastic proliferation and prominent hyperplasia of the alveolar lining-cells.

MISCELLANEOUS DRUGS AND REACTIONS

Many other drugs can cause adverse respiratory reactions of many other kinds. The bronchial tree may be involved in an acute asthmatic reaction of Herxheimer type that may complicate the treatment of tropical eosinophilia by arethylcarb-amazine. The lungs may be involved by the pulmonary oedema that may follow a heroin overdose or, more rarely, other drugs of addiction; 'main-line' drug addicts commonly develop suppurative pneumonia and lung abscess; less commonly they may develop cor pulmonale as the result of pulmonary vascular obstruction caused by repeated intravenous injection of drugs or foreign material in particulate form. The pleura may be involved by localized effusion and underlying fibrosis after the prolonged use of methysergide (there are no reports of mediastinal 'fibrosis' associated with retroperitoneal fibrosis caused by methysergide). The hilar and mediastinal lymph nodes may be involved when drugs cause generalized enlargement of lymph nodes. Hydantoins may cause a picture like lymphoma; phenylbutazone a picture like sarcoidosis; and para-aminosalicylic acid the clinical and haematological features of glandular fever.

The two most common and important diseases of the lung due to a drug are, of course, chronic bronchitis and carcinoma of the bronchus!

REFERENCES

Committee on Safety of Medicines (Report) (1972). *Br. Med. J.* **4**, 912

Doll, W. R. S. (1971). 'Unwanted effects of drugs.' *Br. med. Bull.,* **27**, 25

Martindale Extra Pharmacopoeia. (1972)., 26th edition. Ed by W. Blacow. London: The Pharmaceutical Press

McComb, R. P. (1971). 'Disease due to immunologic reactions in the lungs.' *New Eng. J. Med.* **286**, 1186

Meyler, L. and Peck, H. M. (1968). *Drug Induced Diseases.,* Vol 3. Amsterdam: Excerpta Medica Foundation.

Turner-Warwick, M. (1973). 'Immunology of the respiratory tract.' *Br. J. Hosp. med.,* **9**, 19

9

Some Aspects of Peripheral Neuropathy

Peter Croft

INTRODUCTION

A peripheral neuropathy is a disorder which affects the peripheral part of the neurone, as distinct from the cell body (for example, the anterior horn cell). The terms 'peripheral neuritis' and 'polyneuritis' have been in use for many decades, but they are misleading because the primary pathological process is not usually inflammation. It is now more usual to describe different disorders of peripheral nerves as types of 'neuropathy' so that the underlying cause is not prejudged. However, the term neuropathy is not used consistently. Primary sensory neuropathy (better called primary sensory neuronopathy), in which there is destruction of posterior root ganglion cells, is considered as a neuropathy. Motor neurone disease, in which the anterior horn cell is affected, is not. The word neuropathy has been used even more loosely in describing a condition such as Jamaican neuropathy. This is a disorder affecting West Indians, and in which there is primary damage to the spinal cord producing either a spastic paraplegia or sensory ataxia associated with deafness and optic atrophy.

The term mononeuropathy is used to described an affection of a single nerve — for example, a pressure neuropathy, an entrapment neuropathy (such as occurs in the carpal tunnel syndrome), or an ischaemic lesion of a nerve. In disorders such as polyarteritis nodosa, where various individual nerves may be involved at different times in the course of the disease, the rather clumsy term mononeuropathy multiplex (rather than mononeuritis multiplex) may be used.

SYMPTOMS OF PERIPHERAL NEUROPATHY

Most peripheral nerves contain both motor and sensory fibres, so that the symptoms of peripheral neuropathy are usually mixed. However, in

199

some disorders, such as diabetic or alcoholic neuropathy, symptoms are often predominantly sensory, while in a condition such as porphyria they are motor. The primary motor symptom is weakness, the rate of progression depending upon the underlying cause. The sensory symptoms may be positive or negative. Thus, at first, there may be spontaneous burning or tingling (paraesthesiae) or sometimes pain. Later, as the function of the sensory fibres becomes progressively impaired, sensory loss develops with consequent clumsiness in the use of the hands and feet.

The symptoms in most cases are bilateral, symmetrical and distal, the legs usually being affected before the upper limbs. There are exceptions to this general rule, as in the Guillain–Barré syndrome and porphyria, where the distribution may be more proximal, and sometimes with additional involvement of cranial nerves. The interval between involvement of the lower and upper limbs varies from a day or less in the Guillain–Barré syndrome to weeks or months in more chronic metabolic, toxic or deficiency disorders. Similarly, the rate at which symptoms progress centripetally will vary with the acuteness of the condition.

The diagnosis of peripheral neuropathy should always be reconsidered if the symptoms begin in the upper limbs, or if they remain confined to the lower limbs for long periods. These points will be discussed later in more detail.

SIGNS OF PERIPHERAL NEUROPATHY

As with the symptoms, the signs of peripheral neuropathy tend to be mixed motor and sensory, although the relative proportions vary, and often the extent of objective sensory loss may be quite small in spite of severe paraesthesiae (for example, thalidomide neuropathy).

The motor signs are those of fairly symmetrical distal wasting, with corresponding weakness, but usually without fasciculation. Weakness and wasting are often relatively slight in the upper limbs, although there may be severe bilateral foot drop. In an acute condition, such as the Guillain–Barré syndrome, severe paralysis will be present long before there is any detectable wasting.

Facial palsy, often bilateral, and less commonly other cranial nerve palsies, are frequently encountered in the Guillain–Barré syndrome, porphyria and sarcoidosis.

Distal sensory impairment of 'stocking and glove' distribution may be incomplete and, at times, difficult to define. The relatively ill-defined limit of sensory impairment in neuropathy is quite different from that in hysterical sensory loss where sharply-defined areas of anaesthesia (often capable of being altered by suggestion) are limited by anatomical boundaries such as the wrist or knee.

In an uncomplicated peripheral neuropathy the loss of position and vibration sense will be in proportion to the degree of cutaneous sensory loss. A disproportionate loss of 'posterior column sensation' should suggest co-existing disease of the spinal cord as may occur in subacute combined degeneration of the cord, and sometimes in diabetes.

In modern clinical practice a patient who walks with a high-stepping gait is far more likely to have a peripheral neuropathy than tabes dorsalis, since the former is now a far more common cause of sensory ataxia.

Examination of deep muscle and tendon sensitivity is important, particularly in alcoholic neuropathy where calf tenderness may be exquisite.

The tendon reflexes are diminished or absent, and usually it is the ankle jerks which are first lost, followed by the knee jerks and later the deep reflexes of the upper limbs. The abdominal reflexes are preserved, while the plantar responses are flexor or absent, depending upon the amount of weakness, and the degree of anaesthesia of the sole of the foot.

The peripheral nerves must be inspected and palpated carefully. In cases of mononeuropathy, localized swelling, thickening and possibly tenderness of the affected nerve may confirm the site of the lesion — for example an ulnar nerve lesion at the elbow, median nerve compression in the carpal tunnel, or a lesion of the lateral popliteal nerve at the head of the fibula. In some types of peripheral neuropathy a more generalized thickening of nerves may be detected. Such hypertrophy may be found not only in the rare familial neuropathy of Déjérine and Sottas, but also in the demyelinating type of Charcot—Marie—Tooth disease (peroneal muscular atrophy), in Refsum's disease, and in some examples of relapsing peripheral neuropathy. Hypertrophy is probably the result of repeated segmental demyelination and remyelination. Infiltration of peripheral nerves with consequent thickening, may be detected in such conditions as amyloidosis and leprosy.

INVESTIGATION OF A CASE OF PERIPHERAL NEUROPATHY

In a case of peripheral neuropathy without obvious cause, many investigations may be required to detect possible deficiency states (for example, vitamin B_{12} deficiency), metabolic disorders such as diabetes, exposure to some toxic substance, or the presence of an occult malignant neoplasm. There are, however, a number of investigations which should be carried out in all cases.

Cerebrospinal Fluid (CSF) Examination

In some types of neuropathy, especially the Guillain–Barré syndrome, the amount of CSF protein will be increased. Equally high levels of protein are found in some types of non-metastatic neuropathy (carcinomatous neuropathy) and in diabetic amyotrophy. In other cases, especially where the more distal parts of the nerves are affected, the CSF protein concentration is usually normal.

A rise in CSF cell count is unusual in peripheral neuropathy although sometimes found in cases otherwise typical of the Guillain–Barré syndrome. However, the presence of a CSF lymphocytosis with only a slight increase in protein level may indicate a first episode of multiple sclerosis, sometimes a cause of obscure paraesthesiae without physical signs. In such cases, immunoelectrophoresis of the CSF protein may be helpful since an increase in IgG may give some support for the diagnosis.

Alternatively, in a patient with symptoms confined to the lower limbs, a very high protein level, possibly with a dubious Queckenstedt test, will suggest the presence of spinal compression.

Electromyography (EMG)

This is not the place for a detailed description of the techniques and findings in modern electrodiagnostic investigation of peripheral nerve function, although it is not possible adequately to investigate a case of peripheral neuropathy without the assistance of such methods. These include the findings on electrical stimulation of nerves (motor and sensory), and the study of electric potentials developed when nerves and muscles are active.

Monopolar muscle stimulation to record intensity–duration curves will indicate whether a muscle is being stimulated directly or through its motor nerve. Denervated muscle shows characteristic differences of excitability which may be useful in cases of peripheral nerve injury to assess prognosis, or to demonstrate re-innervation.

Direct electrical stimulation of the peripheral nerves may give much useful information. It is possible to calculate the rate of conduction by motor fibres of the applied stimulus, the results being conduction velocities for the large myelinated fibres; although when the nerve is damaged, the value obtained for conduction velocity is that for the largest surviving fibres. Motor conduction velocity may be reduced in a single nerve locally at a point of injury — for example, the median nerve at the wrist in the carpal tunnel syndrome — or reduced generally in some types of peripheral neuropathy. But not all types of peripheral neuropathy show reduced motor conduction velocities. In general, it may be said that slowing of motor conduction is typical of a neuropathy in which the primary pathological process is one of demyelination. Such a change occurs, for example, in diphtheritic, diabetic, and non-metastatic peripheral neuropathies. Some of the most extreme slowing occurs in the hereditary hypertrophic neuropathy of Déjérine and Sottas where values of 3–5 m/sec have been recorded (normal ranges: 50–70 m/sec in upper limbs and 40–60 m/sec in lower limbs).

By contrast, where the neuropathy is due to a disorder affecting primarily the axone (alcoholic neuropathy, thiamine deficiency, toxic neuropathies due to isoniazid or arsenic, and some forms of Charcot–Marie–Tooth disease), motor conduction velocities may be normal or only slightly reduced. Even when many neurones have been destroyed, the conduction velocity measured in the surviving neurones will be normal.

Thus, a study of motor conduction velocities may help to establish the particular type of neuropathy and thus give some indication of possible causes of the condition.

The study of evoked sensory nerve action potentials — both amplitude and the rate of conduction — is a technique which, although more difficult than the study of motor fibres and muscle action potentials, may be a more sensitive test of impaired peripheral nerve function. This technique may reveal abnormalities even when motor conduction velocities are normal. Similarly, it is possible to distinguish sensory loss due to peripheral neuropathy (with reduced nerve action potentials), from sensory loss due to organic disease of the spinal cord and from hysterical sensory loss.

Electrodiagnostic techniques with concentric needle electrodes inserted into individual muscles, may be used to study the electrical activity of contracting muscle. Muscle action potentials recorded may reveal those occurring spontaneously in relaxed muscle — the small fibrillation potentials particularly characteristic of denervated muscle, and the spontaneous contractions of motor units (fasciculation) seen especially in motor neurone disease. Fasciculation also occurs in spondylotic myelopathy, sometimes in syringomyelia, and occasionally in peripheral neuropathy. It may also be benign, without progressive disease of the nervous system.

Studies of electrical activity of muscle during voluntary contraction are particularly helpful in distinguishing difficult cases of primary muscle disease from those of peripheral neuropathy. In primary muscle disease the characteristic finding is of small polyphasic motor unit action potentials of brief duration seen when some fibres of the motor unit have been lost, the remaining fibres giving visible spikes because synchronization is not possible. On the other hand the interference pattern during maximal contraction is well maintained until a late stage.

In a neuropathy, there are signs of denervation (fibrillation and possibly fasciculation) and the interference pattern is reduced, as fewer units are available to contract in a maximal effort. At lower firing frequencies the individual motor units are of longer duration. Often high amplitude is recorded due to chronic incomplete denervation and subsequent attempts at reinnervation from surviving neighbouring healthy neurones by collateral 'sprouting'.

Nerve and Muscle Biopsy

Modern techniques of study of nerve and muscle biopsy specimens are very complex and now include many histochemical methods. It is sufficient here to note that a nerve biopsy will give an indication of the nature of the disturbance in the peripheral nerve (segmental demyelination or axonal degeneration), and may show evidence of nerve hypertrophy or infiltration and sometimes the nature of such infiltration. Biopsy of the muscle on the other hand will detect changes in the extreme distal fibres of the motor nerve, or in the motor end plates, and thus establish whether the muscle is affected by denervation or is involved in a primary disorder of muscle.

CONDITIONS SIMULATING PERIPHERAL NEUROPATHY

The initial diagnosis of peripheral neuropathy is often simple, even when the cause remains obscure. However, some patients present diagnostic problems which can only be solved by using the special techniques already mentioned.

Myopathies

These do not usually offer difficulty in diagnosis although in some cases of non-metastatic myopathy, both neuropathy and myopathy may be present together. A pure myopathy is free from sensory symptoms or signs, while in the genetically determined muscular dystrophies a family history is obtained. Familial or sporadic cases of muscular dystrophy often show characteristic selective involvement of individual muscles, unrelated to their root innervation. In acquired myopathies and polymyositis, electromyographic tests combined with muscle biopsy, ESR estimation, and study of serum muscle enzyme concentrations, will establish the nature of the condition.

Carpal Tunnel Syndrome

Reference has already been made to the importance of analysing the mode of onset of the symptoms. Sensory disturbances beginning in both upper limbs without affecting the feet are unlikely to be due to a peripheral neuropathy although they were encountered in thalidomide neuropathy. In a case of bilateral carpal tunnel syndrome the symptoms may develop in both hands more or less symmetrically. Characteristically, the symptoms are worse at night — an important diagnostic point. Electromyography will confirm the diagnosis even in the absence of classical physical signs of median nerve damage.

Spinal Lesions

It is sometimes difficult to be confident of a diagnosis where spinal cord lesions cause symptoms very like those of a peripheral neuropathy. Sensory symptoms affecting the upper limbs alone may occur in multiple sclerosis when symmetrical plaques of demyelination develop in the lateral part of each posterior column. When sensory symptoms begin fairly symmetrically in the legs and spread proximally they may be due to spinal cord compression or multiple sclerosis. In spinal compression there will almost inevitably be some evidence of corticospinal tract involvement incompatible with a peripheral neuropathy. In multiple sclerosis the disturbance may be purely sensory and often largely subjective with few objective signs. However, in such cases, the sensory disturbance is frequently asymmetrical, and spreads up the thighs to the hips and often onto the lower anterior abdominal wall. In general, peripheral neuropathy is unlikely to lead to symptoms above the knees unless there is also involvement of the fingers and hands. The extension of sensory symptoms onto the trunk indicates a spinal lesion.

A very important physical symptom or sign is that of Lhermitte — once known also as the 'barber's chair sign', a description with little significance for the modern young doctor not accustomed to the barber's clippers applied closely to the back of his head with the neck fully flexed. The patient experiences sudden electric tingling sensations which shoot momentarily into the limbs and trunk. Most commonly the lower trunk and lower limbs are affected, occasionally all four limbs.

This sensation develops when the head is dropped forward onto the chest and is relieved at once by extending the neck again. Often, the patient will not mention these sensations unless a specific leading question is asked. The Lhermitte symptom is always indicative of organic disease of the cervical cord and is due to slight stretching, during neck flexion, of the posterior columns, most commonly affected by multiple sclerosis. It is a rare symptom in cervical spondylosis, but occurs not uncommonly with cervical trauma and may be present in some cases of cervical cord tumour. It may be an early symptom of subacute combined degeneration of the spinal cord.

Occasionally, a lesion of the conus medullaris may produce motor and sensory symptoms in the lower limbs suggestive of a peripheral neuropathy; there is, of course, no involvement of the upper limbs. Important distinguishing features are early symptoms of sphincter disorder with impairment of urethral and anal sensation, and demonstrable sensory loss over the sacral dermatomes, not found in peripheral neuropathy. In such cases myelography is indicated.

Purely motor disorders such as motor neurone disease can be mistaken for peripheral neuropathy but the weakness and wasting in motor neurone disease more commonly starts in the upper limbs or bulbar muscles, is frequently asymmetrical, is often associated with muscle cramps, and is accompanied by fasciculation and usually by increased deep reflexes.

CLASSIFICATION OF THE NEUROPATHIES

There are several ways in which the neuropathies may be classified. It is less useful to memorize long lists which attempt to include all known causes of neuropathy, than to develop an approach to a clinical problem which may enable one to discover the cause of the disorder and, where possible, an effective treatment for that patient.

Neuropathies may be classified on a neurohistological basis, and may be divided into three groups:

(1)   Those in which the neurone (axone or parent cell body) is affected.

(2)   Disorders damaging the supporting structure of the nerves (Schwann cells with myelin sheath, or connective tissue).

(3)   Conditions affecting the blood vessels of the nerves.

The above classification is made possible by the results of the modern techniques of EMG, nerve biopsy and work on experimental animals, and has advantages in explaining the way in which different types of neuropathy are produced. Thus, toxic and metabolic neuropathies of various kinds are neuronal neuropathies (for example, neuropathies caused by triorthocresyl phosphate (TOCP), arsenic, thallium, isoniazid, porphyria, uraemia and alcoholism) and this group also includes non-metastatic sensory neuronopathy.

Schwann cells are primarily affected in diabetic neuropathy, Guillain—Barré neuropathy, and non-metastatic peripheral neuropathy, and this may lead to demyelination. Connective tissues are involved in amyloid or sarcoid neuropathy and in malignant infiltration of nerves. The vascular supply of nerves is affected in various disorders such as polyarteritis nodosa, SLE, and rheumatoid arthritis.

Of course, not all types of neuropathy fit neatly into such a classification. Some types of diabetic neuropathy are due to a microangiopathy rather than Schwann cell damage. Similarly, in peroneal muscular atrophy investigations indicate that one type is a neuronal disorder while in other cases the disorder is a hereditary demyelinating neuropathy often with some degree of hypertrophy of nerve sheath.

Although this type of theoretical approach is certainly helpful, it is not good enough to consider neuropathies (or indeed other diseases) from a single viewpoint. Clinical, pathological, genetic, biochemical and electrophysiological aspects must all be considered. As with so many other diseases the 'cause' of a neuropathy may be multifactorial.

In considering a patient with neuropathy, it should be remembered that occasionally a mononeuropathy (for example, an entrapment neuropathy or one of vascular origin) may occur in a patient who has a mild and possibly subclinical form of generalized peripheral neuropathy. This may happen, for example, in diabetes or malignant disease where there is increased vulnerability of an already damaged nerve to some additional factor (trauma or ischaemia).

The mode of onset is important — it may be acute, as in the Guillain—Barré syndrome, acute porphyria and acute toxic neuropathy (such as that caused by contaminated cooking oil); subacute (as in subacute combined degeneration of the spinal cord); or more chronic, as in some toxic and hereditary neuropathies.

A neuropathy may be mainly motor (as with lead poisoning, porphyria, diphtheria and the Guillain—Barré syndrome), mainly sensory (diabetes mellitus, leprosy, alcoholism, beriberi, arsenic poisoning and non-metastatic sensory neuronopathy), or of mixed motor and sensory type.

Although most peripheral neuropathies are distal, a more proximal type may be found at times with the Guillain—Barré syndrome and infectious mononucleosis.

In some forms of hereditary peripheral neuropathy there will be, apart from the family history, onset in early life and the presence of foot deformities such as pes cavus. It must be emphasized that sporadic cases without evidence of genetic factors frequently occur. In the rare Refsum's disease (heredopathia atactica polyneuritiformis) other disorders such as ichthyosis, retinitis pigmentosa and deafness may be found.

Toxic Neuropathies

It is essential to make the fullest enquiries about possible toxic factors which might cause a peripheral neuropathy whether by interference with energy production of the neurone (TOCP, arsenic) or by involvement of nutrient vessels (some forms of drug-induced SLE).

Persistent enquiries must include a detailed drug history dealing both with prescribed and unprescribed drugs, including alcohol. The list of iatrogenic causes of neuropathy is almost endless, but includes isoniazid (which in genetically susceptible individuals produces a secondary vitamin B_6 deficiency if no supplementary pyridoxin is given), nitrofurantoin (especially in cases of renal failure) and ethambutol. It must not be forgotten that disulphuram (antabuse), used in the treatment of alcoholism, may occasionally itself cause peripheral neuropathy and so lead to possible diagnostic confusion during the treatment of a chronic alcoholic.

Toxic substances which may be encountered industrially or in the home are also very numerous and much detective work may be necessary to identify them.

A recent celebrated murder trial involving homicide by heavy metals, especially thallium, emphasizes the need to remember the possibility of attempted homicide in some cases of unexplained peripheral neuropathy.

Metabolic and Endocrine Neuropathies

Diabetes is probably the most common cause of peripheral neuropathy and may produce neuropathy in a variety of ways including segmental demyelination, possibly of metabolic origin, and by effects of a microangiopathy. The neuropathy is often relatively mild. Since diabetes is a common disease it does not follow that neuropathy in a diabetic is due to the diabetes. Other causes such as carcinoma or toxic factors must always be sought.

Chronic liver disease and uraemia are causes of peripheral neuropathy which must not be overlooked. Mild peripheral neuropathy may occur rarely in myxoedema (the evidence being electromyographic rather than clinical) but a much more common neurological complication of hypothyroidism is median nerve compression at the wrist.

Deficiency Syndromes

As a cause of neuropathy, deficiency syndromes are relatively rare in Great Britain. It is usual for the central nervous system to suffer as well as the peripheral nerves. Thus, in thiamine deficiency associated with alcoholism, there is frequently evidence of brain damage (for example, fits and Wernicke's encephalopathy) and posterior column damage. There may also be evidence of other deficiency states including anaemia and weight loss.

Vitamin B_{12} deficiency, as in subacute combined degeneration of the spinal cord, does not usually produce a pure peripheral neuropathy and there is evidence of cord damage especially to the posterior columns (with extensive loss of vibration and postural sense) and corticospinal tracts (extensor plantar responses).

Although a megaloblastic peripheral blood picture indicates the need for vitamin B_{12} and folate studies, a normal blood picture does not exclude deficiency of these substances as the cause of a peripheral neuropathy. The spinal cord element in subacute combined degeneration responds much less well than the peripheral neuropathy to treatment with vitamin B_{12}. Hence, it is as essential to estimate vitamin B_{12} and serum folate levels in a case of neuropathy, as it is to carry out serological tests for syphilis in a case of dementia. Delay in treatment of either subacute combined degeneration or neurosyphilis can lead to medical disasters.

Other forms of malabsorption syndromes (for example, post-gastrectomy syndrome) must be considered in addition to true subacute combined degeneration associated with Addisonian anaemia.

Connective Tissue (Collagen) Diseases

Neuropathy is common in polyarteritis nodosa, and moderately common in SLE and rheumatoid arthritis. It is probably due to a vasculitis and often presents as mononeuropathy multiplex, especially in polyarteritis nodosa. Some drugs such as hydrallazine, procainamide or phenytoin sodium may produce SLE with neuropathy.

Neuropathy Associated With Malignant Disease

The diagnostic importance and theoretical interest of the non-metastatic neurological syndromes associated with various forms of malignant diseases justify their consideration in a separate final section.

THE GUILLAIN–BARRÉ SYNDROME
(ACUTE POST-INFECTIVE POLYNEUROPATHY OR POLYRADICULOPATHY)

In this disorder there is a particular emphasis on damage to the spinal nerve roots, and so it is more appropriate to describe these cases as examples of polyneuropathy or polyradiculopathy than peripheral neuropathy.

The classic description by Guillain, Barré and Strohl in 1916 gave a number of diagnostic criteria including weakness, loss of deep reflexes, preservation of cutaneous reflexes, paraesthesiae with slight objective sensory loss, increased muscle tenderness, and a marked increase in CSF protein content without any cellular reaction (the now well-known albuminocytological dissociation). Some of these criteria were modified later by Guillain who also emphasized the favourable prognosis in this condition.

It was later realized that some of Landry's cases of ascending paralysis described more than 50 years before, had fallen into this group. However, the more cumbersome title of Landry–Guillain–Barré, or Landry–Guillain–Barré–Strohl, syndrome has not found general acceptance.

With increasing numbers of case reports, some of which have differed in several respects from the original account, the clinical picture has become somewhat blurred. Cases have been included in which the CSF was normal (or normal in the early stages) or in which there was a rise in the cell count; others are described as part of specific illnesses such as infectious mononucleosis; while others with fatal outcome or relapsing course have been included under the title Guillain–Barré syndrome.

Typical Cases

These show wide clinical variations in severity and distribution of muscle weakness. Mild cases may still be able to walk with difficulty, while severe cases may be fatal because of respiratory paralysis, unless managed by modern methods of assisted positive-pressure respiration. If the patient can be maintained during the phase of bulbar paralysis, the outcome is still favourable even in severe cases. Sequelae are usually minor with perhaps persistent loss of tendon reflexes and some distal weakness in the lower limbs, but in occasional very severe cases power in the limbs does not return. Relapses may occur rarely.

In a third or more of cases the onset is preceded some 1–2 weeks previously by a non-specific infectious type of illness. When the neurological symptoms begin, they are usually progressive for 7–10 days, but in a few patients deterioration may continue for from 3 to 6 weeks.

In a majority of patients symptoms begin in the lower limbs, usually followed rapidly by involvement of the upper limbs. Occasionally the arms, and even more rarely the cranial nerves, are first affected. When the cranial nerves are involved it is the facial nerves which suffer most frequently and often asymmetrically. Involvement of other cranial nerves, including those controlling external ocular movements, is less common but well recognized.

In a few cases, otherwise typical, there may be disturbance of sphincter function, sometimes prolonged.

Diagnosis is not usually difficult although in rare cases without sensory symptoms or signs, anterior poliomyelitis and acute polymyositis must both be considered as alternatives. In the former the typical biphasic illness with inflammatory change in the CSF is helpful, while in the latter electromyography and, if necessary, muscle biopsy will be diagnostic.

Other forms of acute peripheral neuropathy must be considered, especially acute intermittent porphyria and acute toxic peripheral neuropathy. In dyskaliaemic paralysis sensory symptoms are absent, and attacks are usually of brief duration and repeated. Paralysis from diarrhoea or potassium-losing nephritis is more common than familial periodic paralysis.

Cerebrospinal Fluid(CSF)

In the classical case of Guillain–Barré syndrome the patient shows a typical albuminocytological dissociation with CSF protein content increased to 100–400 mg/100 ml or occasionally more, without any rise in cell count. In some otherwise typical case the CSF protein may be normal: this may depend partly on the stage of the illness at which the lumbar puncture is done. The maximum abnormality may not be until the third week of the neurological illness. The severity of the rise in CSF protein in the classical case of Guillain–Barré syndrome does not correlate with the clinical severity of the illness.

Some patients, otherwise typical, may show an increase in lymphocytes in the CSF, though rarely above $20/\text{mm}^3$. This pleocytosis occurs even if cases due to conditions such as mumps and infectious mononucleosis are excluded.

Although the classical case of Guillain–Barré syndrome appears to complicate a non-specific infection or to arise spontaneously without any such infection being apparent, in other cases an identical illness occurs as part of a specific infection – for example, mononucleosis, infective hepatitis, mumps or chicken pox. It may also occur as a sequel to inoculation (post-vaccinal) and, rarely, cases are seen in association with malignant disease.

EMG Studies

These give varying results in different patients. There may be a considerable reduction in nerve conduction velocity indicative of peripheral demyelination. Although such slowing is usually general, it may be maximal at sites of possible nerve compression. In some cases conduction velocity is normal, possibly because the demyelination is mainly in proximal sections of the nerve or confined mainly to the nerve roots.

The EMG interference pattern shows reduction in motor unit activity, and later scanty fibrillation. As recovery occurs polyphasic potentials develop.

Pathology

Fatal cases show pathological evidence of damage maximal in the spinal roots, with first oedema, followed by swelling and irregularity of myelin sheaths and later cellular infiltration with lymphocytes and phagocytes. It is generally accepted that the condition represents an allergic or hypersensitivity reaction to an antigenic stimulus which may vary from case to case.

Treatment

It is logical to treat such patients with steroids or adrenocorticotropic hormone. Many instances are recorded of dramatic improvement after such treatment but assessment of the effects of treatment in a condition with a tendency to full recovery is difficult. Although statistical evidence of the benefit of such treatment is lacking, most neurologists would use steroids or ACTH except in a mild case or one already beginning to improve. There is no justification for classifying cases purely on the basis of their response to steroid therapy.

In very severe steroid-resistant cases immunosuppressant drugs such as azathioprine have been used with apparent benefit.

Prognosis and Classification

In assessing the prognosis in cases of Guillain–Barré syndrome, the main hazards to be anticipated, and where possible treated, are respiratory failure, thrombo-embolic disease and autonomic disturbances (including bouts of tachycardia, flushing, hypertensive and hypotensive crises).

In classifying cases of acute polyneuropathy or polyradiculopathy it is best to identify first those in which the condition is a sequel to a specific pathological disorder, for example, mononucleosis, mumps, or recent vaccination. In the remainder, where the condition fits the criteria of the Guillain–Barré syndrome, this eponym may be used, while in other cases without specific aetiology, and with points of difference from the classical account, especially in regard to the CSF changes, the term acute polyneuropathy or polyradiculopathy is best employed. However, it is likely that these groups share a common pathological process.

PERIPHERAL NEUROPATHY AND MALIGNANT DISEASE

METASTATIC NEUROPATHY

Patients with malignant disease — carcinoma, sarcoma or one of the reticuloses — may have impairment of function of peripheral nerves. Individual nerves or nerve roots may be compressed by local tumour masses, but such cases will not be considered further. Nerves may also be infiltrated by malignant cells extending along the subepineurial lymphatic spaces with consequent demyelination and later axonal damage.

Occasionally, carcinomatous infiltration of cranial nerves supplying the external ocular muscles is encountered. Involvement of these nerves is uncommon in patients with the non-metastatic types of neuropathy, except in some cases of the myopathic–myasthenic syndrome of Eaton and Lambert. Diplopia occurring in a patient with neuropathy and malignant disease suggests the possibility of cranial nerve infiltration.

Diffuse infiltration of peripheral nerves in many parts of the body does not occur with carcinoma, but this condition does occur in patients suffering from the various forms of reticuloses. In such patients symptoms and signs are less regular and symmetrical than those found in patients with non-metastatic peripheral neuropathy.

NON-METASTATIC NEUROPATHY WITH MALIGNANT DISEASE

The term 'carcinomatous neuropathy' has been widely used to describe neuropathies occurring in patients with malignant disease which are not due to metastases. Since the neoplasm is not always a carcinoma, it is more appropriate to describe the condition as a 'non-metastatic neuro-pathy'. The alternative term 'remote effect of malignant disease upon the nervous system' is far too cumbersome for everyday use.

In patients with malignant disease the central and peripheral nervous systems may be affected at all levels. There are, however, two forms of neuropathy distinct both clinically and pathologically, and these will be considered:

(1)   Peripheral neuropathy
(2)   Sensory neuronopathy

We are not concerned here with conditions affecting the central nervous system such as 'subacute cerebellar degeneration', although mention will be made of 'encephalitis with carcinoma'.

It is widely recognized that although more than half of all cases of non-metastatic neuropathy are associated with a bronchial neoplasm, a wide range of other malignant disorders has been found in various individual patients. There is sometimes an association with a particular type of neuropathy: for example, an ovarian carcinoma with subacute cerebellar degeneration, and the malignant lymphomas with progressive multifocal leuco-encephalopathy.

In studies of the incidence of minor degrees of neuropathy in patients with malignant disease, the majority of examples detected were of the proximal myopathic—myasthenic syndromes. As far as the neuropathies being considered here are concerned, true non-metastatic peripheral neuropathy probably occurs in about 2 per cent of cases of bronchial carcinoma. Non-metastatic sensory neuronopathy is much less common — in a large series of cases of non-metastatic neuropathies of all kinds, peripheral neuropathy was nearly five times more common than sensory neuronopathy.

It must be emphasized that cases of non-metastatic neuropathy do not always conform to a 'pure' classical type, and that mixed forms frequently occur. Indeed, the occurrence of such mixed clinical pictures increases the likelihood that an unexplained neuropathy may be due to malignant disease.

Non-metastatic Peripheral Neuropathy (Carcinomatous Peripheral Sensorimotor Neuropathy)

The clinical features of this neuropathy are unremarkable, the onset of typical motor and sensory symptoms and signs being usually sub-acute although occasionally an acute onset is seen. The severity of the neuropathy varies, and sometimes it is no more than a mild disorder adding little disability to a patient in the terminal stages of known malignant disease. In other patients the neurological disability is severe, and in many cases it develops without previous suggestion of malignant disease — indeed this type of neuropathy precedes evidence of malig-nant disease in about 50 per cent of cases. Occasionally the prompt investigation of such a case may lead to the early discovery of a carcin-oma which can be successfully removed. However, careful investigation and follow-up of such patients may not give positive results for months and occasionally for two or more years after the onset of neurological symptoms. It must always be realized that negative results do not exclude the presence of a neoplasm. Indeed, in some patients, the carcinoma is discovered only at autopsy, although long suspected and sought after.

In about two-thirds of cases of non-metastatic peripheral neuropathy a bronchial neoplasm is ultimately discovered, although individual cases occur with a wide variety of malignant disease. In the patients with lung cancer, there is not the high incidence of oat-cell tumours encountered in patients with non-metastatic sensory neuronopathy.

Non-metastatic peripheral neuropathy also occurs in association with the various reticuloses, particularly with myelomatosis, but examples have been reported with many of these disorders including macroglobulinaemia.

Some patients with this type of neuropathy have shown remissions. Sometimes these have occurred after steroid therapy, but at other times they seem to have been spontaneous. Certainly remissions that have been observed do not appear to have been associated with treatment of the primary malignant disease. However, when the development of a neuropathy does lead to the early recognition of a carcinoma, this should be treated on its own merits, and surgery should not be withheld because of the neurological disorder.

Investigations

CSF protein is increased in two-thirds of cases, being more than 100 mg/100 ml in about half, while some patients have 200–350 mg/100 ml. The Lange may be paretic but the cell count is usually normal.

EMG frequently reveals marked slowing of motor and sensory

215

conduction velocities, with muscle action potential patterns indicative of denervation.

Nerve and muscle biopsy show the pathological changes described below.

Other investigations have so far failed to reveal a definite cause for the neuropathy — toxic, metabolic, virological or immunological.

Pathology

The site of damage is in the peripheral nerves with affection of both myelin sheaths and axones. Damage to myelin sheaths is usually more severe than to axones, and in many instances axonal change is slight. Schwann cells are swollen, and in teased nerve-fibre preparations, segmental nodal demyelination has been demonstrated. It cannot be said with certainty whether Schwann cell damage is the essential primary process or whether there is simultaneous damage to Schwann cell and axone. The exact cause of the damage to Schwann cell and/or axone is not established.

Treatment

Apart from the treatment, where possible, of the underlying malignant disorder, steroid therapy is worth a trial in this type of neuropathy, even though the evidence for benefit from such treatment is inconclusive.

Non-metastatic Sensory Neuronopathy (Ganglioradiculitis)

This form of neuropathy, although less common than peripheral neuropathy, is more florid and disabling. 'Sensory neuronopathy' is a better descriptive term than 'sensory neuropathy' because of the primary damage to the posterior root ganglion cell. Onset of symptoms is usually subacute over a few weeks or months — occasionally acute cases are seen. At first there may be distressing spinal and peripheral pains and paraesthesiae which are rapidly followed by the development of a severe sensory type of ataxia which may make the patient quite helpless. There is widespread loss of all forms of sensation, superficial and deep, and the tendon reflexes are lost. In a 'pure' case there is no weakness or wasting in the early stages, but if there is involvement of anterior horn cells (*see* below) lower motor neurone signs may be present from the beginning.

As with non-metastatic peripheral neuropathy, sensory neuronopathy may occur without there being any evidence of malignant disease at first, in about two-thirds of the patients. Discovery of the underlying carcinoma may be delayed for as long as 2 years, or until autopsy.

Bronchial carcinoma is the cause of the neuronopathy in 90 per cent (a much higher figure than for peripheral neuropathy) and, in addition, the growth is usually of the oat-cell type. Another unexplained feature is the disproportionately large number of women patients in cases of sensory neuronopathy — both compared with the sex incidence in non-metastatic peripheral neuropathy, and with the proportion of women with oat-cell types of carcinoma in general hospital series of cases of lung cancer.

Investigations

CSF protein may be increased to more than 100 mg/100 ml and the Lange curve may be paretic. There may also be a slight pleocytosis in the CSF.

EMG: because of the absence of peripheral demyelination, conduction velocities are normal or only slightly reduced at first — sensory potentials are, however, impossible to elicit when the condition is established.

Pathology

In patients who show a clinical picture of sensory neuronopathy the main finding is of degeneration of posterior root ganglion cells, with phagocytosis, and patchy perivascular infiltration by lymphocytes. The distribution of roots involved may be general, but it is at times asymmetrical and some roots may escape. The peripheral nerves, and, very strikingly, the posterior columns of the spinal cord, show prominent Wallerian degeneration of sensory fibres. These cases also show some evidence of loss of anterior horn cells and patchy perivascular inflammatory change in the spinal cord and brain stem.

It is now believed that sensory neuronopathy forms one end of a spectrum, the other being a type of encephalitis in which slight changes of sensory neuronopathy are discovered. The condition can thus be regarded as an encephalomyelitis associated with carcinoma. In different patients the maximal site of damage may be in the limbic system, brain stem, spinal cord or posterior root ganglia. However, we are not concerned here with the cases of encephalitis. It is clear from the very gross neuronal loss which is found in sensory neuronopathy that remissions of the type which have been reported in some cases of non-metastatic peripheral neuropathy, cannot occur.

The Myopathic Myasthenic Syndrome

There are many muscular disorders which may occur in patients with malignant disease — for example, those associated with endocrine disorders and consequent biochemical changes. These cannot be discussed here but mention must be made briefly of the group of patients who develop a syndrome of proximal muscle weakness and wasting, with some myasthenic features including abnormal sensitivity to muscle relaxants. Although a majority show a defect in neuromuscular transmission differing from that of classic myasthenia gravis, some patients with such a proximal muscular disorder have had electromyographic investigations indicative of a motor neuropathy.

Pathogenesis of Non-metastatic Neuropathies

The mechanism of production of the various syndromes occurring as 'remote effects of malignant disease', remains uncertain. Indeed, it is quite possible that different mechanisms are acting in different types of disorder. The role of biologically active substances in the various endocrine disorders associated with carcinoma is well established (for example, inappropriate ADH secretion in the hyponatraemic syndrome). Similarly, the discovery of virus particles in cases of progressive multifocal leuco-encephalopathy has raised the possibility that this rare disorder is due to the action of a virus, not fully identified, in a patient with disturbed immunological reactions. In the case of the neuropathies at present under discussion, while the cases of encephalomyelitis—ganglioradiculitis might also be due to a viral infection, there is no convincing evidence for this as opposed to an alternative immunological explanation. One can only await the results of further virological and immunological as well as biochemical investigations, in the different types of non-metastatic neuropathy associated with malignant disease.

REFERENCES

Calne, D. B. and Pallis, C. A. (1972). 'Electromyography and nerve conduction studies.' *Br. J. Hosp. med.*, **7**, 775

Croft, P. B. (1969). 'Para-infectious and post-vaccinal encephalomyelitis.' *Post-grad. med. J.*, **45**, 392

Henson, R. A. (1970). 'Non-metastatic Neurological Manifestations of Malignant Disease.' In *Modern Trends in Neurology.*, 5th edition. Ed by D. Williams. London: Butterworths.

Marshall, J. (1963). 'The Landry-Guillain-Barré syndrome', *Brain,* **86**, 55

Simpson, J. A. (1968). 'The neuropathies', page 51. In *Symposium: Some Aspects of Neurology.* Ed by R. F. Robertson. Edinburgh: Royal College of Physicians of Edinburgh.

Thomas, P. K. (1969). The Peripheral Neuropathies, page 323. In *Fifth Symposium on Advanced Medicine.* Ed by R. Williams London: Pitman Medical Publishing Co. Ltd.

Wilkinson, M., Croft, P. B. and Urich, H. (1967). 'The remote effects of cancer on the nervous system'. *Proc. R. Soc. Med.* **60**, 683

10

Co-ordinated Care of the Patient with Rheumatoid Disease

A. G. White

INTRODUCTION

The aetiology of the rheumatoid process remains obstinately obscure despite the advances in our understanding of its pathogenesis which the contribution of immunology has afforded us. We know that virus infections such as rubella may cause a transient arthropathy. It has also long been realized that arthritis may result from infections; for example, the tubercle bacillus or the gonococcus. In these examples the duration of the arthritis is limited to the period of activity of the organisms and when they have been eliminated either by the body's own defence mechanisms or through the use of antibiotics, the arthritis remits. The two central problems of rheumatoid disease are to discover, first, what, if any, is the trigger factor involved (and here viruses, mycoplasma and diphtheroid organisms have all been suggested at one time or another), and second, to determine the process by which the arthritis is perpetuated.

Auto-immunity is regarded as the most probable explanation for the long-continued inflammatory response. A number of questions remain unanswered. It may be that antibodies arise following infections and that the antigenic determinants are held in common between micro-organisms and certain body tissues. This would seem to be the case in the relationship between the streptococcus and the carditis of acute rheumatism. It is also possible that auto-antibodies are produced by a disease process which is not primarily immunological in nature but which liberates substances or tissue components which have antigenic properties. The role of the lymphoid cells is the subject of much study

221

at the present time. It has been suggested that the cell-mediated mechanisms concerned in tissue homograft rejection and in the delayed type of hypersensitivity exemplified by the tuberculin reaction, may play a role in producing connective tissue damage, although the stimulus to the altered behaviour of these cells is not established.

While rheumatoid disease is not strictly an hereditary condition there is some epidemiological evidence of clustering of cases in families and of a higher incidence of seropositivity for rheumatoid factor in first degree relatives of rheumatoid patients than in their spouses. Some interpret this as evidence at least for immunological reactivity having a variability which is genetically based. An alternative explanation would be that the first degree relatives were exposed, perhaps in childhood, to a common environmental causative agent but in insufficient degree to cause the overt disease.

The evidence for auto-immunity is clinical, histological and serological. Although there may be lymph node enlargement and, occasionally, splenomegaly in rheumatoid disease – and we know that these structures are important sources of immunologically competent cells – there is no means by which we can distinguish the auto-immune from the hetero-immune response in lymphoid tissue. The presence of lymphocytic infiltration in the synovium of the rheumatoid joint and the demonstration of gammaglobulin in the cytoplasm of cells found in the synovial fluid offer supporting evidence for an immunological disturbance, but again do not indicate its source. Most authorities currently believe rheumatoid factor to be an antibody of IgM type to denatured IgG present in the serum in rheumatoid disease. It is detected *in vitro* by its ability to produce agglutination of red cells or latex particles coated with IgG. However, rheumatoid factor of IgG-type has been demonstrated in synovial fluid and also in the serum of some patients having high titres in the Rose–Waaler test. Although 100 per cent of rheumatoid patients with nodules have positive serum tests for rheumatoid factor its presence in the serum is not entirely diagnostic since there is a gradual increase in positivity with age from 1 per cent at age 15 years to 12 per cent at age 65 in the absence of any arthritis. Cases of tuberculosis and subacute bacterial endocarditis may show transient seropositivity which disappears following eradication of the infection. This suggests that there must be continued exposure to antigen over a long period of time for rheumatoid factor to become consistently present. Killed bacteria can elicit the IgM response in experimental animals. Long-standing cases of rheumatoid disease may become sero-negative and in these the clinical evidence of inflammatory activity is often diminished. It is also true that apparently unrelated conditions such as scleroderma and systemic lupus erythematosus (SLE) may show positive titres of rheumatoid factor.

DIAGNOSIS

The extreme chronicity of a condition in which patients often outlive more than one of their attendant physicians, the relative resistance of the disease to most forms of therapy, and the disabling, yet rarely fatal, nature of the disease, all raise special problems in its management. The importance of a secure diagnosis to the correct management of rheumatoid disease cannot be over-emphasized. The following is intended only as an outline of differential diagnosis to be filled in more fully by case experience and further reading.

When the onset of joint symptoms in a child is acute and large joints are principally involved (but no single joint is affected for more than a short time), *rheumatic fever* must be considered a possibility. Here the history of a previous streptococcal throat infection, a rising antistreptolysin titre and, in some cases, the presence of cardiac involvement, will usually render the diagnosis clear. *Still's disease or juvenile rheumatoid arthritis* may resemble rheumatic fever quite closely, particularly when the arthritis remains active only in a single joint and since cardiac valve damage and rash may occur in both conditions. However, the natural history of the two diseases differs considerably. Iritis is relatively common in Still's disease and the proximity of the inflamed joint to the epiphysis may result in accelerated epiphyseal closure with resultant shortening of long bones. A shortened mandible from this cause may result in malocclusion of the teeth and serious cosmetic disadvantage.

Adult rheumatoid disease is most usually symmetrical in distribution, more than 70 per cent of cases having arthritis of the wrists, metacarpophalangeal joints and proximal interphalangeal joints, ankles and knees. Between 40 and 70 per cent have involvement of the shoulders and elbows. Disease of the hips is rather less common. Rheumatoid arthritis of the terminal interphalangeal joints of the hands is distinctly uncommon whereas in *osteo-arthrosis* it is frequently seen and Heberden's nodes are a common accompaniment. In *psoriatic arthritis,* which may resemble rheumatoid disease closely, arthritis of the terminal interphalangeal joints of the hand is very common and tends particularly to be found in association with nail dystrophy of the same fingers. Although psoriasis and rheumatoid disease are both common conditions and therefore may exist together in one patient, there is now no doubt that psoriatic arthritis has been established as a distinct entity. Other distinguishing features of psoriatic arthritis include the less frequent tendon sheath involvement, the prominence of sacro-iliac joint involvement, and a characteristic 'cup and stem' deformity of the metatarsophalangeal joints of the feet which, on radiological examination, can clearly be distinguished from the erosive changes in rheumatoid disease at this site. The presence of an asymmetrical arthritis in the male should suggest the alternative diagnosis of *ankylosing spondylitis* or of *Reiter's syndrome. Brucellosis, typhoid* and *tuberculosis* should be considered in the differential diagnosis of the single acute joint, especially if there is also evidence of spinal disease. Peripheral joint disease in ankylosing spondylitis most commonly affects the hips and knees, but small joints of the hands are occasionally involved. The radiological appearances of the sacro-iliac joints and spine are characteristic and are distinguishing features, and iritis is common. In Reiter's syndrome the triad of arthritis, conjunctivitis and urethritis will usually be obtained from the history. The arthropathy characteristically affects the ankles and knees, and florid spur formation due to periostitis may be seen in x-rays of the heels although similar but less marked changes are also found in ankylosing spondylitis. Such features are not seen in rheumatoid disease. The resurgence of gonococcal infection has resulted in the reappearance of *gonococcal arthritis.* Here the migratory arthritis, tendon sheath involvement, and isolation of the organism from urethral discharge, from blood culture or occasionally from the joint fluid itself, are diagnostically helpful. The onset of *gout* is so different from that of rheumatoid arthritis that confusion does not usually arise and the appearances of the hot, red, swollen joint are unlikely to be mistaken for those of rheumatoid disease except occasionally in elderly patients where soft tissue rheumatoid disease is the presenting feature, and swelling and redness, particularly of the wrist, may superficially resemble gout. The somewhat ill-defined syndrome of palindromic rheumatism may present in a similar manner. However, the finding of tophi, a raised serum uric acid, or, more particularly, monosodium urate crystals in synovial fluid, enables a clear differential diagnosis to be made. The use of the polarized light microscope will enable the distinction between gout and pseudo-gout due to deposition of calcium pyrophosphate crystals to be made. SLE may produce an arthropathy indistinguishable from that of rheumatoid disease in its early stages. Radiological erosions are, however, absent, and skin nodules are uncommon. Indeed, it was formerly considered that their presence ruled out a diagnosis of SLE but otherwise typical cases with rash and renal disease have been described in which nodules are present but do not have the characteristic histology of a rheumatoid nodule. Although the presence of antinuclear antibodies points to a diagnosis of SLE and the demonstration of rheumatoid factor to one of rheumatoid disease, differentiation is unfortunately not as satisfactory as one would wish (*see* Table 10.1). Antinuclear

TABLE 10.1

Diagnostic Aids and their Limitations

Sheep cell agglutination	*Number of cases*	*% positive*
Rheumatoid arthritis		
Active	2702	60
Inactive	144	22
Osteoarthritis	411	5
Controls – healthy	258	2
SLE	67	46
Dermatomyositis and progressive systemic sclerosis	24	38
LE cells		
SLE		75–80
Dermatomyositis and progressive systemic sclerosis		10–25
Rheumatoid disease		10–25

antibodies are found in 20–25 per cent of rheumatoid disease. Where facilities are available, the immunofluorescent appearances may enable a more precise distinction to be made and the demonstration of anti-DNA antibody by the Farr technique renders the diagnosis of SLE more than 95 per cent certain. The LE cell phenomenon, although positive in 75–80 per cent of cases of SLE, may also be found in 10–25 per cent of cases of rheumatoid disease. Tests for rheumatoid factor, although positive in 100 per cent of cases of nodular rheumatoid arthritis, may be positive in as few as 60 per cent of those without nodules, particularly if only peripheral joints are affected. Some 30 per cent of cases of SLE, polyarteritis nodosa, dermatomyositis and progressive systemic sclerosis may also have rheumatoid factor in the serum, as may some 10

225

per cent of cases of Still's disease in children, particularly those most resembling the adult form of rheumatoid disease. In short, the diagnosis must rest upon the combination of clinical acumen and intelligent interpretation of the investigations available to us, whether radiological or serological, bearing in mind that none of them gives an absolute correlation with any one diagnostic category, and that patients will occasionally be found who show features of more than one disease, and in these cases the insistence on a single diagnosis may lead to inadequate treatment.

NATURAL HISTORY IN RELATION TO TREATMENT

Although statistically it can be shown that when large numbers of patients are considered, rheumatoid disease has a negligible effect upon expected lifespan, there are nevertheless a number of fatalities attributable to complications of the disease or to its treatment. Even patients not being treated with corticosteroids have an increased incidence of pyarthrosis and thus of septicaemia. Patients with a rheumatoid vasculitis may develop gangrene of the extremities or involvement of the viscera with fatal outcome, and it is probable that a greater number of patients than was formerly believed die from atlanto-axial subluxation, a direct consequence of the involvement of the ligaments securing the odontoid process in its correct anatomical position *(see Figure 10.4)*. Although the older physical forms of treatment are probably less effective and undoubtedly less fashionable in the treatment of this disease, it seems likely that a greater number of deaths result from the complications of drug therapy than from the older forms of treatment.

CO-ORDINATION OF LOCAL AND GENERAL MEASURES

Successful management depends upon the realization that it is necessary to treat local manifestations by both local and general means. At the same time our preoccupation with treating the arthritis must not blind us to the systemic manifestions, and indeed to the complications of our treatments, an example of which is the anaemia of gastrointestinal bleeding due to salicylate. In the more severely affected cases we must extend our concept of treatment and, with the help of occupational therapists, try to ensure that it meets the differing needs of each patient in his domestic and working environment. Emphasis on systemic therapy or on local measures alone, or a failure to appreciate the need to make maximum use of a patient's remaining abilities, will result in a failure to relieve areas of the patient's distress.

REST

Rest is the most ancient form of treatment applied for arthritic conditions and its efficacy has been the subject of much controversy. We know that a generalized arthritis, whether osteo-arthrosis or rheumatoid disease, affecting a patient with a paralysed limb, results in less severe involvement of that limb whether or not it be weight-bearing. Conversely, we know that the joints most heavily used, as for instance the index metacarpophalangeal joint of the right hand, are more severely involved in the rheumatoid process than are joints less frequently used. Furthermore, bed-rest in the acute phase of rheumatoid disease is known to produce an improvement not only in the local joint condition but also in the constitutional disturbance, as evidenced by reduction in the erythrocyte sedimentation rate (ESR).The disease of acute onset, primarily affecting large weight-bearing joints and accompanied by fever and loss of weight, tends to improve rapidly when the patient is confined to bed. Such patients do have, perhaps, a better long-term prognosis than those whose condition is of insidious onset and affects many small joints in succession. The latter, when confined to bed, may temporarily improve, only to relapse when discharged from hospital.

For those in the later stages of the disease, when inflammation is less intense and the danger of progressive immobility is greater, stress should be laid upon maintenance of activities rather than upon rest. There will probably always be a small group of severely disabled patients for whom mobility can only be continued with the help of a wheelchair and in some cases its use for part of the day's activities may actually enable residual walking to be prolonged by reducing the stresses on grossly destroyed joints and so preserving remaining function. Selection of an inappropriate chair can be a considerable disaster for the patient and a very great waste of money. The physician who has not acquired the necessary technical information and skill should not be reluctant to seek help.

HEAT AND OTHER PHYSICAL MODES LOCALLY APPLIED

The use of various forms of heat, though time honoured, has little more than transient effect, and in acutely inflamed joints may actually produce an increase in pain, particularly if short-wave diathermy is employed. An exception to this is the use of short-wave treatment of the temporomandibular joints where rapid relief of symptoms may be obtained. The use of warm wax baths may be of value in the mobilization of the small joints of the fingers but only as an adjunct to other forms of therapy. Where the rheumatoid process has been superseded by osteo-arthrosis of secondary type, short-wave therapy or micro-wave treatment may give symptomatic relief; other patients may find ice therapy more effective, particularly in the mobilization of stiff shoulders subsequent to corticosteroid injection. Briefly stated, the functions of exercise in this condition are the maintenance of the range of motion in joints and, more important, the strengthening of muscles whose power is necessary to the stability of weight-bearing joints and in particular of the knee. The use of ultra-violet therapy in the form of general body irradiation or in the form of high intensity Kromayer therapy as a counter-irritant, no longer finds a place in modern therapy. The use of ultrasonic treatment is of very doubtful value in this condition and the use of radiotherapy should not be countenanced.

SYSTEMIC DRUG THERAPY

In the therapy of serious and fatal diseases we are guided consciously or unconsciously by the law of double effect. By this we mean that we balance the good effects we hope for from the drug against the likely harm from unwanted effects. These are just as much an inherent quality of the drug as those effects for which we prescribe it. For diseases of almost certainly fatal outcome, drugs with higher risk are acceptable, but for a condition with an extremely low mortality, drug toxicity becomes a severe limiting factor. It is here that the balance between local and general therapy is particularly important. It may often be wiser to make a concerted attack on one particularly troublesome joint by aspiration, local corticosteroid injection and splintage, than to increase further the level of general drug dosage.

Oral Anti-inflammatory Drugs

Aspirin remains the drug of first choice for general long-term use. It is essential that the patient understands that the anti-inflammatory effect of this drug depends upon high and constant dosage. According to body weight and efficiency of absorption of the aspirin preparation in use, 3–4 g per day will be necessary. The use of buffered or enteric coated aspirin will reduce the gastro-intestinal blood loss, and benory-late (a liquid compound of aspirin and paracetamol) may do so further.

228

Reduction in joint size and improvement in symptoms by day may often be achieved in the early stages with aspirin alone, but night pain and morning stiffness may remain a problem. A night dose of *indomethacin* (25–27 mg in capsule form or 100 mg in suppository form) is often effective. Additional doses may be given during the day as a supplement to aspirin. Dizziness is a problem in some patients, especially when the drug is taken before breakfast. However, it should be borne in mind that large symptomless gastric ulcers may be produced and their presence may only be revealed when frank haematemesis ensues. *Phenylbutazone* is a drug of approximately equal potency but less flexibility of dosage. Present evidence suggests that doses in excess of 300 mg per day carry a greater risk of bone marrow depression. Rash, fluid retention and dyspepsia also occur. While twice as many cases of unwanted effects are reported with indomethacin as with phenylbutazone, the death rate from the complications of phenylbutazone approaches twice that for indomethacin.

Many patients who have gastric intolerance to one of the antirheumatic drugs will have similar problems with others. Here the 'second line' drugs may prove of value. *Mefenamic acid* and *flufenamic acid* are probably less effective than phenylbutazone and indomethacin but patients who can take flufenamic acid in doses in excess of 400 mg/day without troublesome diarrhoea may benefit considerably. *Ibuprofen* is probably as effective as aspirin if given in a dosage range of 600–800 mg/day, and it has a very low incidence of gastric side-effects.

Gold Therapy

The role of gold therapy in rheumatoid disease remains a matter for considerable debate despite many years of use. Many physicians employ it enthusiastically while a few deny that its use can ever be justified. *Sodium aurothiomalate,* injected intramuscularly in doses of 50 mg, is usually given at weekly intervals. Improvement can rarely be expected before three months have elapsed so that previous therapy should not be reduced or discontinued before that time. After a total dose of 1 g has been reached some physicians stop, while others advocate the use of very small doses given monthly over a period of several years. There is no doubt that gold therapy can produce remissions in a proportion of cases and a substantial improvement in others. The physician must weigh against this the hazards of gold toxicity which occurs in up to 38 per cent of cases and is serious in some 5 per cent. Exfoliative dermatitis and gold nephropathy usually improve on withdrawal of the drug but systemic corticosteroids will be required in more severe cases. Dimercaprol (3 mg/kg body weight in 6-hourly doses over 3 days) is of use, especially where the total dose has been high. Bone marrow depression, however, may be irreversible. The view that gold and phenylbutazone, when given together, are more hazardous to the marrow than when given separately, has never been properly substantiated. Some believe that gold should be reserved for those cases of slow insidious onset in females, particularly where there is a strong family history of unremitting disabling disease, and where the simpler measures have failed. It is probably not justifiable for acute onset disease affecting a few large joints in male patients. It may be that its use in this latter group, in whom a high proportion of remissions in any case may be expected, has given it a greater reputation for efficacy than it deserves. Regular white cell counts and examination of the urine for albumin are essential precautions.

Chloroquine

It has been claimed that the potency of this drug is similar to that of gold. Chloroquine has, however, tended to fall into disuse in the U.K. since the recognition of its ocular complications. These include retinal degeneration and band keratopathy. Early hopes that these complications could be avoided by electro-diagnostic tests proved ill-founded. Furthermore, damage to the eye may continue after the drug has been stopped. In the circumstances its use in rheumatoid arthritis can no longer be recommended, despite its continued use in other EEC countries.

Immunosuppressive Drugs

Immunosuppressive drugs have been used in rheumatoid disease on the assumption that a disturbance in immune activity plays a role in the condition. Features which suggest this are the histology of lymph nodes, local reduction in complement levels in affected joints, the appearances of the synovial membrane examined by immunofluorescent techniques, and the improvement in the rheumatoid condition during pregnancy and following hepatic disease or virus infection; in all of these conditions there is some degree of suppression of the immune response. Despite these theoretical considerations, recent work has suggested that, in practice, the effect of these drugs is more an anti-inflammatory one than the result of immunosuppression. While it is certainly true that in carefully organized trials of patients already on corticosteroid drugs, a reduction in the latter can be achieved by the addition of immunosuppressive agents, they have not so far found general acceptance.

Corticosteroids

When, in 1948, corticosteroids were first used in the treatment of rheumatoid disease, the results were startling but the ultimate complications were grave. These drugs have found their place with the passage of

TABLE 10.2

Corticosteroids

Useful effects	Relief of inflammation
Unwanted effects	Fluid retention
	Hypertension
	Facial rounding
	Diabetes
	Osteoporosis
	Aseptic necrosis
	Peptic ulcer
	Hypokalaemia
	Menstrual disorders
	Acne
	Trunk obesity
	Psychosis
	Bruising
	Striae
	Purpura
	Poor healing
	Infection
	Myopathy
	Benign intracranial hypertension
	Epilepsy
	Posterior capsular cataract
	Silent tuberculosis
	Growth suppression in children
	Teratogenicity
	Neoplastic enhancement
	Problems of withdrawal

time and the aim should now be not to exceed a dose of 7.5 mg of prednisolone or its equivalent per day and preferably not to exceed 5 mg for long-term use. At these levels of dosage most patients do not have significant pituitary depression, and provided dose reduction is gradual, withdrawal should be possible. The drug is best given at night when it will usually relieve morning stiffness and may be supplemented by other drugs by day. Bearing in mind the many unwanted effects (Table 10.2) the decision to commence corticosteroids should never be a hasty one. A past history of depression, peptic ulceration or tuberculosis should make one still more cautious. It has not been shown that the use of these drugs improves the likelihood of remission or the eventual level of disability. There is evidence that abrupt reduction of dosage or abrupt withdrawal may precipitate vasculitis and neuropathy. It should also be remembered that these drugs inhibit the healing process and this should be borne in mind when orthopaedic surgery is contemplated.

Adrenocorticotrophic Hormone (ACTH)

As an alternative to oral corticosteroid medications ACTH offers one major advantage and one major disadvantage. On account of its mode of action it can be withdrawn much more abruptly than corticosteroids without the hazard of adrenal insufficiency. On the other hand, it must be given by injection at frequent intervals. So far as complications are concerned, there are those who believe that, when compared with corticosteroids, ACTH causes rather more fluid retention and osteoporosis and rather less peptic ulceration, but these differences are difficult to evaluate. With the advent of purified and synthetic preparations, problems of sensitization to foreign protein have been largely overcome. ACTH has a particular place in the management of Still's disease, the juvenile variant of rheumatoid disease. Here the use of corticosteroids is limited by their tendency to retard growth by pituitary suppression. With ACTH, growth retardation is very much less and it is therefore preferable in this age group.

Penicillamine

When first used for the treatment of rheumatoid disease, it was thought that this drug might have immunosuppressive properties and it was employed solely in those cases with complicated rheumatoid disease whose response to corticosteroids and other drugs had been poor and for whom no other remedy was available. The results at that time were somewhat disappointing. It has subsequently been claimed by some workers that the drug does not act as an immunosuppressive. Others have shown that in doses of up to 1500 mg daily significant reduction of serum IgG and IgM levels occurs and when IgM levels fall to 40 per cent of the level before treatment, latex agglutination titres fall. Its mode of action, therefore, remains unclear. Depolymerization of rheumatoid factor may take place, but it is not certain that this is related to clinical improvement. A recent careful trial of this drug in rheumatoid disease of moderate severity rather than as a last resort, has shown definite benefit in the treated group as compared with controls. It is therefore probable that it will find an increasing place in therapy. One of its disadvantages is the fairly high incidence of side-effects, particularly rash, thrombocytopenia, neutropenia and gastro-intestinal disturbance. Added to this there is a disturbance of the sense of taste. These side effects are reversible on withdrawal of the drug. Occasionally, a nephropathy occurs and it is not yet certain whether this is always reversible. Therefore, any patient who develops albuminuria while receiving the drug should at the present time not receive a second course.

THE PLACE OF LOCAL CORTICOSTEROID INJECTIONS

When joint pain and swelling is insufficiently relieved by regular and adequate doses of anti-inflammatory drugs, rest and splintage, and it is not desired to commence or to increase systemic corticosteroid dosage, the injection of long-acting preparations of hydrocortisone, methyl-prednisolone, triamcinolone or betamethasone into synovial cavities may provide considerable improvement over a period of 4—12 weeks. If strict aseptic technique is observed less than 1 in 7,000 cases results in infection being introduced, and this is an acceptable risk. It is known that too frequent and too large injections of steroid drugs can result in aseptic necrosis, particularly of the hip, and to more rapid deterioration of other weight-bearing joints, especially the knee. For this reason, it is usual to restrict such injections both in dose and frequency. For example, it is probably unwise to repeat a steroid injection sooner than 6 weeks after the previous occasion and the dose should not exceed 80 mg methyl prednisolone or its equivalent. Since tendon sheaths also have a synovial lining and their involvement in the rheumatoid process is frequent, corticosteroid injection has also proved useful in this situation. Soluble prednisolone phosphate is perhaps the better preparation for tendon sheath injections since it leaves no crystalline residues and, being of low viscosity, can be injected along the whole length of the tendon sheath with greater ease.

Detailed techniques for the injection of particular joints will not be described here; they are available in rheumatology texts. However, it is worth considering some of the special situations in which these injections may be employed. Involvement of the temporomandibular joints may cause pain and difficulty in opening the mouth. This is sometimes

233

responsive to short-wave diathermy but an injection of local steroid will often give more rapid and total relief. When injecting the shoulders, an effusion which may not be clinically obvious can be detected by drawing back on the syringe before injecting the steroid. Complete removal of the effusion with a larger syringe should then be carried out, and the injection may then be completed. Since there is at the present time no wholly satisfactory shoulder prosthesis and arthrodesis of the shoulder is to be avoided where possible, the need for injections into the shoulder may be a recurrent one. In the case of the elbows there is a tendency for flexion contractures to develop at quite an early stage in the disease. Reduction in synovial thickening and a greater degree of extension of the elbow will follow steroid injection. Inflammatory lesions of the lateral epicondyle ('tennis elbow') or of the medial epicondyle ('golfer's elbow'), which may form part of the rheumatoid peri-articular inflammation, can also be relieved with intra-articular injection, but in this case a local anaesthetic solution should be mixed with the steroid preparation. Injection of the wrist and of the ankle should similarly be combined with local anaesthetic since when these joints are actively inflamed injection will otherwise be particularly painful. However, there is little advantage to be gained by the admixture of a local anaesthetic when injecting the knee or the hip.

The injection of the small joints of the hands, particularly the metacarpophalangeal and proximal interphalangeal joints, tends to be painful for the patient and time-consuming for the physician, and it is therefore too often neglected. Nevertheless, this is a valuable procedure, particularly in the early stages of the disease when the patient's symptoms may, apart from a few small joints, be well controlled by background medication with salicylate only, and there may be a temptation to launch into more potent and more dangerous drugs at too early a stage. The metatarsophalangeal joints of the feet are even less commonly injected. Nevertheless, if the injection is given into the joint from the dorsal surface of the foot after a thorough cleansing and using very careful aseptic technique, the results can be excellent.

INTRA-ARTICULAR INJECTIONS OTHER THAN CORTICOSTEROID

The search for a more long-acting intra-articular injection than hydrocortisone or methylprednisolone has yielded few results so far with the possible exception of triamcinolone hexacetonide. Thus, attention has turned to other agents having the capability of inhibiting the inflammatory reaction. Local injections of cyclophosphamide have been employed and also of radioactive gold and other isotopes. Although these substances are capable of producing improvement often lasting several months, there are still difficulties in regard to the absorption of these substances from the joints and therefore concerning their effects elsewhere in the body. In the case of cyclophosphamide, general effects including damage to the bone marrow have been reported in a few cases. In the case of radioactive isotopes, it seems probable that the choice of an isotope with a suitable short half-life and strict immobiliz-ation of the joint for 48 hours after the injection may overcome this problem. Clinical trials are at present in progress to assess the usefulness of radioactive isotope injections.

The destruction of the abnormal synovial membrane by chemical agents such as osmic acid has also been employed with some success. There is no doubt that in the experimental arthritis of animals, injec-tion of osmic acid into a joint results in the total removal of abnormal membrane and this is followed by regrowth of normal synovial mem-brane. However, in the human disease this does not always occur, and the regrowth of synovium may be equally affected by the rheumatoid process. Furthermore, the injection is extremely irritant and causes much pain to the patient. This is also true of the cytotoxic drug mus-tine which has similarly produced benefit. In both these instances patients who have received one such injection are not always willing to tolerate the pain and discomfort a second time and the usefulness of these two substances is therefore very limited.

High viscosity silicone oil had a brief vogue as an artificial joint lubricant for the stiff arthritic knee. Long-term results were disappoint-ing. Similar oil of higher viscosity may offer some advantage but a synthetic lubricant having the non-Newtonian characteristics of synovial fluid is awaited.

SURGERY IN RHEUMATOID DISEASE

A fundamental requirement for successful co-ordinated management of rheumatoid disease is close co-operation between physician and ortho-paedic surgeon. Although to some the idea of joint consultation clinics may seem novel, we know that they were taking place as long ago as the latter part of the eighteenth century in what is now the Royal National Hospital for Rheumatic Diseases, Bath. It is essential that the physician referring patients for surgery has a clear idea both of what is possible and what is practical for a particular patient. It is equally essential that he should prepare the patient so as to reduce as far as possible the risks of surgery. In long-standing cases, flexion and extension views of the cervical spine must be taken to exclude the possibility of atlanto-axial subluxation. Corticosteroid dosage must be reduced gradually over a period of time to the minimum requirement. Evidence of joint infection must be sought and excluded and anaemia corrected. Since the operative risks may be increased by ischaemic heart disease, hypertension or other general conditions, high standards of care of these must be maintained up to the time of surgery and afterwards, so that the physician must involve himself both in the initial decision-making as to the correct operative procedure and in the post-operative phase. It is important to warn the surgeon of the presence of arteritis since this will reduce tourniquet time and hence in some cases limit the extent of the procedure. Gangrene of digits or occasionally of the whole limb can occur after episodes of ischaemia of a duration which would cause no ill effect in a patient with normal vessels. If in doubt, arteriography is of value.

The principal objects of surgery in rheumatoid disease are the relief of pain, the arrest of local disease and an improvement in function. Factors which affect the decision to operate or not in a particular case are rather different from those encountered in other situations. For example, the patient of advanced years and inactivity would be considered less favourably for general surgery, whereas in rheumatoid patients the disease is likely to be less active in the elderly and repairs and prostheses are unlikely to be subjected to the stresses and strains which would obtain in the younger patient. Such patients, if otherwise fit, may therefore benefit more than the active younger age-group. However, the extent of the disease can be an important factor as, for example, when several joints are involved in both lower limbs. The replacement of a hip joint may permit a patient to become ambulent when before she was chairbound, but this in itself creates a problem of added strain upon joints formerly subjected to little use. These joints, in turn, may then require surgery. If a well-planned series of potential disasters is to be avoided, a full assessment of the likely outcome must· precede intervention. Not only must the motivation and the economic need of the patient to return to work be taken into consideration, but also the domestic and working environment, including travel. Arthrodesis of the right knee, which would be most convenient if the patient were a car driver, may render getting into the passenger seat a great problem for the non-driver for whom the other knee should be fixed.

Different stages of the disease require different forms of surgery and it is usual to divide procedures available into early and late. There has been increased emphasis on the value of synovectomy in early stages of the disease not only as a highly effective means of pain relief but also as a means of maintaining function and minimizing deformity. The procedure is applicable to the wrist, the metacarpophalangeal joints of the hands, sometimes to proximal interphalangeal joints, and to the elbow, where it is often accompanied by excision of the head of the radius. It is not applicable to the shoulder for anatomical reasons. Likewise, in the lower limbs the hip is unsuitable for this procedure. It has been used fairly extensively in the knee but not elsewhere in the lower limbs. It must be explained to the patient that only the joint actually operated upon will show improvement as some patients offer themselves for surgery under the misconception that its performance upon one joint will influence the disease in others (nevertheless they are sometimes correct in this belief since in a few cases any operation seems to be followed by a temporary remission akin to that which may occur in pregnancy or following hepatitis). The patient must also understand that although the duration of benefit is likely to be two years or more, it may well not be permanent and further surgery to the same joint may become necessary later. The results in the wrist, the elbow and the metacarpophalangeal joints of the hands are particularly favourable provided that the operation is carried out early enough. On direct examination at operation, the extent of erosive damage in a joint is usually greater than that which was apparent radiographically. It is thus much better to operate when erosions first become visible rather than to wait until much more gross destructive change has taken place. In the earlier years of the disease the patient may pass from the first to the second of these

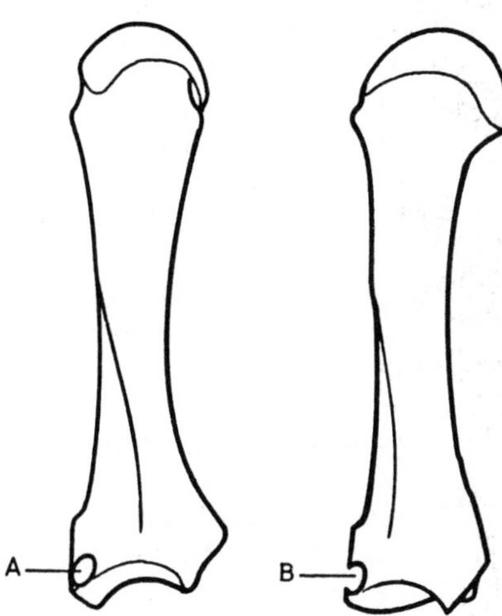

Figure 10.1. Rheumatoid erosions may not be visualized radiologically in the conventional views of the hands if they are set within the contour of the bone, as in A. When rotation is produced as in Norgaard's views of the hand the same erosion, B, becomes visible

stages in a matter of months; thus serial x-rays taken at three-monthly intervals of a joint for which surgery is contemplated are extremely valuable. 'Ball-catching' or Norgaard's views of the hands and similar views of the feet reveal unsuspected erosions *(Figure 10.1)*.

In selected cases synovectomy of the wrist may need to be extended to include removal of the ulnar styloid process. In those cases where there is gross erosive change at this site, removal of the styloid process will not only result in relief of pain but will also remove the risk of attrition rupture of the extensor tendons to the fourth and the fifth fingers which the roughened bone edge so often causes. If the pre-operative assessment has revealed carpal tunnel syndrome it may be necessary to undertake a decompression procedure as a further extension of synovectomy of the wrist. Although synovectomy of the knee in the early stages of the disease has found favour in some centres, there is occasionally loss of full extension of the knee and more frequently some loss in the range of flexion. Although in many cases the relief of pain is satisfactory, at least during the first year, there is in a proportion of cases a return of pain subsequently and treatment of these cases then proves difficult. It is believed that in some instances there is a reduction in the joint space available for the reaccumulation of synovial fluid with the regrowth of abnormal synovium and that the steep rise in pressure which therefore results occasions the pain. Nevertheless, where stability is preserved and pain and effusion are persistent and severe, early synovectomy probably has a limited place. The presence of a Baker's cyst in the knee is not in itself an indication either for its removal or for a synovectomy. It is now believed that these cysts, which communicate with the joint cavity by a one-way valve mechanism, offer some measure of pressure release and the extent of joint damage in a large series of knees with Baker's cysts, has been shown to be inversely proportional to the size of the cyst. This accords well with the view that articular cartilage destruction is accelerated in the presence of high joint pressure on flexion of the knee. However, if the cyst ruptures and irritant synovial fluid passes into the calf with symptoms and signs closely mimicking those of a deep vein thrombosis, synovectomy and removal of the cyst should either be undertaken when the swelling of the leg has subsided or should the condition recur after an adequate period of conservative treatment.

The procedure of arthrography, in which a radio-opaque agent such as Conray 280 is injected into the joint, is valuable in demonstrating the site, extent and point of leakage of these cysts before operation is undertaken *(Figure 10.2)*. Although synovectomy of the hip joint is not a practical proposition, there are those who advocate the use of pain-relieving osteotomy at a relatively early stage in the disease and certainly before it advances to the point at which hip replacement becomes necessary. The results of osteotomy are variable and osteotomy has not become universally accepted for the rheumatoid hip in the way that it has been for osteo-arthrosis.

When the disease has been present for a number of years but is still obviously active, the condition of the joints may be such that the value of synovectomy is in doubt. For example, in the wrist there may be advanced erosive change and much synovial thickening. It is often necessary for the surgeon to decide at the time of operation whether he

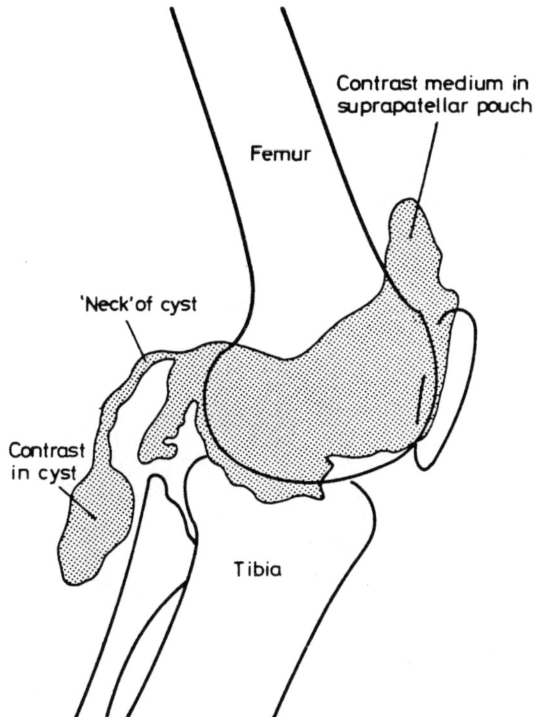

Figure 10.2. Arthrogram of rheumatoid knee. Lateral view showing appearances following injection of 20 ml Conray—280. The popliteal cyst and its communication with the joint cavity are visualized

should still undertake synovectomy alone or whether it would be more sensible to perform an arthrodesis of the wrist. This will have the advantage of giving more complete relief of pain but at the cost of complete loss of movement. Thus, the greater the limitation of movement and of pain, the more likely is the patient to accept this procedure. Patients with much pain and only very slight residual movement, who have had the operation performed on one wrist, will frequently ask for it to be done on the opposite side. The position in which the wrist is fixed is of importance not only for the function of the limb as a whole, but also for its effect upon ulnar deviation. Radial angulation of the wrist during arthrodesis will result in an increase in the degree of ulnar deviation of the fingers, while ulnar deviation of the wrist will tend to correct this deformity. When synovectomy of the metacarpophalangeal joints of the hands is undertaken at a time when ulnar deviation has already commenced, a number of ingenious procedures have been developed for correcting the ulnar deviation by means of the realignment and reinsertion of tendons. At the elbow, ulnar nerve entrapment may complicate synovial thickening and flexion contracture. In this instance, synovectomy, removal of the head of the radius, and transposition of the ulnar nerve to an anterior position at the elbow, will relieve pain, improve the range of movement, and eliminate the risk of further damage to the ulnar nerve. At the shoulder, the removal of an

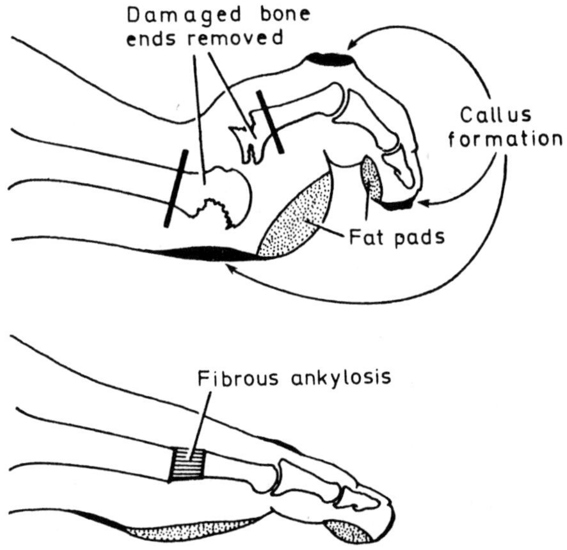

Figure 10.3. The rheumatoid foot. Severe involvement of the feet with erosion and subluxation (upper view) results in pressure being taken by skin unprotected by fat pads. Fowler's operation removes the source of pain and restores weight-bearing to correct areas (lower view)

inflamed bursa, may reduce pain and improve the range of movement. Careful post-operative physiotherapy is essential if stiffening of the shoulder is to be prevented.

Late-stage surgery now has a great deal to offer the rheumatoid patient. Patients who have persistently painful feet and gross destructive erosions of the metatarsophalangeal joints, often complicated by subluxation, benefit greatly from Fowler's operation in which the base of the phalanges and the heads of the metatarsals are removed *en bloc* *(Figure 10.3)*. Triple arthrodesis of the painful ankle is the only measure available for this joint. In the presence of mobile hips, unaffected by the disease, and especially when the disease process is believed to have become inactive, arthrodesis of the knee is still valuable but bilateral arthrodesis of the knee can rarely be recommended.

A number of arthroplastic procedures for the knee have been developed but at present none can be said to be wholly satisfactory. Of those in routine use the Walldius prosthesis probably offers the best success rate. The alternative type of hinge arthroplasty (the Shier's prosthesis), although simpler and cheaper, requires a greater removal of bone from the femur and tibia and also the removal of the patella. Should the prosthesis have to be removed and arthrodesis subsequently performed, gross shortening of the leg results. A number of other prosthetic replacements for the knee are at the experimental stage and so it would now seem sensible to adopt a conservative approach wherever possible pending the production of a more satisfactory prosthesis.

In the hip the situation is different, as there are now several excellent prosthetic replacements including the all-metal McKee ball-and-socket type and the Charnley (metal-on-high-density polypropylene). Although the Charnley prosthesis has a number of theoretical advantages, both prostheses give excellent results in practice.

Replacement surgery for the large joints of the upper limb is not yet perfected although hinge joints at the elbow have found some acceptance. A prosthetic replacement for the shoulder has been developed in the University of Leeds and is currently under preliminary trial. A number of implant replacements of the small joints of the hands have now been in use for several years. These may be of polypropylene, silastic or metal. A recent symposium suggested the following guides for finger joint arthroplasty:

(1)   Destruction of the MCP and PIP joints on any finger except the thumb in which only one joint, the finger, must be significantly affected.

(2)   Joints which are fixed or nearly fixed or grossly destroyed with resulting palmar subluxation or ulnar deviation.

(3)   Increased function should be the aim rather than cosmetic improvement.

(4)   Elimination of other defects such as intrinsic contraction,

tendon rupture or a weak wrist, should be done before or at the time of operation on a finger.

(5)   No evidence of arteritis other than skin nodules should be present.

(6)   There should be absence of severe osteoporosis.

(7)   The rheumatoid disease process should be relatively inactive.

(8)   The arthroplasty must not be liable to excessive strain as, for example, from the use of crutches.

(9)   The patient should have a suitable personality.

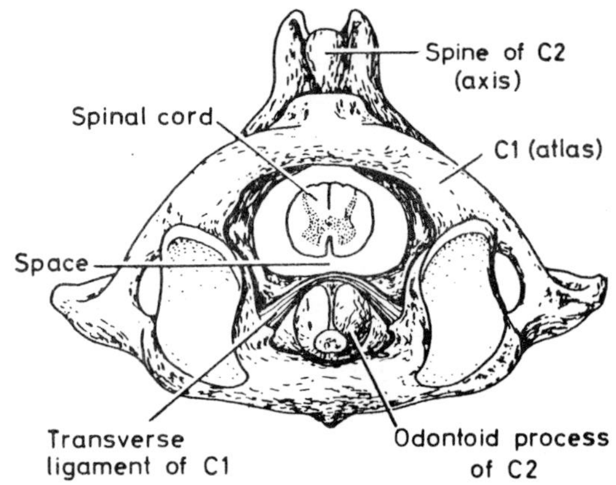

Figure 10.4. The normal anatomy of the first cervical articulation, showing the ligament which maintains apposition between anterior portion of C1 and odontoid peg of C2 and the degree of 'space' surrounding the spinal cord

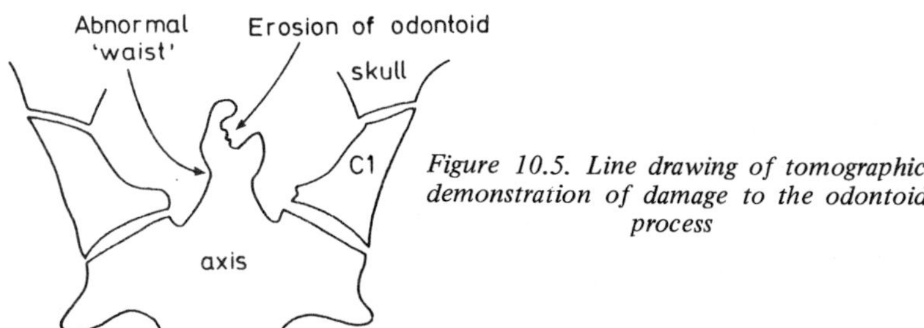

Figure 10.5. Line drawing of tomographic demonstration of damage to the odontoid process

Items 5, 6, 7, 8 and 9 are clearly applicable to replacement surgery as a whole. The ideal implant replacement has not yet been developed, but such a prosthesis would have to be simple and efficient in design, easy and cheap to manufacture, sterilize and use, be resistant to stress and deterioration, and provide a simple and durable fixation, at the same time as being biologically and mechanically acceptable to the host tissues. One of the advantages of prosthetic replacement surgery is the range of movement afforded. Although arthrodesis gives stability and relief of pain, the cost in terms of immobility may often be too high. Furthermore, other joints, free at the time of operation, may later become fixed, rendering the activities of daily living increasingly impossible.

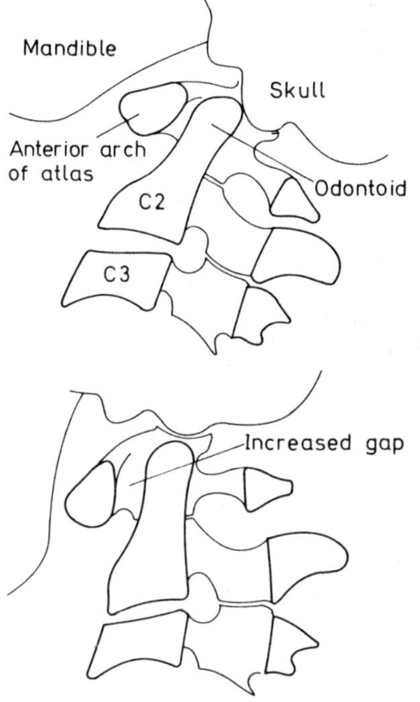

Figure 10.6. Atlanto-axial subluxation of rheumatoid disease. (a) This was drawn from a lateral tomograph of the atlanto-axial articulation in extension and shows a normal anatomical relationship. (b) In this view, taken in flexion, the increased gap due to forward luxation of the skull and C1 upon C2 is clearly seen.

Atlanto-axial subluxation is now recognized as relatively common in advanced rheumatoid disease. A separation of greater than 4 mm between the anterior surface of the odontoid process and the arch of the atlas is abnormal and follows destruction of the ligaments supporting the odontoid process in its normal position *(Figures 10.4. 10.5* and *10.6).* Compression of the upper segments of the spinal cord and kinking of the vertebral arteries result in neurological signs and symptoms and in transient dizziness or loss of consciousness from vertebrobasilar insufficiency. The natural history of this condition is not yet clearly established and there is evidence that some cases stabilize with time and conservative measures in the form of restrictive collars. However, those cases with progressive neurological signs will require surgery if paraplegia or sudden death are to be avoided. Both anterior and posterior spinal fusion procedures are available. When, as is often the case, subluxations are also present at mid-cervical level, fusion of the cervical spine from the occiput to C34 may be necessary. Close attention to the maintenance of mobility of other joints during the prolonged period of bed-rest which follows this operation is essential.

SYSTEMIC FEATURES OF RHEUMATOID DISEASE AND THEIR MANAGEMENT

Anaemia

One of the most common general manifestations of the disease is anaemia. A number of factors contribute to rheumatoid anaemia, a common one being gastrointestinal bleeding from the drugs employed. Here aspirin and indomethacin are the chief culprits. Rheumatoid patients are predominantly female and many will already have a blood loss anaemia from menstruation with loss of reserves of iron. Average red cell life is reduced by up to 7 days suggesting some haemolysis. In addition, as with a number of chronic infective conditions, there is a defect in the re-utilization of iron liberated from destroyed red blood corpuscles. Sequestration of iron in the reticulo-endothelial system and probably also in the synovial membrane itself, takes place. Iron given intravenously is cleared more rapidly from the circulation in rheumatoid subjects than in controls, presumably because it takes these abnormal pathways. The finding of a very low serum iron with a normal iron-binding capacity is a frequent one in rheumatoid disease and when patients' investigations are followed serially, a fall in serum iron is often noted to take place shortly after serum globulin levels have become high. In these cases the prescription of oral iron is frequently ineffective. Iron given intramuscularly may be effective, and the use of corticosteroids may cause a steep rise in haemoglobin concentration, even when iron is not prescribed. Although the majority of rheumatoid anaemias are normocytic or microcytic, macrocytosis is sometimes found. While it is true that some patients have a dietary folic acid deficiency it is probable that the majority in whom folic acid deficiency seems to be a factor have a defect in its utilization, the nature of which is not entirely explicable. A group of patients exists with a malabsorption syndrome either from amyloidosis, from very long-standing disease or, of a lesser extent, from more obscure causes. Anaemia in these cases may be due to malabsorption of iron, of folic acid, or of vitamin B_{12}. It must be borne in mind that pernicious anaemia may be found coincidentally in a patient suffering from rheumatoid disease, as may other anaemic states. It is doubtful if there is actually a higher incidence of pernicious anaemia in rheumatoid subjects than in controls, although cases certainly exist in which a number of organ specific antibodies may be found in the serum in addition to rheumatoid factor, and some of these cases will have an anaemia indistinguishable from pernicious anaemia.

Felty's Syndrome

The association of leucopenia, splenomegaly and rheumatoid arthritis, described by Felty in 1924, is sometimes accompanied by weight loss, fever and skin pigmentation. In some cases there is a depletion of the whole white cell series and a thrombocytopenia and improvement of the haematological condition, but not of the arthritis, may follow splenectomy. It is curious that a number of patients with an apparently dangerously severe leucopenia survive in good health for many years and the necessity of splenectomy is therefore not proven. Enlargement of regional lymph nodes with or without splenomegaly is common. There is some evidence that those lymph nodes draining the joints most actively involved tend to be those most increased in size. It may be impossible to distinguish them from the enlarged nodes of a reticulosis or other malignant process and in these circumstances biopsy is justified. However, the histology usually shows reactive hyperplasia, some increased iron deposition and, occasionally, typical rheumatoid histology.

Amyloidosis

The development of amyloidosis of the secondary type tends to occur in cases of long duration as is also true in ankylosing spondylitis and tuberculosis. This complication is important mostly in so far as it contributes to renal failure and to loss of weight. The diagnosis may usually be made by rectal or gingival biopsy. Renal biopsy is occasionally positive when these are negative. Although the histology of a liver biopsy may also give the diagnosis, the procedure is not advisable if amyloidosis is suspected because of a higher complication rate. The Congo Red test is now no longer used because it is hazardous.

The Kidney

Apart from amyloidosis, the kidney is known to be the subject of damage, rarely from phenylbutazone, and more often gold and analgesic nephropathy. It is commonly believed that the agent concerned in analgesic nephropathy is phenacetin, but aspirin itself is not wholly free from suspicion when taken in large quantities over many years, as is usual in the management of rheumatoid patients. Recent work suggests that concurrent ingestion of aspirin and phenacetin results in a greater production of 2-hydroxyphenetidin, which is nephrotoxic, than when phenacetin is taken alone, due to a displacement of intermediate metabolism into an alternative pathway. Studies of renal function show reduced glomerular filtration in many patients, but, in addition, obliterative endarteritis, focal glomerulonephritis, and a reduced concentrating capacity, are suspected as further complications of the rheumatoid process although their delineation from other concurrent renal disease presents difficulties. It also seems likely that an increased incidence of pyelonephritis may be due to steroid treatment. Since the blood urea is an insufficient guide to a patient's renal state, it is essential that a creatinine clearance test be undertaken before gold therapy is commenced. Regular examination of the patient's urine for albumin is advisable when any of the nephro-toxic drugs are in use.

Rheumatoid Involvement of the Cardiovascular System

Focal myocarditis and arteritis of myocardial vessels may occur. Rheumatoid granulomata of the valves and conducting tissue may give rise to valvular defects and to abnormalities of conduction. Acute pericarditis, while found in Still's disease, is uncommon in rheumatoid arthritis of adults, but chronic pericardial effusions are more frequent than usually suspected, particularly in those cases where pleuro-pulmonary involvement occurs. Ultrasonic scanning may aid diagnosis if pericardial effusion is suspected. The aortic incompetence found in ankylosing spondylitis and sometimes in Reiter's syndrome is very uncommon in rheumatoid disease. It should not be assumed that the patient with rheumatoid disease who is found to have oedema of the ankles and legs necessarily has renal or cardial failure unless definite evidence of these conditions is to be found. Hypo-albuminaemia from malabsorption, the effects of anaemia and of such drugs as phenylbutazone, corticosteroids and ACTH, may all produce oedema which may be aggravated by immobility of the limbs in chairbound patients. Furthermore, there has now been shown to be a capillary defect in rheumatoid disease which may be fundamental to the development of many of its other features and which, by leakage of fluid into the interstitial tissues from defective capillary walls, leads to oedema.

Skin and Bone

Rheumatoid disease also produces changes in the skin elasticity and in bone matrix leading to increased fragility of both of these. Unduly transparent skin, the presence of purpura and pigmentation, and a tendency to spontaneous fractures may all be seen, even in patients not being treated with corticosteroids, and the addition of these drugs tends to accelerate these conditions.

Lungs and Pleura

The incidence of pleuro-pulmonary manifestations bears a clear relationship to the presence in the serum of rheumatoid factor, an abnormal chest x-ray being found in 23 per cent of sero-positive rheumatoid disease compared with only 8 per cent in sero-negative cases. Pleurisy and effusion are six times as common in rheumatoid arthritis as in osteo-arthrosis. The majority of cases of rheumatoid pleurisy are found in male patients over the age of 45 years. Features of the pleural fluid lending support to the diagnosis are low sugar level, and a positive Roses test, often in a titre higher than that found in serum — also raised acid phosphatase and LDH enzymes where these are determined. Many rheumatoid effusions settle spontaneously; aspiration may be helpful and the installation of local corticosteroid may accelerate their resolution. A number of patients with diffuse interstitial fibrosis of the lungs are found to have rheumatoid factor in their serum. Some of these later develop rheumatoid arthritis while others never do. There is also a chronic fibrosing pneumonitis of rheumatoid disease and both these conditions carry a rather poor prognosis, being by no means always helped by corticosteroids. The development of rheumatoid nodules in the lung is not uncommon and may give rise to unusual radiological appearances. The association of rheumatoid disease and massive pulmonary fibrosis is known as Caplan's syndrome and it seems probable that the immunological disturbance which gives rise to rheumatoid nodules in the lungs is in some way accentuated by the presence of silica dust. Attempts have been made to relate the onset of rheumatoid disease seasonally to the occurrence of episodes of lower respiratory tract infection. These findings, though offering an attractive aetiological theory, have not so far been repeated outside the original centre which reported them.

Rheumatoid Involvement of the Nervous System

There are several sites at which peripheral nerves are particularly subject to compression in rheumatoid disease and hence to segmental demyelination. The most common is carpal tunnel syndrome in which the median nerve at the wrist is subject to compression from the flexor retinaculum under which it passes, as a result of synovial thickening in relation to the carpus and adjacent tendons. In the early stages this may respond to splintage of the wrists in the neutral position at night, is sometimes aided by the use of oral diuretics, and is more frequently relieved by local injection of corticosteroid beneath the flexor retinaculum. Where there is doubt concerning this diagnosis the finding of a prolonged motor or sensory latency using standard electrodiagnostic techniques, gives supporting evidence in many cases. Normal results, however, should not deter one from making the diagnosis and, indeed, those cases with normal latency measurements have the best prognosis. If conservative measures prove ineffective, surgical decompression should be recommended, since the addition of a median nerve palsy to a hand already disabled by inflammatory joint disease adds an unnecessary further burden of disablement. Another common site of nerve compression is that of the ulnar nerve at the elbow. The best treatment of this is transposition of the ulnar nerve to a more anterior position. Here again, electrodiagnostic techniques may be most valuable in accurately localizing the site of compression where doubt exists. Nerve conduction neasurements may similarly be helpful when a patient with rheumatoid disease presents with a foot drop or sensory loss when a lateral popliteal nerve has become damaged due to the pressure of splints or plasters or occasionally, due to trauma against some portion of the wheelchair. In this connection it is worth bearing in mind that some cases of ulnar nerve palsy result from the pressure of crutches of the gutter type upon the elbow. In cases of this kind, it is advisable to examine not only the patient but also the appliances and how he uses them. In addition to these nerve entrapment and compression syndromes, there is a digital sensory neuropathy which has a patchy distribution over the fingers. It may well be that this is a complication of rheumatoid vasculitis with involvement of the digital vessels. However, this particular neuropathy carries a fairly good prognosis compared with the mixed type of sensorimotor neuropathy which tends to be progressive and is often associated with a poor prognosis for the disease in general. Occasional patients are seen with mononeuritis multiplex in which several peripheral nerves are involved in sequence and finally there is some evidence of autonomic dysfunction, as evidenced by palmar erythema and palmar sweating, commonly found in long-standing cases of rheumatoid disease or those in whom the disease has recently become more active. The nature of this disorder is not fully understood. It is now fairly well established that the sensorimotor neuropathy in particular and possibly digital sensory neuropathy, like the vasculitis of this disease, may be precipitated by abrupt withdrawal or sudden reduction of dosage of corticosteroid.

The Eye

The eye may be affected in rheumatoid disease in several ways. It is important to be aware of ocular complications since treatment is available for some of them. Iritis occurs, though less commonly than in juvenile rheumatoid disease. Disease of the sclera, sometimes termed episcleritis, is not uncommon, and in its more serious form (scleromalacia) may cause rupture of the contents of the anterior chamber of the eye through the sclera and may lead to blindness. Both these conditions in their early stages are amenable to corticosteroid eyedrops. Conjunctivitis may occur as part of keratoconjunctivitis sicca either by itself or as part of Sjögren's syndrome (*see* below). Long-term systemic corticosteroid medications may lead to posterior capsular cataract. Other drugs, including indomethacin, may cause similar temporary changes but these are reversible. Chloroquine, as mentioned above, has serious effects upon the eye, but with a diminution in its use fewer cases should be seen. Dryness of the eyes, keratoconjunctivitis sicca, may occur by itself, in association with rheumatoid arthritis or sometimes with other rheumatic diseases, and there is frequently an associated dryness of the mouth, xerostomia, the triad being known as Sjögren's syndrome. The dryness of the eye may be confirmed by Schirmer's Test in which a specially prepared length of blotting paper is hooked over the lower eyelid and the distance the tears travel along it is then measured. The ophthalmologist may also wish to examine the eye using fluorescein or other agents to detect corneal erosion, consequent upon the cornea being insufficiently protected by the tear film. The frequent installation of eyedrops of hygroscopic type are sometimes effective but if symptoms persist, sealing of the lachrymal punctum by cautery may prove necessary. Some 50 per cent of patients with keratoconjunctivitis sicca with or without xerostomia have rheumatoid arthritis. Ten to 15 per cent of patients with rheumatoid arthritis have this syndrome. These cases invariably have a positive Rose's test and long-standing rheumatoid disease, although not necessarily active synovitis. It should be noted that up to 20 per cent of patients with the sicca syndrome (dry eyes and dry mouth) will be found to have one of the following: SLE, polymyositis, scleroderma, or Hashimoto's thyroiditis. It is only when the sicca syndrome is found in a patient with a connective tissue disorder that it is properly called Sjögren's syndrome. The failure of tear and salivary secretion is consequent upon the pathological changes in the lachrymal and salivary ducts. In the early stages the glands may show some, enlargement which may be clinically visible. There is peri-duct infiltration with plasma cells and lymphocytes and oedema of the parenchyma. In the later stage there is atrophy of the acini, fibrosis and stenosis of the ducts, sometimes with sialectasis. In the eye the lack of tears tends towards conjunctivitis, corneal erosion, and sometimes fibrillary keratitis. Changes also occur occasionally in the genito-urinary tract leading to atrophic vaginitis and dyspareunia, and in the respiratory tract to sinusitis and dryness of the tracheal mucosa. There is occasionally an associated renal tubular defect leading to hyperchloraemic acidosis. A number of other symptoms are found less commonly of which lymphadenopathy and splenomegaly are perhaps the most frequent. There is probably an increased incidence of reticulum cell sarcoma and non-thrombocytopenic purpura has been described. Peripheral neuropathy has been attributed to this condition and there is an increased incidence of allergic reactions to penicillin and other drugs.

Rheumatoid Disease and Voluntary Muscle

Muscle wasting is a frequent accompaniment of severe disabling joint disease and there is no doubt that pain inhibition is a real factor. When joints become fixed, muscle wasting follows. However, there is some evidence of minor abnormalities in muscle function as determined by electromyography in a proportion of rheumatoid patients who do not have obvious wasting. These occasionally resemble polymyositis but are usually not of great significance. However, when patients are treated with corticosteroid drugs, particularly those whose molecule contains fluorine such as triamcinalone, a definite myopathy may emerge. Thus, it is also seen occasionally with dexamethazone and betamethazone but very much less commonly still, with prednisolone. In addition to the characteristic electromyographic findings there will be creatinuria although the muscle enzymes creatine-phosphokinase and aldolase are not universally elevated in these cases. There is gradual return to normal if the steroid medication implicated can be withdrawn or replaced with prednisolone.

REFERENCES

Burry, H. C. (1971). 'Renal disorders in rheumatoid arthritis'. *Rheum. phys. Med.*, **11**, 2

Calnan, J. S. and Holt, P. J. L. (1969). Workshop on artificial finger joints'. Supplement to *Ann. rheum. Dis.* **28**

Cosh, J. A. (1972). 'The heart and the rheumatic diseases'. *Rheum. phys. Med.*, **11**, 267

Fowler, A. W. (1959). 'A method of forefoot reconstruction'. *J. Bone Jt Surg.*, **41B**, 507

Gardner, D. L. (1972). *The Pathology of Rheumatoid Arthritis* London: Arnold

Glynn, L. E. (1968). 'The chronicity of inflammation and its significance in rheumatoid disease'. *Ann. rheum. Dis.* **27**, 105

Heathfield, K. (1973). 'Neurological complications of the rheumatic diseases'. *Rheumatol. and Rehab.* **12**, 2

Kessler, I. and Vainio, K. (1966). 'Posterior (dorsal) synovectomy for rheumatoid involvement of the hand and wrist'. *J. Bone Jt Surg.*, **48A**, 1085

Norgaard, F. (1969). 'Earliest roentgen changes in polyarthritis of rheumatoid type; continued investigations'. *Radiology.* **92**, 299

Smiley, W. K. (1969). 'The eye in arthritis'. *Ann. phys. Med.* **10**, 157

11

The Bullous Dermatoses

C. M. Ridley

INTRODUCTION

This chapter should be regarded as a simplified and somewhat didactic account for non-dermatologists. It does not claim to be comprehensive; rare conditions which are of interest only to dermatologists are omitted. Some rare conditions, however, are discussed since they are of considerable clinical and academic importance.

Definitions

A bulla (Latin — blister) may be defined as a circumscribed elevated fluid-containing lesion greater than about 0.5 cm in diameter. A similar lesion, smaller in size, is generally called a vesicle, or a pustule if it contains pus. The word blister itself may be used of either type of lesion but is probably more often used of the larger variety, that is of a bulla.

It is important to remember that a lay person's view of a blister may not be that of a doctor. Patients often speak of solid lesions as blisters; a history of 'blisters' without confirmatory evidence should always be checked by means of questions directed at establishing the presence or absence of fluid.

The consideration of bullous diseases by definition excludes that of vesicular conditions, whether non-infective (such as eczema) or infective (such as tinea, herpes zoster, and herpesvirus hominis). The distinction, in fact, is usually straightforward. Bullous dermatoses form a group which is clearly distinguishable on clinical grounds, though aetiologically diverse, and which comprises some very common and some very rare conditions. However, for the sake of exactness it should be noted that in some cases of eczema, notably acute allergic contact dermatitis, the vesicles may approach the size of bullae. Similarly,

TABLE 11.1

The Bullous Dermatoses

Main causative factors	*Diseases and skin conditions*
Physical agents	Blisters from cold, heat, etc.
Infections	Impetigo Some cases of toxic epidermal necrolysis Some cases of erythema multiforme
Drugs	Some cases of toxic epidermal necrolysis Some cases of erythema multiforme Fixed drug eruptions, and other drug-induced bullous eruptions
Metabolic disorders	Porphyria Diabetes
Congenital disorders	Epidermolysis bullosa, Congenital syphilis, etc.
Coma	
Idiopathic bullous diseases with clinical and histological resemblances	Pemphigus, Pemphigoid, Dermatitis herpetiformis, etc.
Bullous variants of normally non-blistering dermatoses	Urticaria pigmentosa, Lichen planus, etc.

some conditions which are usually vesicular, such as eczema or insect bites, may become bullous on the legs, particularly in the elderly (presumably as a result of stasis); and, in children, bullae rather than vesicles may follow insect bites at any site, or may mark the position of acari in scabies.

254

PRINCIPLES OF DIAGNOSIS

The history may help; the presence or absence of itching is often useful although, since any skin condition may itch and any may not, this feature should not be made of prime importance. The family history, age and race should be carefully noted. Infections or the ingestion of drugs, within the relevant period, may be significant.

The whole body should be inspected, not forgetting the mucous membranes, and further examination of other systems carried out where appropriate. The inspection should be carried out in a good light. The pattern of the eruption may be important — whether, for example, the lesions are confined to light-exposed areas, or are symmetrical on the limbs, or scattered on the trunk.

The individual lesions comprising the rash must be examined carefully and, as regards the blisters, a note made not only of their distribution but also of their size, tension, contents, and the skin at their base, the presence or absence of scarring, whether or not they are ruptured and, if so, whether there is a smooth erosion or crusting.

Where the situation is not straightforward, and where there is a possibility of prolonged therapy that is not itself without risk, histological examination should be made. Conventional histology and, later, electron microscopy, have enabled us to separate many of the entities to be discussed. Immunofluorescence techniques are now also adding valuable information.

The bullous dermatoses may be classified in terms of aetiology where it is known (Table 11.1).

PHYSICAL AGENTS

Experimental induction of bullae by physical and chemical irritants is a valuable source of information on the mechanism of blister formation. Similar lesions may be observed in a non-experimental setting in blisters following burns, treatment (of warts, for example) by carbon dioxide snow or liquid nitrogen, in artefactual lesions induced in various ways by the patient, and in the dramatic bullous patterns drawn on the skin by the combination of plant phototoxins (furocoumarins) and light in phytophotodermatitis ('meadow dermatitis').

INFECTIONS

Impetigo

Impetigo is a common and highly contagious superficial skin infection, occurring at any age but most often encountered in children.

It is caused by a *Staphylococcus pyogenes* (usually phage type 71), by a streptococcus (usually Lancefield group A), or by both together. The prevalence of each type varies from time to time and place to place.

Blisters form within the epidermis, just below the horny layer. They contain bacteria mixed with polymorphs and serum. These blisters are easily ruptured – particularly in streptococcal or mixed infections – and they may be small. Intact large blisters usually indicate a staphylococcal aetiology. When rupture has occurred, the lesion is covered by a golden crust. No scarring is left on healing. Lesions may extend peripherally or coalesce with others. Any area of the skin may be affected.

There may be underlying and predisposing lesions such as bites, scabies, herpesvirus infections, pediculosis, trivial injuries, and occasionally eczema. When impetigo is secondary to other dermatoses the process is referred to as impetiginization.

Impetigo Neonatorum

This is a staphylococcal impetigo of the newborn. Pemphigus (Greek: pemphis – blister) neonatorum is an older and less apt name. The infecting organism is usually of phage type 71. Both host-resistance and bacterial pathogenicity are involved. Male infants are more commonly affected. The bullae may spread rapidly and lead to generalized exfoliation (Ritter's disease – *see* below). As mortality is high, with pyogenic lesions involving other systems, it is of prime importance to trace the source, often a medical or nursing attendant.

Differential Diagnosis

The differential diagnosis of impetigo usually presents no difficulties because the typical pus-filled blisters or golden crusting are characteristic. An underlying condition, however, unless its possibility is borne in mind, may easily be missed.

Treatment

Bacteriological investigations should preferably act as a guide. The staphylococci are usually resistant to penicillin and often also to tetracycline.

In severe forms at any age, in the new-born, and where a nephritogenic strain (*see* below) may be involved, systemic treatment is indicated. Milder cases can be treated by local antiseptics or antibiotics. When the latter are used, care must be taken to avoid agents which readily sensitize the skin, such as penicillin and neomycin.

Complications of Impetigo

Acute post-streptococcal glomerulonephritis may complicate impetigo or respiratory infection. When nephritogenic strains infect the skin they are usually of M-type 49 though other types may sometimes be responsible. Acute post-streptococcal glomerulonephritis, following respiratory infections, is usually related to organisms of M-type 12 although, again, others have been implicated. The M-antigen is a protein in the streptococcal cell wall and determines virulence; it is capable of inhibiting phagocytosis, thus enabling the cell to survive and divide. When M-antibody is produced it seems to coat the cell and make it vulnerable again. M-antigen possibly occurs in streptococci of strains other than group A, conceivably as a result of transfer between strains. Such nephritogenic strains have not yet been reported with certainty in this country but they are of great importance elsewhere, notably in parts of North and Central America and Trinidad (where skin infections are a commoner cause of acute post-streptococcal glomerulonephritis than are respiratory ones). There is no difference in the renal disease, however it is produced.

In some affected areas, for example Trinidad, it has been shown that there is a streptococcal skin infection throughout the year with occasional outbreaks of acute post-streptococcal glomerulonephritis, whereas in other areas, for example Alabama, the skin infection and the acute post-streptococcal glomerulonephritis are alike seasonal. The infection is often spread by flies from skin to skin.

Although it has not been proved that prompt and thorough treatment, preferably systemic, of the skin lesions will prevent the development of acute post-streptococcal glomerulonephritis in these cases, it would seem safer to act in that belief. Such treatment would, moreover, lessen the risk of spread of dangerous strains from person to person.

Staphylococcal impetigo may be associated with toxic epidermal necrolysis (sometimes referred to as Lyell's disease). Since staphylococcal impetigo or staphylococcal infections in any form are only part of its story, the disease will be considered under a separate heading.

DISEASES WHICH MAY BE DRUG-INDUCED OR INDUCED BY INFECTION

Toxic Epidermal Necrolysis

Toxic epidermal necrolysis is characterized by a peeling off of necrotic epidermis (hence 'necrolysis'); so although a bulla, as such, is not seen, or is seen only transiently, kinship with the bullous diseases is close.

In one group of cases a staphylococcal skin infection, usually of phage type 71, is frequently associated. This group is sometimes called Ritter's type of toxic epidermal necrolysis. Recent experimental work in mice suggests that the responsible agent is diffusible, probably a protein, and not identical with staphylococcal alpha- or delta-toxin or hyaluronidase.

In the other group, the condition may be drug-induced or remain idiopathic.

The level of the split in the skin is intra-epidermal in the staphylococcal group and sub-epidermal in the other.

There is extensive, often almost universal, erythema and peeling, extreme tenderness (hence the term 'scalded skin syndrome'), and considerable systemic disturbance.

In the staphylococcal group the patient is often a child or an infant. There is a preceding staphylococcal infection, usually of the skin and frequently in the form of impetigo; there may also be a history of staphylococcal infections in the family. On culture, the staphylococcus, usually of phage type 71, is found only in the primary lesion. In infants, the picture is that which used to be called Ritter's exfoliative dermatitis and considered to be a severe form of impetigo neonatorum (*see* above). The illness is dramatic but mortality is low. No scarring ensues.

In idiopathic or drug-induced toxic epidermal necrolysis, drugs are very often apparently responsible, particularly sulphonamides, pyrazolone derivatives (for example phenylbutazone) and barbiturates; some cases remain unexplained. The mortality is high, as one would expect in such a serious illness, often in an elderly person with pre-existing ill-health.

Differential Diagnosis

The fully-developed picture is unlikely to be confused with any other condition — except scalding itself, consideration of which may be of medico-legal importance. However, some cases, particularly those where a drug is suspected, may show mucous membrane involvement and may be difficult to distinguish from the severe form of erythema multiforme known as the Stevens–Johnson syndrome (*see* below) and often also drug-induced.

Treatment

In the staphylococcal group systemic antibiotics must be given. Nursing care is of great importance.

In the idiopathic or drug-induced group, any drug which might be responsible must be stopped and any then given must be chemically unrelated. Corticosteroids may help, a dosage of 60–100 mg of prednisolone being indicated. Good nursing care may be life-saving.

Erythema Multiforme

Erythema multiforme is a distinct and fairly common entity characterized by a typical histology, morphology and distribution, although of variable severity. The term should not be used loosely to describe erythematous eruptions which do not show these specific features. The Stevens–Johnson syndrome is a severe form of erythema multiforme.

The aetiology often remains unknown. However, erythema multiforme may be provoked by many drugs, notably phenylbutazone, sulphonamides, and barbiturates. It may also be initiated by many infections. Herpesvirus hominis (herpes simplex) lesions are a fairly common cause of erythema multiforme, although erythema multiforme is a rare complication of this infection. There have been conflicting reports but the balance of evidence suggests that the infective agent is not to be found within the erythema multiforme lesions themselves. There is usually an interval of one to three weeks between the primary infection and the erythema multiforme. Cases have been reported in association with neoplasms and radiotherapy.

The mechanism of provocation is not known. However, once precipitated by a drug or an infection, the erythema multiforme tends to recur with further exposure to the agent. Any suspected drug should therefore never be given again.

There is marked dermal oedema, inflammation and degeneration, epidermal degeneration or necrosis, and a tendency to liquefaction degeneration at the dermo-epidermal interface. Bulla formation therefore occurs between the dermis and the epidermis.

The lesions are symmetrical and usually confined to the limbs, particularly distally and on extensor aspects. Occasionally the face and trunk are involved. They appear as erythematous macules which become oedematous and palpable and show rings of different shades of red. Such lesions are often referred to as iris (rainbow) or target lesions. Clinically, bullae are not always seen but when they are present they develop at the centre of these lesions. In severe cases the lesions are florid and the oral, genital and ocular mucous membranes are involved. There is considerable systemic disturbance, with sometimes pulmonary or even renal involvement. It is this serious type which is called the Stevens–Johnson syndrome; it has a high mortality. The condition is self-limiting and lasts a few weeks. No scarring remains. Recurrences due to precipitation by any relevant drug or infection may be seen and the idiopathic form also tends to recur.

Differential Diagnosis

A typical case is easily recognizable by the distribution of the rash and the iris- or target-like lesions; as already stated, the term should be kept for such cases. Pemphigoid (*see* below) may cause difficulties but the rash usually has a different distribution. The Stevens–Johnson syndrome can be difficult to distinguish from idiopathic or drug-induced toxic epidermal necrolysis, but this is fortunately not of practical importance.

Treatment

Any drugs likely to be responsible must be withdrawn and if substitutes are necessary they must be chemically unrelated. Open areas left by the rupture of bullae must be protected, and treatment as necessary given for secondary infection. Systemic corticosteroids probably help in the severe forms: a dose of prednisolone of about 40–60 mg daily is likely to be needed initially. Good nursing care is important, particularly for the mucous membrane lesions.

In erythema multiforme precipitated by herpesvirus infection, it appears that partial suppression of the virus infection by idoxuridine will not prevent the eruption. However, when complete eradication of the virus has been achieved, as it sometimes may be by repeated use of idoxuridine in the attacks, the erythema multiforme seems not to recur. To be effective, the idoxuridine should be applied as far as possible 3-hourly for the first two days of the infection and made up in dimethyl sulphoxide. The more easily available preparation designed for use in the eye is of limited value.

DRUG-INDUCED BULLOUS ERUPTIONS

The Fixed Drug Eruption

Drugs, as has been noted, may cause toxic epidermal necrolysis or erythema multiforme; the fixed eruption is a further lesion which may be drug-induced and bullous. This eruption recurs at the same site or sites after readministration of the drug concerned.

Whenever the question of a drug eruption is raised, the only safe assumption is that any drug may produce any type of rash. However, the drugs which most readily cause a fixed eruption are phenazone, phenolphthalein, barbiturates, sulphonamides, dapsone, quinine, and tetracyclines. Their relative frequency will vary with prescribing patterns. The mechanism is obscure. Provocative tests are usually, but not invariably, positive where clinical evidence is convincing. It has been shown that the drug involved is probably not taken up preferentially at the involved sites. The bulla is sub-epidermal.

There may be one or more lesions but usually few in all. Mucous membranes may be involved; the penis, lips and hands are common sites. Each lesion shows as a more or less round patch, red or brown when quiescent and becoming oedematous and often bullous in the active phase.

Other Bullous Eruptions Related to Drugs

Bullous eruptions not clearly falling into the above categories have been reported. Bromides and iodides may produce a few scattered thick-walled bullae. A further example is the occurrence of bullae in light-exposed areas as a result of the photo-sensitivity sometimes induced by nalidixic acid.

BULLAE IN METABOLIC ABNORMALITIES

Porphyria

In this group of diseases porphyrins, or their precursors, are produced in excess; delta-aminolaevulic acid synthetase, important at an early stage in production, is increased in all forms.

Bullae on light-exposed areas are a feature of most types of porphyria. The exception is acute intermittent porphyria where there is no light-sensitivity. In the light-sensitive types the mechanism of bulla formation is unknown but is probably related to the effect of light on the porphyrins accumulated in the skin — an effect which is thought to lead to lysosomal and hence to tissue damage. The PAS positive material round the capillaries probably results from repeated damage of this sort which involves the vessels. The bulla is subepidermal and below the basement membrane, with disintegration of the subjacent corium.

The clinical features vary somewhat according to the type of porphyria.

Congenital Erythropoietic Porphyria

In this rare disease, inherited as a recessive character, there is a defect of haem synthesis in the red cell corpuscles and light-sensitivity is extreme. Bullae may occur from an early stage on exposed areas, but they tend to be overshadowed by the other cutaneous manifestations of the disease which lead to gross scarring and tissue loss. Unfortunate patients suffering from the condition may have given rise to the stories of night-prowling werewolves.

Erythropoietic Protoporphyria

This is much more common and is inherited as a dominant character. The main, abnormality concerns porphyrin metabolism in the erythrocytes. In later life liver disease may, on occasion, be associated. The patients, usually children, complain of intense pain and burning of the exposed areas when in sunlight. The symptoms may be dismissed as psychogenic, since there is little or nothing to be seen in the skin. In the course of time, however, small pitted scars appear in these areas. Occasional blisters are seen but are relatively insignificant.

Porphyria Variegata

This is a form of hepatic porphyria, common in white South Africans, and is inherited as a dominant character. In this type of porphyria cutaneous and systemic manifestations are combined, as the name implies. Cutaneous changes are commoner in men. In women, systemic and light sensitivity reactions may be induced by pregnancy or the oral contraceptive. Bullae on exposed areas are a prominent feature although not as a rule until adult life. Associated with the bullae there is fragility of the skin, hypertrichosis, and scarring.

Porphyria Cutanea Tarda

Porphyria cutanea tarda is usually non-hereditary and is induced by the effect of alcohol or toxic substances on the liver, though perhaps only in genetically-predisposed subjects. Oestrogens or chloroquine may precipitate it. The patient is usually in middle life and bullae appear on exposed areas, leaving, as they heal, scars and milia (small hard white keratin cysts). The skin is fragile, pigmented and hypertrichotic.

Similar changes were found in Turkish children when hepatic porphyria was induced by a toxic agent (hexachlorbenzene) used on wheat some years ago.

Treatment

With congenital erythropoietic porphyria and erythropoietic protoporphyria, no active form of treatment is of proven value, although the use of oral beta-carotene in erythropoietic protoporphyria holds out some promise. In other types, avoidance of drugs which may precipitate exacerbations, and of alcohol in the case of porphyria cutanea tarda, may help. Venesection is effective in porphyria cutanea tarda. In as far as treatment is successful, the skin changes will improve. Otherwise, light-barrier creams are of some benefit although the wavelengths responsible for the damage (about 400 nm) are such that adequate protection is difficult to achieve.

Diabetes

Bullae are a rarely noted, but perhaps not really rare, cutaneous manifestation of diabetes.

The cause is obscure and does not appear to be coma, trauma, infection, or neuropathy. The bulla has a distinctive appearance, being intraepidermal and without acantholysis (a term defined in the discussion of pemphigus — *see* page 266).

Large but sparse blisters are seen, usually on the feet or hands.

CONGENITAL BULLOUS DERMATOSES

Epidermolysis Bullosa

This is a rare, genetically determined, and, except in mild cases, congenital condition existing in a variety of forms.

In general, those inherited by way of dominant genes are less marked and disabling than those with recessive inheritance.

There is a separation at or below the dermo-epidermal junction, except in the mildest (simplex) form where it occurs between epidermal cells, though without acantholysis. With advances in electron microscopy it may be possible to distinguish the various forms more precisely.

The common feature is a tendency for bullae to develop as a result of minor trauma. The mildest forms show themselves only in summer or after much walking, and there is no scarring. A more severe form shows scarring, with milia, nail dystrophy and occasional mucosal involvement.

The recessive forms may be lethal at birth, or lead in infancy and childhood to severe scarring and deformity. There may be oesophageal strictures. In the past these children often died but with systemic steroids they may survive. Plastic surgery can help considerably in restoring function to the grossly contracted hands which often appear as if sealed in a case of skin.

Congenital Syphilis

This may occur in a bullous form; the bullae are widespread, flaccid and arise on an erythematous base.

BULLAE IN UNCONSCIOUS STATES

These blisters are of uncertain aetiology but have long been recognized in a variety of unconscious states.

Histological evidence is not always available but such studies as there are show epidermal and eccrine sweat gland necrosis. The necrotic reaction recalls that in toxic epidermal necrolysis.

The bullae are usually scattered, sparse, tense, and large. They may heal with or without scarring which, when it occurs, may be keloidal.

Study of individual cases suggests that the blisters are related to local pressure or to apposition of skin surfaces, or both, but not always to sites of maximal pressure.

It is generally agreed that they may occur in unconscious patients who have taken no drugs — for example those with severe brain damage, strokes or hypoglycaemia. Nor is it disputed that they may occur in patients who have taken overdoses of barbiturates and many other drugs, and that there is no evidence of any allergic reaction to the drugs in question. Some say that the blisters are so much more a regular feature of barbiturate overdosage than of overdosage with other drugs that they may be used as a diagnostic feature, but this is contested.

By the nature of the clinical situation, histological findings and pharmacological proof of the drugs taken are not always available. Pressure and hypoxia are undoubtedly important features; but the dermal and epidermal metabolism of the drug may also be important, and barbiturates have been shown to reduce oxygen consumption of the skin more than do some other sedative drugs.

THE IDIOPATHIC BULLOUS DISEASES

It is now convenient to discuss the important group of idiopathic bullous diseases. Some have been distinguished from one another only in the last 20 years or so, on histological grounds. Electron microscopy and immunofluorescence techniques have now, in general, confirmed these distinctions.

Pemphigus Vulgaris

A rare and dread disease, always fatal if untreated, pemphigus is mainly a disease of middle life, in either sex, and has a predilection for Jews. It is characterized by extensive blistering, often affecting mucous membranes.

There is much evidence to suggest auto-immune processes. Auto-antibodies, directed against the intercellular substance of epidermal cells, have been found in the serum of patients with pemphigus vulgaris, and immune complexes between the cells are demonstrable *in vivo* by immunofluorescence. Although it is still not known whether or not the antibodies are secondary or primary, the antibody titre varies with the clinical state and may be helpful in assessing progress.

The essential histological feature is acantholysis. In this process the individual epidermal cells appear to lose the prickles which join them to their fellows (Latin: acanthus − prickle). They therefore separate and float in a cleft produced as a result of their detachment. This change can be followed in considerable detail with electron microscopy. The bulla of pemphigus is therefore intra-epidermal, the epidermo-dermal junction remaining intact. Difficulties in interpretation may occasionally occur where the skin is examined after intensive treatment. When formal biopsy for any reason is difficult, for example when the lesions are confined to the mouth, help may be obtained by examining stained scrapings from bullous areas and looking for acantholytic cells (the Tzanck test).

A circumscribed area of easily-ruptured bullae, often in the mouth, may precede the widespread eruption by many months. Eventually the mucous membranes and all the body surface may be involved, becoming eroded and exquisitely painful and tender. The bullae tend to arise from apparently normal skin. When, on treatment, healing takes place there is usually pigmentation but no scarring. Nikolsky's sign − the demonstration of epidermal dissolution in apparently normal skin by sideways pressure with the finger − is positive; but it should not be regarded as diagnostic of pemphigus vulgaris since a somewhat similar sensation can be elicited in other bullous diseases. The patient is extremely ill. The serum albumin falls but other biochemical changes are inconstant. Post-mortem examination reveals no significant lesions in other systems.

Differential Diagnosis

Lesions confined to the mouth must be differentiated from aphthous ulcers (small, discrete), benign mucous membrane pemphigoid (*see* below) (associated with scarring) erythema multiforme (different in its course), and lichen planus (usually showing a typical white tracery as well as ulceration). Skin lesions may initially suggest impetigo or eczema but when fully developed the main differential diagnosis is from pemphigoid (*see* below). The distinction can usually be made on the pattern and morphology but atypical cases occur and the diagnosis is so important that histological examination is essential in all cases.

Treatment

Death in pre-steroid days was inevitable. High doses of corticosteroids are needed to gain control. A common error is to start with too low a dose. An initial dose of 150–200 mg prednisolone would be expected to be effective but if control is not achieved within a few days the dose should be raised by 50 per cent. In desperate cases intravenous ACTH can be added and may be life-saving, though the mechanism is obscure. When the lesions have been controlled the dose can be lowered but only after at least a week on the effective dose; the rate of reduction should become slower as the probable maintenance dose (15–30 mg daily) is reached. Obviously, care must be taken to check the urine and blood pressure in such cases. Enteric-coated prednisolone or alkalies with each dose may help if there are symptoms, or a history, of peptic disease.

In view of the immunological findings, methotrexate and azathioprine are now used. Methotrexate has serious adverse side-effects, mainly on the marrow and liver, and azathioprine is preferred. It is very important to remember that azathioprine seems to establish its effects slowly, often only after two or three weeks, and it is not therefore suitable for initial treatment; but it is useful in maintenance because of its steroid-sparing effects and many patients can be kept well on a fairly small dose of each drug. Even with adequate treatment, mortality (often from side-effects of the drugs) is still about 40 per cent. Jewish patients seem to fare worse than those of other races. A few patients may eventually go into remission but most cases appear to need maintenance treatment indefinitely.

There are several variants of pemphigus vulgaris which need not be discussed here in any detail. Pemphigus erythematodes, however, should be mentioned briefly. The patients are younger than those with pemphigus vulgaris and the condition has no predilection for Jews.

The pathology shows acantholytic bullae higher in the epidermis than those of pemphigus vulgaris. As in pemphigus vulgaris auto-antibodies to the intercellular substance have been demonstrated. In addition, there are immunological changes in the skin suggestive of lupus erythematosus. Moreover, the condition has been associated, probably significantly, with thymoma, myasthenia gravis and lupus erythematosus itself. Clinically, the lesions are often confined to the face and show moist scaling which can sometimes be difficult to differentiate from frank lupus erythematosus or seborrhoeic dermatitis. It may be that pemphigus erythematodes represents a combination of pemphigus vulgaris and lupus erythematosus.

Pemphigoid

Pemphigoid is much more common than any form of pemphigus. It has been differentiated relatively recently from pemphigus (hence its name) mainly on histological grounds; cases regarded in the past as pemphigus with a benign course were probably pemphigoid. It affects the elderly as a rule, of both sexes, and has no racial predilection.

The aetiology is unknown. The relationship of pemphigoid to malignant diseases has been the subject of much speculation. Cases have been reported associated with malignant melanoma and with carcinomata of various organs but in general the course of the malignancy does not correspond to that of the skin lesions. The significance of the association is difficult to evaluate in a disease occurring mainly in the elderly. Possibly the rare cases of pemphigoid with mucous membrane involvement are those most likely to be significantly associated with malignancy. Auto-immune processes are involved. Auto-antibodies to the basement membrane and complexes at that site can be demonstrated; there is no involvement, as there is in pemphigus, of the epidermal intercellular zones.

The bullae are subepidermal and may contain eosinophils. Acantholysis is not seen. Regeneration may result in an apparently intraepidermal bulla, so recent lesions must be examined.

For a variable period there may be only a nonspecific rash. The typical eruption, however, consists of bullae which are tense and often on an erythematous base. As in pemphigus, only a small area may initially be involved. Later the rash becomes widespread, with somewhat urticarial plaques studded with blisters. The rash usually itches. The mucous membranes are rarely affected. When healing occurs, there is no scarring.

Differential Diagnosis

Pemphigoid may be distinguished from pemphigus by the lack of mucosal involvement, the tense bullae on an erythematous base, the itching, and the differences in age and race. However, not all cases are absolutely clear-cut and histology is of great importance. Pemphigoid may usually be distinguished from erythema multiforme by the more widespread rash, the absence of target lesions, and the clinical course; here again in doubtful cases the histology is decisive.

Treatment

Corticosteroids — usually 60–100 mg of prednisolone daily at first — are effective. The maintenance dose tends to be about 10–20 mg daily. Azathioprine is of value though it is slow to take effect. As in pemphigus, it has a steroid-sparing effect.

The general outlook is good although the frail elderly patient may succumb to the disease or to its treatment. A certain proportion of cases will go into a spontaneous remission, some within a year, whereas some will continue to require treatment for many years. Valid figures are hard to obtain as patients may die from unrelated causes.

Benign Mucous Membrane Pemphigoid

This is a rare condition characterized by subepidermal bullae which leave scarring. There is no evidence of auto-immune phenomena in the skin. Its importance lies in its predilection for mucous membranes. Adhesions and obliteration of natural spaces may lead to blindness, dysphagia and difficulty in micturition.

Herpes Gestationis

This is a rare disease of pregnancy characterized by widespread subepidermal bullae. Clinically and histologically the picture resembles pemphigoid. It may occur for the first time in the puerperium and will then recur in subsequent pregnancies at an earlier stage. Progestogens have been suspected as aetiological factors and certainly recurrences in the non-pregnant patient may be triggered off by the contraceptive pill.

Dermatitis Herpetiformis

Dermatitis herpetiformis is uncommon and usually affects the young or middle-aged, men more than women.

The aetiology is unknown though immune processes may be involved (*see* below).

The bulla is subepidermal, without acantholysis, and contains eosinophils. There is an eosinophilic and polymorphonuclear dermal inflammation and often blood eosinophilia.

The rash is symmetrical and pleomorphic, consisting of vesicles, bullae, erythematous papules, and urticarial plaques. Sites usually affected are the buttocks, scalp, shoulders, and extensor elbows and knees. The mucous membranes are rarely affected. Itching is typically intense and often results in excoriated bullae and consequent difficulty in obtaining histological evidence.

Differential Diagnosis

The diagnosis of dermatitis herpetiformis is often difficult to make. Scabies can be confused but it is rarely that a burrow cannot be found to diagnose it positively; patchy eczema may be distinguishable from dermatitis herpetiformis only by histological examination. Erythema multiforme and pemphigoid can usually be distinguished by their course and pattern as well as by their histology.

Treatment

Corticosteroids systemically are of doubtful value, although locally they may help to allay itching. Dapsone is effective; so much so that it may be used as a diagnostic test. The drug may cause mild methaemoglobinaemia and haemolytic anaemia. It has been shown not to be taken up preferentially by the skin, and the mechanism of its action is unknown. The doses of dapsone required to treat dermatitis herpetiformis are of the order of 50–150 mg daily — very much larger than those used to treat leprosy. The dose required varies considerably from patient to patient; the explanation of this finding may lie in the widely differing serum levels which have been found. Sulphapyridine is of some use if dapsone cannot be tolerated. The course is chronic.

Dermatitis Herpetiformis and Enteropathy

Over the last few years it has been established that at least 70 per cent of patients with dermatitis herpetiformis have histological evidence of an enteropathy, more marked in the upper than in the lower small intestine. The mucosa is flat or convoluted as in coeliac disease; microscopic evidence of lymphocytic infiltration may be a more valuable and sensitive indicator than macroscopic changes. The enteropathy is by no means always associated with symptoms, but many patients tend to be underweight in relation to their height. As one would expect, there is often evidence of a deficiency in folate and iron. Moreover, both histological and blood changes improve on a gluten-free diet, and diarrhoea, if it has been present, abates. The enteropathy has been demonstrated in patients who have never had dapsone, so this drug cannot be the cause. Coeliac disease itself, however, is rarely accompanied by a rash and very few patients with dermatitis herpetiformis have symptoms or signs typical of fully developed coeliac disease.

The general view is that the enteropathy and the rash are not causally related and that the link may be genetic. An opposing view suggests that the enteropathy causes the rash and its supporters claim that the rash improves with a gluten-free diet though only over a long period. Not all workers, however, agree that such improvement occurs. Moreover, dermatitis herpetiformis has been known to appear for the first time in a patient on a gluten-free diet, and in one patient on such a diet milk seemed to provoke the disease.

Recently, immunological studies have been brought to bear on the question. Thyroid microsomal auto-antibodies and perhaps gastric auto-antibodies and antinuclear antibodies are found in a significant proportion of patients with dermatitis herpetiformis, and serum IgM levels tend to be low. Antireticulin antibodies have been found in the serum in dermatitis herpetiformis and in coeliac disease. Furthermore, IgA immunoglobulin deposits have been found in the dermal papillae (probably on the reticulin) in uninvolved skin or almost all dermatitis herpetiformis patients tested, but in scarcely any patients with coeliac disease or in control patients. The hypothesis has therefore been put forward that reticulin in dermatitis herpetiformis is abnormal in skin and gut, and in coeliac disease only in gut; reticulin cross-reacts with gluten, thus accounting for the skin lesions of dermatitis herpetiformis. This would seem a useful and stimulating hypothesis. However, it has been challenged by, among others, those who think that the primary abnormality in the gut, at least in coeliac disease and perhaps, therefore, in dermatitis herpetiformis, is in the basement membrane rather than in the reticulin which may be only secondarily involved. These and other immunological findings await clarification.

The practical problem is how far one should investigate a patient with dermatitis herpetiformis but without bowel symptoms or obvious signs. The investigations are not altogether pleasant, and a gluten-free diet is expensive and difficult to follow. On the other hand, there is an increased risk of neoplasia in untreated coeliac disease, which, as we have seen, is indistinguishable from the enteropathy of dermatitis herpetiformis. Moreover, reticulum cell sarcoma of the gut has recently been reported in dermatitis herpetiformis treated with dapsone only.

BULLOUS VARIANTS OF NORMALLY NON-BULLOUS DERMATOSES

Urticaria Pigmentosa

This condition is one example of cutaneous mastocytosis. The melanin in the epidermis is increased and collections of mast cells are seen in the dermis. Histamine, and possibly other substances, are released with friction or spontaneously and cause increased vascular permeability and consequent accumulation of fluid. Bulla formation, when it occurs, is therefore primarily subepidermal.

There are widespread reddish-brown nodules and macules, tending to urticate on friction. Occasionally there is evidence of systemic masto-cytosis. There is a childhood and an adult form; the former tends to clear spontaneously, the latter to persist. Bullae, when they occur, do so mainly in children.

Lichen Planus

This fairly common condition is of unknown aetiology. Similar or identical appearances, however, can be provoked by various drugs. It may be a reaction pattern set off by various agents.

There is epidermal thickening, particularly in the granular layer, with a dense upper dermal infiltrate. The infiltrate extends up to the epidermis and there is often liquefaction degeneration of the basal cell layer. Consequently, bulla formation, when it occurs, takes place between the epidermis and dermis.

Usually there is a characteristic eruption of shiny, violaceous, flat-topped polygonal papules, often confluent and forming annular or reticulate patterns. Sometimes white dots or streaks can be seen on the surface of the papules. Lesions may occur along scratch marks. The condition often also affects the mucous membranes, particularly the oral mucosa, where a milky-white network is seen.

The course of the condition is variable. It may last for months and then clear, to return later on occasion.

Bullae are uncommon but are seen in a few cases and may even dominate the picture.

CONCLUSION

It will now have become apparent that, in this heterogeneous group of conditions, bullae may resemble one another to the naked eye and yet differ histologically. They may have broadly similar appearances on light microscopy and yet be the end result of widely differing pathological processes. The dynamic aspects of such processes may sometimes now be made clear by immunofluorescence techniques and by electron microscopy which can, for example, distinguish between several mechanisms of dermo-epidermal separation. The same considerations apply to the vesicular dermatoses, which have not been discussed here, in that the vesicles are produced by several different mechanisms.

However, for practical purposes, most common and important bullous dermatoses can be adequately distinguished by clinical appearances, with or without histological examination.

A further useful point to bear in mind is that common things commonly occur: thus in infants and children one's first thoughts would be of impetigo and insect bites; in adults of insect bites, erythema multiforme and drug eruptions; and in the elderly of pemphigoid.

REFERENCES

Rook, A., Wilkinson, D. S. and Ebling, F. J. G. (1972). *Textbook of Dermatology.*, 2nd edition, Vol 2, Chapter 42. Oxford: Blackwell Scientific Publications.
Braun-Falco, O. (1969). 'Pathology of Blister Formation.' In *Year Book of Dermatology* Ed by A. W. Kopf and R. Andrade. Chicago: Chicago Year Books Medical Publishers.

12

Serum Enzymes in Diagnosis

T. L. Dormandy

INTRODUCTION

For some time in the early 1960's serum enzymes promised — or threatened — to eclipse all other diagnostic tests in clinical chemistry. That enzymic activity in serum could be used for diagnosis had of course been known for decades — the serum amylase test dates back to the beginning of the century — and the field is still open. But the time is now gone when every week produced its serum-enzyme novelty and when the possibility was seriously entertained that a clutch of these tests would eventually pinpoint the site, severity, nature and prognosis of every disease. This is, of course, the way of all fashion. What is more remarkable is that after such a period of concentrated interest the nature and meaning of these measurements is still widely misunderstood.

No attempt will be made here to review all the serum-enzyme tests that have been described, promoted and abandoned; they number over 100, discounting innumerable technical variations. It is still worth looking at some common principles, however, and considering how they apply — or should apply — to the currently standard repertory.

GENERAL PRINCIPLES

The Function of Serum Enzymes

Most plasma constituents whose concentration one measures in the laboratory have some definite physiological or pathological function; and clinical pathologists are occasionally asked what the function of serum enzymes is. Unlike most questions about enzymes this one can be answered in a word. So far as is known they have none. Serum enzymes

273

are exhaust products which have retained some of the specific catalytic properties but none of the catalytic functions of intracellular enzymes. The exceptions to this rule are, of course, the enzymes which act on blood itself — for example, those concerned in clotting, fibrinolysis and transport. They are best treated separately. The enzymes commonly grouped under the heading of diagnostic enzymology have but one role; they are tools in laboratory diagnosis.

The Origin of Serum Enzymes

That the cells of the body (with few exceptions) are continuously destroyed and renewed is a familiar fact. It is less well known generally that the proteins which largely make up these cells are also — and at a much faster rate — continuously broken down and replaced. Why this should be so is a question of great philosophical but little practical interest; the death of human beings and their replacement by individuals who must look indistinguishable through an intergalactic microscope is presumably governed by the same principle of creative extravagance. What matters from the practical point of view is that normal serum-enzyme activity is essentially a reflection of this intracellular molecular turnover. In cells whose life-span as morphological entities may be 100 days the life-span of a single phosphatase molecule may be only a few hours. Its useful life-span as a catalyst may be less. Enzymes, like cells, tissues, organs, and individuals, suffer from constant wear and tear, and, as with larger units, nature deals with the problem by replacement rather than by repair. This is the basis of diagnostic enzymology. What one measures in the laboratory are the time-worn enzymic discards which, to a varying degree and for varying lengths of time, carry into extracellular fluid their intracellular catalytic past.

The Mechanism of Raised Serum Enzymes

The diagnostic value of serum enzymes is limited today not by a shortage of tests or imperfections in techniques; nor even by a lack of skill and money. It is limited by a failure to understand how abnormal results arise and therefore what in pathological terms they mean. The mechanism originally envisaged — that of disintegrating cells spilling their enzyme content into the extracellular fluid — had the merit of simplicity but none other; it soon became clear that spectacular increases in serum-enzyme activity could accompany minimal (if any) demonstrable cell destruction. A modification of the doctrine was then propounded; that cells need only be damaged by disease to develop an enzyme 'leak'. This notion, too, is contradicted every day both at the

274

bedside and at the bench, yet it is still copied from textbook to text-book.

Let it be supposed that one wanted to raise the serum transaminase in an experimental animal by an intravenous drip, and that one wanted to maintain the raised level for several days (in imitation of a myocardial infarction). If one used healthy heart muscles as the source material it would be necessary to destroy many *whole* hearts to extract sufficient transaminase to complete the experiment. Even more hypothetically one might conceive a state in which the plasma membranes of an otherwise normal myocardium suddenly became totally permeable to transaminase. Calculations based on indirect evidence suggest that the consequent rise in serum transaminase would be slight and transient, yet a tenfold increase sustained over many days is common in clinical practice and is still attributed to leakage from a minute portion of the heart.

It has already been suggested that normal serum enzymes are the exhaust products of normal cells. The sustained steep increases in disease can have only two explanations. In a few instances the rise undoubtedly depends on more cells turning over the enzyme (the raised serum acid phosphatase in carcinoma of the prostate can serve as an example). But in most cases the raised serum enzyme reflects a vastly increased *rate* of molecular turnover in the parent tissue. The point is so fundamental and yet so rarely made that it seems permissible to revert to the childish analogy of a car engine. Even the most economical and best-maintained machine will waste potential fuel in its exhaust. A damaged or run-down machine will waste more. But the main variable which determines wastage is not the state of the engine but the speed at which it is running. The same principle applies to cells. Damaged cells may lose marginally more intracellular proteins than undamaged ones; but from the point of view of serum enzymes this is relatively unimportant. What sends extracellular enzyme activity soaring is the fact that under certain conditions intracellular molecular turnover increases ten-, twenty-, or one hundredfold.

The Causes of Increased Molecular Turnover

When a noxious agent — physical, chemical or biological — acts on living tissue, the response pattern can be arbitrarily divided into stages of stimulation, irritation, injury and death. During the stages of stimulation and irritation, cell activity — and in particular molecular turnover — increases enormously. Activity slows down as prolonged stress leads first to reversible and then to irreversible cell damage, and it ceases abruptly with cell death. Some diseases, including many virus infections, do not progress beyond the early stages, but even when the outcome is cell death there is an initial phase of vigorous counteraction. Only rarely does a devastating chemical, immunological or toxic insult extinguish a whole organ virtually outright. This accounts for the fact that the occasional case of fulminating pancreatitis or acute yellow atrophy of the liver kills rapidly with little or no rise in serum enzymes. With most lesions, moreover, there is a gradient of severity over an area as well as over a period. At the core of an infarct may be a few dead cells. Around them, often undetectable even with a microscope, is an area of irreversible damage. Around this is a much larger area of cellular hyperactivity, the response to irritation and stimulation. Some manifestations of this — for example, the redness or the oedema — are striking and familiar, but the cellular basis of the changes is an increased rate of intracellular molecular (including enzyme) turnover. It is this hyperactivity (not the few dead and damaged cells) which is responsible for the rise in extracellular enzymes. Because cells take time to respond to stress — just as an engine takes time to accelerate — the rise is characteristically delayed.

The changes in bone alkaline phosphatase after fractures are of little diagnostic use but they illustrate better than most naturally occurring diseases the underlying mechanism. A traffic accident causing multiple fractures clearly marks the moment of maximum tissue destruction. Yet not only is there no immediate rise in serum enzymes but usually several days or weeks must elapse (during which damaged cells might be presumed to be at their leakiest) before the rise begins. This rise, moreover, depends both on the type of fracture and on the treatment. Multiple fractures of long bones are usually treated with immobilization, and it is rare, despite the relative severity of injuries, for the alkaline phosphatase to reach a high peak. By contrast, multiple fractures of the ribs, a painful but comparatively trivial injury, cannot be effectively immobilized; and after 5–7 days they will often lead to a sharp increase in the serum enzyme. The pattern clearly reflects not cell damage but osteoblastic stimulation and activity.

Quantity Versus Activity

In one respect serum enzyme tests differ from other conventional clinical chemical estimations; they measure not quantities but activities. In Gowland Hopkin's memorable phrase, an enzyme is where it acts; and it is only by its action that one can demonstrate its presence. Since this action is that of a catalyst — that is, an accelerator of a specific chemical reaction — all enzyme estimations require a relatively complicated series of experiments. First, a control system is needed in

276

which a known biochemical transformation is allowed to proceed without the aid of an accelerator/enzyme/catalyst. Second, to a series of standards, more-or-less purified enzyme is added in varying concentrations. Third, the experiment is performed with a known amount of plasma added to the same reaction mixture. In all these one has to measure either the time it takes for a fixed amount of substrate to be transformed into the reaction products or the amount of substrate transformed during a fixed period of time. In neither case is it possible to measure the actual amount of enzyme in plasma as one measures plasma sugar, sodium, carbon dioxide or even plasma hormones. The practical implications are not always appreciated.

If plasma were a simple enzyme solution (comparable to the enzyme standards) or if enzymic reactions depended only on the substrate and enzyme concentrations, the clinical chemist's task would be easy. In fact, most enzymic reactions are exceedingly complex; they are influenced by such physical variables as temperature or ionic strength and they are critically affected by trace concentrations of chemical activators and inhibitors. Plasma in particular contains not only the enzyme one hopes to estimate but also a multitude of substances – some known and some not – any or all of which might influence the enzyme reaction. Of course, diagnostic enzyme tests are so designed that as many as possible of these variables are either standardized or eliminated (so that differences in reaction rates can be confidently ascribed to the enzyme), but nature and medical science combine to set a limit to such attempts at streamlining. Powerful new drugs are powerful for the very reason that they interfere with enzymic reactions in cells; and what they can do in cells in the living they can also do in plasma on the bench. This can lead both to false alarm and groundless optimism.

Because enzyme tests are such sensitive indicators of the effects of chemical poisons, they are rightly used in drug trials – for example, to detect incipient liver damage when a new antihypertensive is tried. A rise in serum transaminases will then be accepted as adequate reason – indeed often as an absolute indication – for stopping treatment. This may be the correct decision; if in doubt it is always better to err on the side of caution. But the drug or one of its metabolites circulating in plasma could also be an enzyme activator; and the *enhanced* transaminase reaction would automatically be reported and interpreted as an *increased* transaminase level.

Conversely, a drug may be hailed as an important advance on similar questionable evidence. The course of acute pancreatitis is notoriously difficult to assess on clinical findings alone; and the serum amylase is therefore widely used to monitor progress. When an enzyme inhibitor is introduced as a form of treatment – not unreasonably since many of the complications of the disease may be caused by enzymic 'auto-digestion' — the test can become a snare. There is no merit in inhibiting the serum amylase reaction as such (which most of these inhibitors do); one is merely throwing away a useful diagnostic tool. It certainly does not mean that more destructive enzymic digestion elsewhere is similarly inhibited. And yet a precipitous drop in serum amylase has been advanced as evidence for the efficacy of some of these drugs.

The widening gap between the bedside and the laboratory is largely to blame for such errors. Chemists measure ostensibly standardized reactions, unaware of the extraneous chemicals that have been fed into their system; and clinicians confidently interpret results whose doubtful origin remains shrouded in laboratory mystique. But neither can be absolved from responsibility. Clinicians cannot expect to be familiar with the chemical details of enzyme tests; but they can reasonably be expected to grasp the basic difference between an absolute quantity (for example, the blood urea) and measuring the catalytic influence of an unidentified molecule on an imperfectly characterized biochemical reaction.

The Fate of Serum Enzymes

No details are known about the degradation and elimination of intracellular proteins, and, since all enzymes are proteins, this applies to enzymes. Nor need clinicians be particularly concerned with this problem — except in the context of a comparatively common error. Whether their patient is in renal failure or has biliary obstruction, it is always unsafe to attribute a rise in serum enzymes to abnormal retention. Complete anuria by itself causes only a minimal increase, and, contrary to many textbooks, the same is probably true of complete obstruction to bile flow.

For collectors of rare biochemical syndromes (and verbal monstrosities) an exception may be mentioned. Amylase is among the smallest enzymes — its molecular weight is around 45000 — and much of it is therefore excreted in urine. In macroamylasaemia it is retained in serum either bound to a specific immunoglobulin or perhaps as a polymer. The condition is not associated with any clinical abnormality but does not, of course, exempt individuals from developing a surgical abdomen. The high serum amylase — it may be several thousands of Somogyi units — may then mislead the surgeon into diagnosing pancreatitis. A normal urinary amylase with a raised serum level should give the diagnostic clue.

Names and Units

Clinical chemists are much attracted by the precise language of organic chemistry, and one must regret that their inclinations often exceed their means. After a period of expansion diagnostic enzymology in the 1960's was — or seemed to be — ripe for terminological reform. Eponymous units proliferated. King, Armstrong, Bodansky, Gutman, Shinovara, Jones, Bassey and Lowry are but a pick of the names which had become associated with the alkaline phosphatase test alone. And commercial firms, marketing their expensive but labour-saving kits, were quick to add their quota of fancy. Many of these units were based on methods reproducible only by their inventors and sometimes not even by them; and that deplorable cliché, 'a slight modification of', was their only saving grace or disgrace. One must therefore admire the international commissions (or at least not begrudge them their fun) who strove long and hard to bring logic and uniformity to the subject. Unfortunately, serum enzymes are not pure chemical preparations and the conditions under which they must perform in clinical laboratories do not lend themselves to rigorous standardization. The new system took no account — indeed it could not — of local skills, idiosyncrasies, loyalties and prejudices. Clinicians not unreasonably preferred woolly but simple terms to precise but incomprehensible definitions; and even by the debased standards of chemical latin much of the new coinage was a linguistic outrage. Nevertheless, a system of international units expressed in terms of litres of plasma (but which plasma?) now exists and is regarded by some as a significant advance. Others continue to use King, Bodansky, Armstrong, or various home-made combinations; and (so far as the present writer is concerned) long may they flourish.

Isoenzymes

Isoenzymes are a somewhat ill-defined concept and for everyday use they are probably best defined in methodological terms. They are a family of enzymes which are indistinguishable by their biochemical action — that is, they are isodynamic — but more-or-less easily distinguishable by their physical properties. To this one must add a half-apology. It may be remembered that there are at least a dozen phosphatases in every cell (whether acid or alkaline simply depends on the pH at which they are at their catalytic best) and literally thousands in the body. It is therefore unlikely that the few isoenzymes which separate on gel electrophoresis are truly homogeneous at the molecular level. Nor is it, strictly speaking, true that isoenzymes are indistinguishable by their biochemical action; it would be better to say that, beyond a certain point, it is technically easier to identify them by their physical properties – their molecular size, their electrophoretic mobility, their sedimentation constant, or their heat stability – than by subtle differences in their catalytic performance. Generally speaking enzymes which promote the same (or a similiar) reaction but which are derived from different species, different cells, or different parts of the same cell, are potentially at least identifiable as different molecules; and, when they are, they can be dignified by the name of isoenzyme.

In practice, the separation of isoenzymes has a limited but real diagnostic value. It can give differential measure of the alkaline phosphatases derived from bone and from liver respectively when one or other organ is not obviously diseased or when both may be abnormal, and it will occasionally reveal a large (and still largely unexplained) increase in 'intestinal phosphatase'. A placental isoenzyme appears in late pregnancy. Isoenzyme techniques are used to measure prostatic and breast acid phosphatase specifically, to distinguish pancreatic from parotid amylase, and to select a heart-specific lactate dehydrogenase. The last is one of 5 isoenzymes which represent different combinations of two basic monomers – the only instance so far where the distinction is based on insight into molecular structure.

THE CURRENT REPERTORY

Serum Amylase

This is the oldest and still one of the most useful serum enzyme tests. It would, perhaps, be even more useful if its diagnostic value in mumps were more widely recognized. The level begins to rise in contacts several days or even weeks before the parotid swelling – in time, that is, to enable one to cancel the holiday cottage. In emergency surgery the test is, of course, virtually diagnostic of acute pancreatitis. It is true that the serum amylase can increase as a result of a penetrating or perforating gastroduodenal ulcer, in acute cholecystitis or in any condition causing upper abdominal (and therefore pancreatic) irritation; and a raised level as such is not therefore synonymous with primary pancreatic disease. Emergency laboratory tests should, however, be used to arrive at therapeutic decisions, not to make precise diagnoses. The normal serum-amylase level is less than 150 Somogyi units (less than 300 iu/l). In a patient admitted with the classical features of an acute abdominal catastrophe from a perforation or cholecystitis the serum amylase is often raised to 400–500 units but almost never higher. If the symptoms and signs are due to pancreatitis and if, therefore, an emergency operation is contra-indicated, the serum amylase is rarely less than 1000 units.

Serum Enzymes in Myocardial Infarction

Many serum enzymes are raised in myocardial infarction, and the latest test is generally claimed to be the best. Best in this context usually means most specific, or earliest to show a rise, or both. It rarely means — as it should — most easily reproducible from one laboratory to another and therefore most reliable in the average hospital. The enzymes most widely used are the aspartate transaminase (normal: 4–15 iu/1), formerly glutamic oxalo-acetic transaminase or GOT (normal: 9–32 units), the lactate dehydrogenase (normal: 60–150 iu/1), the 'heart-specific' lactate dehydrogenase isoenzyme (normal: 50–150 iu/l), and the phosphocreatine kinase (4–60 iu/l). The last is said to show a rise a few hours before the rest. Two enzyme tests are often better than one, and three may be marginally better than two, but if one, two or three are equivocal it is unlikely that six will provide a clear answer. The differential diagnosis on the basis of serum enzyme results is usually between myocardial infarction on the one hand and either liver disease or a pulmonary infarction on the other. In liver disease virtually all known serum enzymes tend to be raised; and in proportion the 'heart enzymes' are usually less raised than the others. For example, the isocitric dehydrogenase, 5-nucleotidase, the slow-moving lactate dehydrogenase isoenzyme (LD_5) are relatively higher than the aspartate transaminase (GOT) or the fast-moving lactate dehydrogenase iso-enzymes (LD_1 and LD_2). In pulmonary infarction the lactate dehydrogenase is usually markedly raised whereas the aspartate transaminase (GOT) is either normal or only slightly raised (an underused chemical test in this differential diagnosis is the serum bilirubin which often shows a transient but early rise in pulmonary but not in cardiac infarction).

Serum Enzymes in Skeletal Muscle Disease

The serum phosphocreatine kinase has now supplanted the serum aldolase as the enzyme test most commonly used in skeletal muscle disease. It is said to be a particularly sensitive index of the Duchenne type hereditary dystrophy and *may* detect clinically unaffected carriers or affected siblings before obvious clinical signs. The pathological process recorded by serum enzyme tests, however, must be remembered; one is measuring not cell degeneration but cell reactivity. This means that the result may be normal in a chair-ridden chronic invalid and grossly abnormal in a mild but widespread myopathy (it often shows an abnormal rise in the comparatively mild myopathy of myxoedema). It should also be remembered that it takes 6–12 hours before enzyme levels in the serum begin to reflect stress in the tissues. It is therefore a misguided effort – though misguided in the right direction – to try and provoke a response in a borderline case by making the patient run up and down stairs immediately before the blood sample is collected. It is more reasonable to try and collect blood after a day of strenuous physical activity.

Serum Alkaline Phosphatase in Bone Disease

The alkaline phosphatase released into serum by bone is the product of osteoblasts and an abnormal rise reflects increased osteoblastic activity. Bone destruction alone does not cause a rise. An increase from the normal 3–13 King–Armstrong units (this equals 1–4 Bodansky units) to about 40 units, is common in a variety of skeletal disorders – for example, rickets, hyperparathyroidism, or the healing stage of fractures. A great increase – and the level may exceed 100 units – is almost diagnostic of Paget's disease. A further sharp spurt may signal sarcomatous change in Paget bone. Secondary carcinomatous deposits, especially in the long bones and vertebral column, often cause a slight to moderate rise so long as the patient is active and ambulant. The level may fall after admission for a pathological fracture or for some other complication which confines the patient to bed. If treatment with cytotoxic drugs, hormones or irradiation is started at the same time the fall may be attributed to regression of the tumour. The real reason in most cases is removal of mechanical stress.

The expression 'abnormal rise' must be qualified in the case of children; during periods of fast skeletal growth the serum-enzyme level may reach 20–25 King–Armstrong units. Reliable information about patients at the other extreme of life is scarce and contradictory (as is true for most serum enzymes). Work in progress in the geriatric unit at this hospital suggests that an otherwise unexplained rise in alkaline phosphatase in the elderly is usually caused by the 'liver' enzyme. The bone enzyme rises in osteomalacia, a condition in which poor mineralization puts extra strain on the osteoblasts. In osteoporosis, in which the osteoblasts themselves are defective, the bone enzyme is normal.

Bone alkaline phosphatase is the only serum enzyme which has diagnostic value when absent (or at any rate abnormally low). In the rare hereditary disorder of hypophosphatasia the patient presents with a rickets-like condition and an unexpectedly low or undetectable serum alkaline phosphatase. There is a corresponding increase in the concentration of phosphorylethanolamine (and other presumed substrates) in the urine.

Serum Acid Phosphatase

As with most serum enzymes one can construct a long list of conditions in which an occasional rise in the serum acid phosphatase had been reported. Such compilations are meaningless at best. In clinical practice when the estimation is done by a reliable laboratory the enzyme is virtually specific for carcinoma of the prostate. The proviso is necessary because interfering acid phosphatases can, and should, be eliminated by pre-treating the serum. The normal range is 0'5–3 King–Armstrong units. A level of 5 units or above is diagnostic of prostatic cancer. Conversely, a normal result excludes the diagnosis – with three reservations. First, there must be a true increase in the number of cells which elaborate the enzymes. In other words no rise can be expected from those microscopic growths which are said to be common when looked for specifically in unselected post-mortem series on elderly men. Second, at the opposite extreme from these minute and clinically insignificant lesions, the most undifferentiated and fastest-killing sarcomatous tumours may not produce specific enzymes. Third, treatment with oestrogens will suppress cell activity and the serum acid phosphatase will drop and may even return to normal. This does not mean actual regression of tumour.

These comments apply to men only. In women a breast-specific serum acid phosphatase may rise in carcinoma of the breast; but the test has found little favour in routine diagnosis.

Serum Enzymes in Liver Disease

No organ in the body has a biochemical repertory remotely comparable to that of the liver; it is not therefore surprising that liver disease has become the *locus classicus* of the use and misuse of serum enzymes. Repetition of a few basic principles may help to guard against the latter.

First, unlike most other liver-function tests – for example, thymol turbidity, serum albumin, serum bilirubin – serum enzymes measure the active response of liver cells to a variety of harmful or potentially harmful stimuli; and the intensity of this response bears only a tenuous relation to the severity or prognosis of the disease. A virus hepatitis is usually a comparatively mild though disagreeable illness from which most patients recover. Yet, for the very reason that most hepatic viruses irritate but do not kill their host cells, they can provoke a steeper rise in serum enzymes than many drastic or even fatal poisons.

Second, because serum enzymes reflect cell response, not cell damage as such, the levels begin to rise and may even reach their peak before the disease becomes clinically manifest. More precisely, the peak is often reached before jaundice gives the diagnosis away. In general practice serum enzyme tests could often lead to earlier diagnosis and prevent the indiscriminate prescription of 'anti-nausea' remedies, many of which are hepatotoxic.

Third, because serum-enzyme tests in liver disease do not measure the amount of tissue destroyed a chronic cirrhotic can die for sheer lack of liver with near-normal enzyme results. On the other hand, in a smouldering illness the enzymes can provide a seismographic (if somewhat delayed) record of repeated minor insults. They will, if required, faithfully monitor a medium-sized hangover.

The 'liver enzymes' which are still most widely used are the transaminases. Except on rare occasions when a relatively greater rise in aspartate transaminase (GOT) compared to alanine transferase (GPT) points to the myocardium rather than to the liver as the site of disease, there is little point in performing both. The isocitric dehydrogenase (normal: 1–7 iu/l) and a number of other enzymes provide roughly the same information; the so-called liver alkaline phosphatase and the serum 5-nucleotidase deserve special mention.

The 'Liver' Alkaline Phosphatase

The 'liver' alkaline phosphatase is still often described as a measure of biliary obstruction on the hypothetical ground that it is excreted in bile and retained when bile-flow is blocked. The enzyme is largely a product of the biliary epithelium and its rise in serum reflects over-activity, hyperplasia or neoplasia of this tissue. It is true, of course, that obstructive lesions almost always affect the duct system and therefore cause a rise; there is, however, no direct correlation between the enzyme level and the depth of jaundice as measured by the serum bilirubin. The highest levels are seen in carcinomas which actually arise from biliary epithelium, 100 units or over being virtually diagnostic. High levels can also be reached after repeated attacks of ascending cholangitis punctuated by attempts at surgical correction and long spells of in-dwelling tubes. In this syndrome each acute episode leaves the patient with a higher resting level than the one before; and eventually 60–80 units may come to represent a base line during quiescent periods, even in the absence of jaundice.

The hepatotoxic effect of most drugs is due to interference with the metabolic activity of liver cells and is sensitively reflected by a rise in the serum transaminases. Some drugs, however — chlorpromazine being the best-known — affect the biliary epithelium rather than the hepatic parenchyma. The reason for the difference is unknown. Microscopically there is cellular proliferation of the lining of the bile canaliculi; this is accompanied by a rise in the serum alkaline phosphatase. Jaundice may be a comparatively late development and can sometimes be warded off by stopping the drug in time. Even after treatment has been discontinued, however, the serum enzyme may take weeks or months to return to normal.

The Serum 5-Nucleotidase

The serum 5-nucleotidase (normal: 2–15 iu/l) has had a quick rise to fame but now seems to be falling from favour (neither trend is necessarily related to its diagnostic merits and limitations). Like the liver alkaline phosphatase the enzyme reflects disease of the biliary tract rather than of the liver cells, but the results of the two tests do not usually move in parallel. This is not altogether surprising since the alkaline phosphatases are a large family of heterogeneous and mainly cytoplasmic enzymes, whereas the 5-nucleotidase is relatively specific and derived mainly from the cell nucleus. The principal role originally assigned to the latter was to help to decide whether an obscure rise in alkaline phosphatase is of hepatic or of bony origin; but this particular question can be more reliably answered by the separation of the alkaline phosphatase isoenzymes. A better recommendation is that occasionally the 5-nucleotidase is the only — or the earliest — test to point to some hepatobiliary abnormality.

Serum Cholinesterase

This enzyme was originally known as pseudocholinesterase and introduced (not very successfully) as a liver-function test. It is now used to detect a rare inborn error of metabolism. A number of derivatives of succinyl-choline are used in anaesthesia as muscle relaxants. After a period of paralysis (due to interference with chemical neuromuscular transmission) the drug is normally inactivated by the enzyme cholinesterase. The activity of the enzyme is low in liver disease. More important the enzyme is defective in about one out of every 4000 people; and when the customary dose of the relaxant is given to such individuals their paralysis is prolonged and may end in death. It is, perhaps, arrogant to call the condition an inborn 'error' and the enzyme 'defective'; nature could hardly have foreseen the routine therapeutic administration of potentially lethal arrow-poison. The current method for detecting the abnormality is to expose the serum enzyme to the quaternary ammonium compound dibucaine and measure its effect on enzyme activity. The enzyme of abnormal homozygotes is inhibited by 20 per cent dibucaine (dibucaine number 20), whereas the inhibitory concentration in normals is 80 per cent or over (dibucaine number 80). Heterozygous carriers give intermediate values. The enzyme is also inhibited *in vivo* by a number of organophosphorus insecticides used in agriculture and industry.

CONCLUSION

In many ways serum enzymes epitomize the advances and paradoxes of modern laboratory diagnosis. They have great potential value for recording disease *activity* but, because activity is an elusive concept, their actual value depends on close understanding between the wards and the laboratory. This is becoming more, not less, difficult.

For full advantage to be taken of the versatility of serum enzymes they ought to be studied in combinations appropriate to individual cases. Yet these tests are now generally available as a result of widespread automation, and automated mass-production and individual service are as incompatible in clinical chemistry as they are in any other enterprise.

Lastly, serum enzyme tests are often alone in showing up disease processes which do not fit the overall picture — or at least the labels which have become attached to them. This can lead to better and earlier diagnosis but it can also lead to much unnecessary and officious investigation.

13

Multiple Choice Questions and Case Presentations

THE MEMBERSHIP EXAMINATION

THE MEMBERSHIP EXAMINATION

The appropriate regulations should be obtained from the Royal College of Physicians, St Andrews Place, London NW1, since changes take place from time to time.

Part 1

This consists of 60 multiple choice questions. Each question is composed of an initial statement or 'stem' followed be a number of possible completions or 'items' identified by A, B, C, D etc. The number of true or false items for each stem will vary but although, as a rule, some of the items are true and some false, it is possible for all items to be true or for all to be false.

Part 2

This part of the examination is in three sections, the first being a written test, the second an oral test, and the third a clinical test.

The Written Section

This consists of case histories, interpretation of data, and slide interpretation.

(1) *Case Histories.* In this section candidates are offered five case histories, and are asked to answer questions on three of them. At least one of the cases is paediatric. The questions are designed to test problem-solving ability requiring the application of general principles.

(2) *Interpretation of Data.* Candidates are asked to identify abnormalities and answer specific clinically-orientated questions on ECG's and laboratory data, etc.

(3) *Slide Interpretation.* Candidates are shown a series of slides projected on a screen and are asked to identify abnormalities and answer specific questions on them. The slides include x-rays, clinical photographs and other material.

The Oral Examination

This is designed to assess the candidate's understanding of basic principles and his capacity to deal with clinical situations including emergencies. He is expected to be able to devize a plan of management for a given clinical situation.

The Clinical Section

In this section the candidate has one hour in which to examine a long case and should take a full history with a careful physical examination. He should try to assess the clinical problem as a whole taking into account the patient's personality and social background. It is a good policy to have decided on a differential diagnosis and plan of management of the case before meeting the examiner. These are questions on which the candidate would have reached some conclusion from the result of his findings.

The short cases offer an opportunity to elicit and interpret physical signs and are a test of clinical acumen and experience.

The multiple choice questions, and case histories in this chapter can be regarded as typical. It is a mistake to look for 'catches'; the questions are designed to test knowledge in as straightforward a manner as possible. In most instances the questions and case histories are related to the content of the chapters. Answers begin on page 303.

MULTIPLE CHOICE QUESTIONS

1. THE FOLLOWING DRUGS MAY BE USED
    THERAPEUTICALLY TO LOWER SERUM CHOLESTEROL:
    A. L-thyroxine
    B. Procainamide
    C. Clofibrate (Atromid-S)
    D. Cholestyramine
    E. Nicotinic acid

2. THE SERUM CHOLESTEROL IS USUALLY RAISED IN:
    A.   Nephrotic syndrome
    B.   Hypothyroidism secondary to hypopituitarism
    C.   Xanthoma tuberosum
    D.   Myelomatosis
    E.   Diabetic ketosis

3. DIFFUSE PULMONARY FIBROSIS MAY BE THE RESULT OF:
    A.   Exposure to tin
    B.   Exposure to aluminium
    C.   Exposure to cadmium
    D.   Treatment with methotrexate
    E.   Treatment with methyldopa
    F.   Treatment with nitrofurantoin

4. ASTHMA IS A RECOGNIZED COMPLICATION OF:
    A.   Treatment with indomethacin
    B.   Treatment with a β-adrenergic receptor stimulant
    C.   Treatment with sodium fusidate
    D.   Systemic lupus erythematosus (SLE)
    E.   Pulmonary embolism
    F.   Infestation with echinococcus granulosus

5. IN ACUTE POST-INFECTIVE POLYNEUROPATHY
    (GUILLAIN–BARRE SYNDROME):
    A.   There is clinical evidence of meningeal irritation
    B.   Objective sensory loss may be mild in degree
    C.   CSF protein may be normal early in the neurological illness
    D.   Death may occur from disturbances of function of the
         autonomic nervous system
    E.   Cranial nerve palsies are rare
    F.   The pathological process affects mainly the distal portion of
         the peripheral nerves

6. PATIENTS WITH NON-METASTATIC (CARCINOMATOUS)
    PERIPHERAL NEUROPATHY:
    A.   May have high CSF protein levels
    B.   Often have diplopia
    C.   May show spontaneous remissions
    D.   Frequently have slowing of motor and sensory nerve
         conduction velocities
    E.   May have the neurological disability for months before a
         malignant disorder can be discovered
    F.   Usually have more damage to axones than to myelin sheaths
         and Schwann cells

7. A MAN OF 55 HAS HAD DIABETES FOR 10 YEARS. HE HAS INTERMITTENT PROTEINURIA. HE SUDDENLY LOSES VISION IN ONE EYE.
    A. The loss of vision is probably due to a retinal haemorrhage
    B. A renal biopsy will probably show Kimmelstiel–Wilson lesions in the glomeruli
    C. Neurological examination will probably reveal a reduction of vibration sense in the legs
    D. He probably needs insulin to control the diabetes
    E. He is likely to have a family history of diabetes

8. CANNON WAVES ARE COMMONLY SEEN IN THE NECK IN:
    A. Atrial flutter
    B. Ventricular tachycardia
    C. Second degree AV block
    D. Complete (third degree) AV block
    E. Junctional tachycardia

9. THE FOLLOWING FINDINGS ARE SUGGESTIVE OF VENTRICULAR RATHER THAN ATRIAL TACHYCARDIA:
    A. Variable intensity of the first heart sound
    B. Wide splitting of the heart sounds
    C. Slowing of the heart rate with carotid sinus pressure
    D. Slight irregularity of the ventricular complexes on the electrocardiogram
    E. A pre-excitation pattern on the electrocardiogram after reversion to sinus rhythm

10. INTOXICATION WITH DIGOXIN:
    A. Is potentiated by hypokaliaemia
    B. Is potentiated by hypocalcaemia
    C. Causes anorexia
    D. Is likely in the presence of a plasma digoxin level of 1.0 ng/ml
    E. May cause a junctional tachycardia

11. IN THE NEPHROTIC SYNDROME IN ADULTS:
    A. The plasma volume is expanded
    B. There is a tendency for intravascular thrombosis to occur
    C. Highly selective proteinuria is an indication for corticosteroid therapy
    D. A blood urea of 200 mg/100 ml indicates a 'nephritic' as well as a 'nephrotic' component to the glomerular disease
    E. A low serum complement might favour a diagnosis of post-streptococcal glomerulonephritis

12. A MAN OF 60 PRESENTS WITH ADVANCED CHRONIC RENAL FAILURE. A POSSIBLE DIAGNOSIS OF CHRONIC GLOMERULONEPHRITIS IS STRENGTHENED BY FINDING:
    A. His urine contains protein ++++
    B. High dose intravenous pyelogram (IVP) reveals smooth symmetrical kidneys 13 cm in length
    C. The blood pressure is normal
    D. There has been no abdominal or loin pain
    E. There are many red blood corpuscles (RBC) and white blood corpuscles (WBC) in the urine
    F. There is a family history of 'kidney trouble'

13. ERYTHEMA MULTIFORME:
    A. May involve mucous membranes
    B. Has more than one cause
    C. Is commoner in Jews than in others
    D. Affects mainly the trunk
    E. Is characterized by blisters arising from normal skin

14. DRUGS MAY PRECIPITATE OR CAUSE THE FOLLOWING BLISTERING DISEASES:
    A. Pemphigoid
    B. Erythema multiforme
    C. Pemphigus vulgaris
    D. Toxic epidermal necrolysis
    E. Impetigo

15. IN ISCHAEMIC DISEASE OF THE COLON:
    A. The hepatic flexure is commonly involved
    B. Histological examination of a random rectal biopsy will usually reveal abnormalitites
    C. Barium enema should be performed within the first few days to reveal characteristic 'thumbprinting'
    D. Angiography will show occlusion or stenosis of the inferior mesenteric artery in most cases
    E. Up to a third of patients may develop a stricture at the site of damage

16. DIVERTICULA OF THE COLON:
    A. May give rise to bleeding having previously been asymptomatic
    B. Are associated with an increased risk of volvulus of the sigmoid colon in the elderly
    C. Will eventually give rise to symptoms in the majority of patients

    D.   May present with peritonitis in previously asymptomatic patients

    E.   When causing symptoms of diverticular disease, are best treated by a low residue diet

17. **REVERSE SPLITTING OF THE SECOND SOUND MAY BE FOUND IN:**

    A.   Left bundle branch block

    B.   Ischaemic heart disease

    C.   Ventricular septal defect

    D.   Hypertensive heart disease

    E.   Patent ductus arteriosus

    F.   Aortic stenosis

18. **PULSUS PARADOXUS MAY BE FOUND IN:**

    A.   Pericardial constriction or tamponade

    B.   Pulmonary embolism

    C.   Cardiac amyloidosis

    D.   Atrial septal defect

    E.   Obstructive airways disease

    F.   A flabby myocardium

19. **ENZYMES:**

    A.   Are essential components of both the cytoplasm and the nucleus of all cells

    B.   Are essential trace constituents of the diet

    C.   Are mainly nucleoproteins

    D.   Often incorporate a heavy metal as an integral part of the molecule

    E.   Require a cell or some other organized biological structure for activity

20. **A SERUM AMYLASE ACTIVITY OF 2800 SOMOGYI UNITS (= 5000 + iu/l) CAN BE REASONABLY ACCOUNTED FOR BY:**

    A.   Appendicectomy for an acutely inflamed unperforated appendix 12 hours previously

    B.   Acute epidemic parotitis (mumps)

    C.   Acute glomerulonephritis with oliguria and a rising blood urea for 3 days

    D.   Amyloid disease

    E.   A recent course of tetracycline for recurrent otitis media

21. **THE LATEX TEST FOR RHEUMATOID FACTOR IN THE SERUM IS POSITIVE IN SOME 10 PER CENT OF CASES IN:**

    A.   Psoriatic arthropathy

    B.   Subacute bacterial endocarditis (SBE)

C. Sarcoidosis
D. Still's disease
E. Sicca syndrome
F. Normal persons more than 65 years old

22. IN THE THERAPY OF THE RHEUMATIC DISEASES UNWANTED EFFECTS UPON THE BONE MARROW ARE A RECOGNIZED COMPLICATION OF:
A. Flufenamic acid
B. Azathioprine
C. Ibuprofen
D. Sodium aurothiomalate
E. Phenylbutazone
F. Corticosteroids

23. ADVANCED BONE AGE MAY BE FOUND IN THE FOLLOWING CONDITIONS IN CHILDHOOD:
A. Cushing's syndrome due to bilateral adrenal hyperplasia
B. Congenital adrenal hyperplasia
C. Hypothyroidism
D. Growth hormone deficiency
E. Precocious puberty
F. Administration of oestrogens to the mother during pregnancy

24. CRETINISM IS CHARACTERISTICALLY ASSOCIATED WITH:
A. Increase in linear growth
B. Prolonged jaundice in the neonatal period
C. Abnormality of the chromosomes
D. Mental retardation if untreated
E. Diarrhoea
F. Goitre

CASE HISTORIES

1

A retired car salesman, aged 69, was referred to hospital because of increasing unsteadiness on walking. He was a widower and lived on his own, doing his own shopping and cooking. He smoked 30 cigarettes a day but although, at one time, he had drunk spirits heavily, he now restricted himself to a pint of beer in the evenings.

Fifteen years ago he had experienced epigastric pain at night, culminating in a severe haematemesis. This failed to respond to transfusions and conservative treatment and so an emergency partial gastrectomy was performed. Twelve years ago he developed diabetes; his father had suffered from the same disorder. Although he tried to observe a diet for a time, the nature of his occupation made this impossible, though he never overate and always avoided sugar. He took tolbutamide (500 mg t.d.s.), but soon gave up testing his urine for sugar when the initial specimens were found to be sugar-free. Five years ago he had experienced difficulty in passing urine and was admitted to hospital for a prostatectomy; the diabetes was easy to control during the post-operative period. Subsequently, he was still troubled with frequency and urgency from time to time but never retention.

During the last 2 years his health had deteriorated. He had lost over a stone in weight, he tired easily, and was breathless on exertion. His bowels were open frequently, sometimes 5 or 6 times a day, and the motions were loose and bulky. His legs felt heavy and stiff, as though they did not belong to him, and his walking had become unsteady.

On examination he looked pale, tired and thin. The urine sample contained 1 per cent sugar, and 30 mg/100 ml protein but no acetone. His chest was emphysematous with generalized rhonchi. BP: 190/100. Heart sounds were distant but regular, and there were no bruits. JVP was not raised. Examination of the fundi revealed discrete white exudates on both sides. Neck movements were painful and restricted; in particular there was practically no lateral flexion. Arm reflexes were obtainable but more sluggish on the left. There was marked wasting of the first dorsal interossei muscles in both hands. In the legs, the thigh muscles were wasted with loss of power. Although tone seemed increased, the knee and ankle reflexes could not be obtained. The right plantar response was extensor, the left equivocal. There was loss of sensation to pin-prick, cotton wool, and vibration sense in both legs. Cranial nerves were normal.

Questions

    (1)   Suggest 5 likely causes for the unsteadiness of gait
    (2)   Name 5 investigations likely to help in the diagnosis

2

A 26-year-old woman who was undergoing treatment with amitriptyline for depression, went to a party at which she had a lot to eat and drink. That night, at 4 a.m., she awoke feeling intensely nauseated, and vomited copiously. This was followed at once by pain across the upper chest radiating down both arms. The pain steadily increased in severity and so she dialled 999 and was taken to hospital by ambulance. By the time she reached hospital 20 minutes later the pain had gone. The casualty officer could find no abnormal physical signs that he considered significant but, as a precaution he ordered a chest x-ray which showed no abnormality. He therefore sent her home. On the way home the pain recurred and so she returned to hospital. This time she was admitted to the ward. The physician found her to be tall at 184 cm (5 ft 10½ in) and thin (9st 2 lb); she was afebrile. She had a depressed sternum. Apart from a pulse rate of 88 with regular rhythm he found no abnormal physical signs.

Questions

(1)   What 3 conditions should be included in the differential diagnosis?

(2)   What special points should be elicited in the history?

(3)   What special points should be looked for on clinical examination?

(4)   What investigations should be ordered?

3

A 60-year-old male canteen assistant was referred because of malaise, pins and needles in the hands and feet, and weakness of the upper limbs. There was no significant family history. He smoked 1 oz of pipe tobacco daily, and had drunk up to 8 pints of beer each night until stopping work 2 months earlier — after this he drank beer only at weekends.

Six months before admission he had noticed that as he walked he would tend to go more and more slowly. This symptom was inter-mittent and he could not explain what was slowing him down — it did not appear to be pain. Two months previously he had given up work because he felt unable to cope with it, although his only symptom seemed to have been a general malaise. He developed an aching across both shoulder blades, and down both arms. This pain was worse at night and there seemed to be 'trigger spots' in the neck. He experienced pins and needles and numbness of the fingers of both hands with difficulty in holding small objects, especially in the left hand. His walking was described as shaky. He lost a few pounds in weight before admission to hospital.

He was found to have a normal temperature and pulse, his blood pressure being 170/100. There was no clubbing. Examination of the respiratory and cardiovascular systems, including peripheral arterial pulses, showed no abnormality. The liver edge, which was soft, was felt one finger breadth below the costal margin and was not tender. His fundi showed a marked retinopathy with widespread haemorrhages and microaneurysms. The pupils reacted normally and the other cranial nerves were normal. He had a severe weakness of both upper limbs, more marked proximally in the right arm and distally in the left. There was no wasting or fasciculation in upper or lower limbs. In the lower limbs he had slight general weakness. He had slight distal blunting of sensation to pin-prick and cotton wool in all four limbs. Vibration sense was lost in the feet. Position sense was impaired in the fingers and toes. Deep pain sensation in his calves was reduced. All the tendon reflexes were absent and both plantar responses were flexor. He walked with a waddling type of gait due to weakness of the pelvic girdle muscles, and, in addition, his walking was very unsteady. The urine contained large amounts of sugar, but no ketones.

Questions

(1) Suggest up to 4 possible causes for the neurological symptoms
(2) Suggest 6 investigations which might prove helpful in diagnosis

4

A 69-year-old woman, recently widowed, complained of pain in the left wrist, the fingers of both hands, the right hip and the knee. She had experienced this for the past 4 months. She also described episodes of stabbing pain extending down the whole length of the right leg to the foot. Lately, she had felt more tired, had taken longer to dress in the mornings, and had found her feet to be swollen by the end of the day. She had experienced no chest pain at any time and had not been breathless. She denied having any indigestion or disturbance of bowel habit but had lost a little weight without any attempt at dieting.

She had suffered no serious illness in the past and had no family history of arthritis of any kind. Her letter of referral mentioned that a latex test for rheumatoid factor had been negative.

On examination she was anxious and tearful. Clinically she did not appear anaemic; there were no enlarged lymph nodes or subcutaneous nodules but an area of silvery scaling of the scalp was noted just above the hair-line, the skin elsewhere being normal. The hands showed swelling and limited flexion of both the distal and proximal interphalangeal joints. The finger nails were normal. The left wrist was tender on pressure and there was some swelling of the adjacent tendon sheaths. The right knee contained a small effusion, there was limitation of rotation of the right hip, and straight leg raising on that side caused pain in the back. The range of movement in the spine seemed reasonable for the age of the patient and other peripheral joints were normal. Examination of the cardiovascular, respiratory and central nervous systems, and of the abdomen, revealed no abnormalities.

Questions

(1)   What is the most likely cause of her joint symptoms?
(2)   Give up to 3 other conditions present
(3)   Give up to 4 investigations which would be likely to clarify the diagnosis

5

A Jewish man of 70 went to his doctor with an itching rash of the arms and legs which had been present for about 2 weeks. He had experienced no skin trouble before, although there was a strong family history of eczema and asthma and his granddaughter, living in the same house, had 'nettlerash'.

Apart from mild diabetes, controlled by chlorpropamide, he was fairly well. He had recently been given ampicillin for a chest infection. Following that infection he developed cardiac failure and was given frusemide; in spite of this he had mild stasis oedema increased by his tendency to sit for long periods musing or playing with his cat.

On examination he was found to have grouped erythematous papules and vesicles, with large blisters round the ankles. The rash was almost confined to the legs and the flexor aspects of the forearms. The hands were spared. Some of the blisters on the ankles had ruptured and were crusted; some were quite deeply eroded. Such blisters as remained intact were tense and arose from normal skin. The mucous membranes were not involved. The remainder of the examination was normal and there were no signs of heart failure apart from the residual stasis oedema.

Questions

(1)   Suggest 3 dermatoses which should be considered in the differential diagnosis
(2)   Suggest one therapeutic measure for each of the likely causes

6

An Italian, aged 56, had been well until 5 years previously when he began to notice reduction in his exercise tolerance. Since then he had experienced episodes of severe breathlessness and had required admission to hospital on several occasions. He gave a history of intermittent haemoptysis for some weeks. There was no history of rheumatic fever. On direct enquiry he had orthopnoea (3 pillows), and had had intermittent swelling of the ankles. He was being treated with digoxin and diuretics.

Past medical history: he had been investigated 3 years previously when an x-ray had shown an interlobar effusion in the right mid-zone. Bronchoscopy was negative. Because of past exposure to chemicals a diagnosis of industrial lung disease was made, but there did not seem to be any evidence for this now. Four months previously he had sustained myocardial infarction.

On examination he was overweight and breathless on mild exertion, but not anaemic or cyanosed. The cardiovascular system was as follows: pulse: 80, regular, reduced amplitude, normal quality. BP: 130/90. JVP: raised 4 cm. Clinically, there was no cardiac enlargement. On auscultation, there was a grade 2/4 high frequency pansystolic murmur heard at the lower left sternal edge and apex. P2 was slightly accentuated but moved normally with respiration. There were no diastolic murmurs, even after exercise. There was no ankle oedema. Abdomen: the liver was palpable two fingers below the right costal margin, and was firm and tender. Respiratory system: no clubbing; trachea central; good expansion; breath sounds vesicular; no adventitious sounds.

A straight x-ray of the chest showed enlargement of the heart and of the pulmonary arteries, dilatation of the upper lobe veins, and a perihilar haze. The ECG showed sinus rhythm with left atrial hypertension.

Questions

(1)   Give up to 4 possible causes of his cardiac condition
(2)   Give up to 4 investigations that would help in the differential diagnosis

7

A 68-year-old woman was recovering from an acute chest infection. She gave a history of occasional indigestion, her only other complaint being one of increasing deafness over the past 2 years. As she was thought to have had a significant intake of alcohol in the past liver function tests were performed. The results were:

Serum bilirubin : 0.8 mg per cent
Thymol turbidity : 3 units
Serum aspartate aminotransferase (GOT) : 8 iu/l (normal: 4–15)
Serum alkaline phosphatase : 98 King–Armstrong units (normal:3–13)
Serum lactate dehydrogenase : 200 iu/l (normal: 60–250)
Total serum proteins : 6.9 g per cent (albumin:4 g per cent)
Electrophoretic strip : normal
Prothrombin time : 15 sec (control:13 sec)

Questions

(1) What are the likeliest causes which will explain these results?
(2) What further tests might be of value?

8

A 66-year-old retired commissionaire was admitted in a confused state
with a 12-hour history of nausea, vomiting, abdominal pain and diarrhoea containing dark red blood. He attributed all his present ills to his
having stopped drinking beer a year earlier when chronic bronchitis had
forced him to retire from both his work and his visits to the pub. Since
then he had become increasingly constipated and on the day before
admission he had taken twice his usual dose of two cascara tablets.
During the past year he had experienced lower abdominal discomfort
relieved by defaecation when, after much straining, he would pass a
hard dry stool. He had occasionally noticed blood on the paper but
never in the stool.

The man had experienced increasingly severe bronchitis progressing
over 15 years and necessitating hospital admission on 5 occasions in the
last 8 years. The first of these had been complicated by myocardial
infarction and atrial fibrillation and in subsequent admissions the acute
chest infection had precipitated congestive cardiac failure. Despite being maintained on digoxin, thiazides, potassium, bronchodilators and
expectorants, his exercise tolerance was limited to walking around his
flat.

His weight was unchanged at 12 st and he had had a poor appetite
for many years. He smoked 30 cigarettes per day.

On examination, he appeared unwell, cyanosed, and in pain which
made him breathe rapidly. He could not give a very coherent history
without the help of his wife. He had a temperature of 38°C with BP:
130/80 and atrial fibrillation of about 110/min. His legs were cold and
no foot pulses were felt but he was not in heart failure. There was poor

expansion in his emphysematous chest and widespread rhonchi only were heard.

His abdomen was tense, more so on the left side where there was marked tenderness and guarding, though no mass could be felt. Bowel sounds were heard but there was no splash or bruit.

On rectal examination, no mass could be felt but there was altered blood on the glove. Proctoscopy confirmed the presence of non-prolapsing internal haemorrhoids. Sigmoidoscopy showed a normal mucosa with blood coming from above 25 cm.

Questions

   (1)   Give up to 3 possible causes for the rectal bleeding

   (2)   Give up to 3 investigations which would be helpful in diagnosis

9

A 33-year-old unmarried secretary presented with a 6-week history of tiredness, pains in her limbs, dyspnoea and swelling of her legs. She had first felt unwell about one week after returning from a holiday in Tunisia. There was a past history of 'cystitis' at intervals since her teens. There was no family history of renal disease but her father, aged 65, had become deaf in recent years.

On examination she was clinically anaemic. T: 38°C. BP: 120/70. JVP: 3 cm. The heart was not enlarged but a soft mid-systolic murmur could be heard at the left sternal edge. The spleen was just palpable and there was pitting oedema of the ankles.

Investigations: Hb: 6.0 g per cent; WBC: 7,000; ESR: 62 mm at 1 h; urine protein +++; RBC +++; sterile; blood urea: 85 mg/100 ml; serum albumin: 2.3 g/100 ml; 24 h urine protein excretion: 7 g. Five days after admission the urine output began to fall and the blood urea to rise.

Questions

   (1)   Suggest 3 possible diagnoses

   (2)   Suggest 4 further *blood* tests that should be carried out

   (3)   What other important investigation should be performed prior to starting treatment?

10

A man of 68, crippled with rheumatoid arthritis but otherwise symptom-free, slipped in his garden and was admitted with a fracture of the shaft of his femur. Two days after closed reduction and treatment with immobilization the following results were received from the laboratory:

Serum calcium : 10.9 mg per cent
Serum inorganic phosphate : 4.8 mg per cent
Serum alkaline phosphatase : 10 King–Armstrong units
Serum acid phosphatase : 29 King–Armstrong units
Serum proteins : 5.9 g per cent (albumin 3.1 g per cent)
Electrophoretic strip : slight decrease in albumin, diffuse increase in gamma-globulin
Blood urea : 68 mg per cent
Serum electrolytes : normal

Questions

(1)   What is the likeliest explanation for these findings?
(2)   What treatment should be started at once?

11

A man of 57, a banker by profession, was admitted for investigation having experienced during the previous 3–4 weeks difficulty in swallowing in which solid food seemed to stick at the level of the lower end of the sternum. Three days after admission he had an oesophagoscopy under general anaesthetic and the following night he developed a severe pain in the left shoulder region. A few hours later he developed a severe central chest pain which radiated into the back.

In the few months prior to admission he had been attending his general practitioner with effort dyspnoea and angina pectoris when walking to the station (especially in the winter mornings). His blood pressure, which had ranged from 190/120 to 170/110, was controlled each morning with bendrofluazide (5 mg) and guanethidine (30 mg) and this resulted in a level which varied from 150/80 to 160/100.

On examination, during the attack of severe pain, he was sweating. His respiratory rate was 24/min and his blood pressure ranged from 100/60 to 110/70. Pulse rate was 108/ min and regular. There was no evidence of jugular venous congestion or peripheral oedema though there were some basal crepitations in the lungs. No abnormalities were detected in the abdomen or central nervous system.

The man remained in a shocked condition despite attempts at resuscitation and about 24 hours later he developed a right hemiplegia and died a few hours afterwards.

Questions

(1)   Give 3 likely causes for the chest pain

(2)   Give 3 additional signs for which you would look especially

(3)   Give 3 investigations which would help to elucidate the cause of the pain

12

A 6-year-old girl was referred by her general practitioner with a history of increasing size of her breasts over the past 6 months. The mother thought that the child's growth rate had increased rapidly over the past year but the woman had no measurements to substantiate her impression. The child was the biggest in her class at school and was embarrassed by her height. The mother had no other complaints about the child, whose previous medical history was normal. She was well; there was no vomiting or diarrhoea, nor were there headaches or visual disturbance. There was no history of vaginal bleeding. The parents of the child were divorced, the father having lived abroad for the past 5 years. No history of disease was obtained in either of the parents. Birth and previous medical history were not contributory. There were no siblings. There was no history of anyone in the household having used oestrogen-containing medicine or creams.

On examination the girl appeared to be a well-nourished child, large for her age. Her height was 130 cm (4 ft 1 in), 7 cm above the 97th percentile, and her weight was 29.4 kg, 4.4 kg above the 97th percentile. She had approximately 100 light to dark brown patches of irregular shape varying in size from a few millimetres to 3 centimetres in diameter distributed over her trunk and limbs. BP: 90/60. She had stage 3 breast development. The vulva and clitoris appeared to be normal, but the surface of her vagina appeared to be oestrogenized. There was no evidence of pubic or axillary hair. Her thyroid was not palpable. Rectal examination was normal, and her ovaries could not be felt on bi-manual palpation. There were no CNS abnormalities. Small white plaques were present on the retinae.

Questions

(1)   What causes would you consider to account for the early breast development of this girl?

(2)   What investigations would be helpful in establishing the aetiology?

302

ANSWERS TO MULTIPLE CHOICE QUESTIONS

1.	C,	D,	E.		13.	A,	B.
2.	A,	C,	E.		14.	B,	D.
3.	B,	D,	F.		15.	C,	E.
4.	A,	E,	F.		16.	A,	D.
5.	B,	C,	D.		17.	A, B, D, E, F.		
6.	A, C, D, E.				18.	A, B, C, E, F.		
7.	C.				19.	A,	D, E.
8.	B,	D,	E.		20.	B.	
9.	A,	B,	D.		21.	B, D, E, F.		
10.	A,	C,	E.		22.	B,	D, E.
11.	B,	E.			23.	B,	E.
12.	A,	D,	E.		24.	B,	D.

CASE HISTORIES – GENERAL COMMENT AND ANSWERS

1a

Likely Causes

The most obvious cause of the central nervous system (CNS) disorder is diabetes. Even *mild diabetes can be associated with neuropathy and amyotrophy* and this could explain the sensory loss, muscle wasting and extensor plantars. However, other explanations must be explored. Malabsorption of vitamin B_{12} may develop after partial gastrectomy and is usually the result of intrinsic factor deficiency or, rarely, of bacterial overgrowth in a stagnant loop. This may lead to megaloblastic anaemia and *subacute combined degeneration.* This possibility is important because the condition is amenable to therapy. The neck stiffness in a man of his age raises the possibility of *cervical spondylosis* and cord ischaemia, a common cause of long tract involvement in the elderly. He has smoked cigarettes heavily and a lung cancer with a *malignant neuropathy* is a further possibility. Finally, many of the features are consistent with *tabes dorsalis* and this should be excluded.

Urinary disorders and looseness of the bowel are often features of diabetic autonomic neuropathy. Diarrhoea may be due to malabsorption or associated with the previous gastrectomy.

Investigations

These should include:

(1) X-ray: chest; cervical spine; barium meal and follow through
(2) Blood sugar studies
(3) Full blood count and film; serum vitamin B_{12} level
(4) Wassermann reaction
(5) Faecal fat excretion and urinary indicans

2a

General Comment (Including Answers to Questions 1, 2 and 3)

The onset of pain after vomiting suggests the possibility of *rupture of the oesophagus.* In that condition pain is usually felt at the lower end of the sternum (in spontaneous rupture of the oesophagus the tear is always at the lower end of the oesophagus); if the pain radiates it does so through to the back rather than down the arms. It is usual to find *subcutaneous emphysema* at the root of the neck (a consequence of mediastinal emphysema), and it may be possible to detect signs of a *left pneumothorax* (a very common complication). The chest x-ray would show a left pneumothorax or hydropneumothorax and it might be possible to detect mediastinal emphysema.

The woman's physique suggests the possibility of a *dissecting aneurysm* complicating Marfan's syndrome. There might be a family history of the syndrome and the characteristic clinical features should be apparent. The pain is usually maximal at the onset and does not increase as in this case. Recurrence of pain, as in this case, is common. The pain may radiate centrifugally, and symptoms and signs of impairment of blood supply to different organs (for example, the brain or the kidneys) may appear. On examination *absence or inequality of peripheral pulses* is a common finding. *Aortic incompetence* is a common complication. The chest x-ray may show *broadening of the aorta* and its bronchus.

Pulmonary embolism is a likely possibility. When questioned, the patient admitted to taking a combined contraceptive pill for 18 months which much increased the chances of this. The history of 2 episodes of pain suggests that there may have been 2 emboli, and pulmonary emboli are more often multiple than single. An unusual feature is the absence of *hyperventilation,* often the most prominent symptom. The absence of signs of *peripheral venous thrombosis* in no way rules out this possibility. Tachycardia is usually more pronounced than in this case but a *triple rhythm and a rise of JVP* might have been expected. The normal chest x-ray is quite compatible with pulmonary embolism without infarction.

Investigations

An ECG showed a S_1, Q_3, T_3 pattern with evidence of incomplete right bundle branch block (RBBB); these are characteristic findings. Abnormal *serum enzymes* would have been expected if the ECG changes had been due to myocardial infarction, but they were not found (LDH and bilirubin only rise if pulmonary embolism is followed by pulmonary infarction). A lung scan with radioisotope labelled macro-aggregates of human albumin showed a striking absence of perfusion of the lower half of the left lung. *Pulmonary angiography* and *cardiac catheterization* were not thought necessary. A diagnosis of massive pulmonary embolism was made. She was treated with heparin and warfarin, made an uneventful recovery, and discontinued the use of the combined contraceptive pill.

3a

Comment

The loss of weight, glycosuria, and retinopathy suggested that the patient had *diabetes mellitus* and this was confirmed by blood sugar studies. The loss of tendon reflexes and distal sensory loss suggested the presence of a peripheral neuropathy. However, the weakness was more marked in the upper than in the lower limbs, with considerable proximal weakness, and some asymmetry. Such findings are unlikely to be due to a diabetic neuropathy, which is usually mainly distal and sensory in type. In diabetic amyotrophy proximal weakness in the lower limbs may occur, often with severe pain, but there is not usually such predominant and severe weakness in the upper limbs.

Four Possible Causes of the Neurological Symptoms

A *cervical cord lesion* must be considered as an alternative diagnosis to peripheral neuropathy but the general loss of tendon reflexes and flexor plantar responses makes this unlikely.

In spite of the confirmation of diabetes, other causes of peripheral neuropathy must be considered. The relatively slight symptoms in the lower limbs and the absence of exquisite calf tenderness made *alcoholic peripheral neuropathy* unlikely. The 'mixed' clinical picture of peripheral neuropathy and proximal weakness is suggestive of *non-metastatic neurological disorder,* due to malignant disease.

The *Guillain–Barré syndrome* should also be considered, especially in view of the proximal weakness noted in the upper limbs. However, this patient had been gradually developing symptoms for several months before seeking medical advice and this type of history is quite unlike acute post-infective polyneuropathy.

Investigations

Investigations which were indicated in this patient included a full blood count and ESR estimation, chest x-ray, glucose tolerance test, sputum cytology, lumbar puncture, serum B_{12} and folate estimation, EMG, and possibly liver biopsy.

Results

Diabetes mellitus was confirmed in this case and an initial chest x-ray showed no definite abnormality. The CSF protein was high (200 mg/100 ml), and EMG showed slowing of motor and sensory conduction velocities. Treatment of the diabetes was not followed by any substantial improvement in the neurological disorder. Three months after he was first seen his condition deteriorated, and he experienced constant low grade fever, loss of weight, a rise in the previously normal ESR, and an increase in the size of the right lung hilum. Bronchoscopy with biopsy confirmed the presence of a non-keratinizing squamous cell carcinoma.

Final Diagnosis

Carcinoma of the Bronchus; non-metastatic peripheral neuropathy; associated diabetes mellitus.

4a

General Comment

Symmetrical involvement of the proximal interphalangeal joints of the fingers of both hands, of the wrists and adjacent tendon sheaths, and a knee, in a patient with both constitutional disturbance in the form of fatigue and weight loss and difficulty in dressing due to morning stiffness, strongly suggests *rheumatoid disease.* The presence of a moderate degree of anaemia (in this case 12 g/100 ml in association with an ESR of 112 mm/h) is in favour of this diagnosis and, together with the capillary defect of rheumatoid disease, would explain the swelling of the feet.

Although *psoriatic arthropathy* should be considered as an alternative diagnosis it is unusual for it to present for the first time at this age. A widespread arthropathy is more frequently an accompaniment of extensive psoriasis and is often preceded by nail dystrophy. Although the distal interphalangeal joints of the fingers are often involved in psoriatic arthropathy the adjacent nails are particularly likely to show changes in such cases. In this patient there was no nail dystrophy. In this age-group *primary generalized osteoarthrosis* may be superimposed on rheumatoid disease or, as in this case, osteoarthrosis may pre-exist leading to swelling of the distal finger joints and also to pain in the hip. Rheumatoid arthritis of the hips is not uncommon but osteoarthrosis is even more frequently seen. In the case described the radiological findings were those of loss of articular cartilage and upward and lateral displacement of the head of the femur in relation to the acetabulum, together with formation of osteophytes at the acetabular margin — features characteristic of osteoarthrosis. Films of the lumbar spine showed loss of disc space at L5 and S1; additional views in flexion and hyperextension revealed a spondylolisthesis.

The finding of a negative test for rheumatoid factor in the serum in the early months of rheumatoid disease, and in the absence of nodules, should not deter one from making the correct diagnosis since it is not an uncommon finding and a second specimen taken a few months later may prove positive. If the Rose–Waaler test is chosen and proves positive this is more specific than the latex and thus of greater diagnostic value. In this instance rheumatoid factor was demonstrated in the synovial fluid removed from the knee. The fluid contained no crystals but contained 26,000 cells/mm^3, 90 per cent of which were leucocytes, a very usual finding in rheumatoid fluid. Although the radiographs of the hands showed no erosions the appearance of these may be delayed for some months despite soft tissue swelling of marked degree.

Answers

   (1)   Late-onset rheumatoid disease

   (2)   Additional conditions present are (a), psoriasis (b), primary generalized osteoarthrosis, and (c), lumbar disc degeneration

   (3)   Investigations should include (a), haemoglobin, white cell count, ESR (b), radiology: hands and wrists, lumbar spine and pelvis (c) synovial fluid analysis: cells, crystals, Rose's test and (d), repeat Rose's test on serum

5a

Three Possible Dermatoses

Pemphigoid, erythema multiforme (idiopathic or precipitated by his chest infection or by a drug), or a *reaction to bites,* are the most likely diagnoses. Pemphigus and dermatitis herpetiformis are not likely in view of his age and the distribution and character of the rash.

Comment

The morphology of the rash suggests a reaction to bites. The 'nettle-rash' of the child in the household may be relevant as it may represent papular urticaria; the family history of eczema and asthma is, however, irrelevant. The crusted lesions are probably infected. The ankle lesions are bullous because of hypostasis, and may progress to ulceration if the oedema is not controlled.

Therapeutic Measures Indicated

Pemphigoid would be treated with systemic steroids. Erythema multiforme, if sufficiently severe, would also need to be treated with systemic steroids. In the case of reaction to bites appropriate treatment of the cat and its haunts is indicated.

6a

Comment

There was evidence of pulmonary arterial hypertension and pulmonary venous congestion, and a history of recurrent haemoptysis.

The differential diagnosis, therefore (question 1), was between:

(1)   Thrombo-embolic pulmonary hypertension
(2)   'Silent' mitral stenosis
(3)   Left atrial myxoma
(4)   Cor triatriatum
(5)   Pulmonary veno-occlusive disease

Investigations which Proved Conclusive

(1)   Screening with the image intensifier showed a heavily calcified mitral valve

(2)   Echo-cardiography showed a thickened mitral valve with reduced diastolic closure rate

(3)   Right heart catheterization showed a pulmonary artery pressure of 90/45

(4)   Left heart catheterization showed a large diastolic pressure gradient across the mitral valve

(5)   LV angiograms showed no mitral regurgitation

Final Comment

The diastolic murmur from a very tight mitral stenosis was inaudible because of poor blood flow

7a

Likely Causes

Although hepatocellular damage due to alcoholic cirrhosis cannot be excluded on the laboratory evidence provided, nothing in the results gives positive support to the diagnosis. The most likely explanation of the isolated and very high serum alkaline phosphatase is unsuspected *Paget's disease of bone.* This could also be the cause of the increasing deafness.

Further Tests

A normal *serum 5-nucleotidase* would support the interpretation that the raised serum alkaline phosphatase is of bony origin. More specifically, this can be confirmed by the separation of the alkaline phosphatase isoenzymes by *gel electrophoresis.*

If the raised serum alkaline phosphatase should unexpectedly prove to be of 'liver' origin, the most likely diagnosis is a carcinoma arising from the biliary epithelium, either within the liver (cholangiocarcinoma) or from the extrahepatic duct system.

8a

Possible Causes and Appropriate Investigations

Barium enema on the day after admission showed narrowing and 'thumb printing' of the colon from the splenic flexure to the sigmoid. He improved on conservative treatment but a follow-up barium enema

6 weeks later showed a long area of tubular narrowing at the site of the previous changes of *ischaemic colitis.*

Other diagnoses which would be considered would be *diverticulitis* and *carcinoma of the colon.* Other investigations which might be undertaken are *plain x-ray of the abdomen* and *selective arteriography.*

9a

Comment

The patient shows a combined nephritic and nephrotic picture which is almost certainly due to glomerulonephritis with 'proliferative' histology. The symptoms of tiredness and limb pain together with the fever, splenomegaly and anaemia out of proportion to the degree of nitrogen retention suggest a systemic disease.

Possible Diagnoses

A connective tissue disease, notably *systemic lupus erythematosus* (SLE) is the likeliest diagnosis but *rapidly progressive glomerulonephritis,* in which anaemia is often a prominent feature, is a distinct possibility. *Subacute bacterial endocarditis* (SBE) is a potentially curable condition and must be excluded.

Blood Tests

Although the murmur is probably related to the anaemia, and a nephrotic syndrome and oliguric renal failure are uncommon complications, *blood culture* is an important investigation here as well as in all patients with oliguric renal failure. A *blood film* is important in helping to characterize the anaemia which could be micro-angiopathic, haemolytic, or due to unrelated iron deficiency. An *ANF test* (and an anti-DNA antibody test, if available) will be necessary. The *serum complement* level may help differentiate SLE and rapidly progressive glomerulonephritis.

Additional Important Investigation

A *renal biopsy* (preceded by IVP and coagulation studies, including a platelet count) is the most discriminating additional investigation.

Results

The patient had SLE with an auto-immune haemolytic anaemia, a strongly positive ANF and low serum complement, and lupus glomerulonephritis with numerous crescents at renal biopsy. Happily, she had a remission, albeit incomplete, on high dose steroid and cyclophosphamide therapy. Other connective tissue disorders such as Wegener's granulomatosis and Henoch Schönlein purpura (in spite of the absence of a history of rash) could have given a similar clinical picture. The renal disease in the haemolytic uraemic states tends to be less nephrotic and more nephritic than in this patient.

10a

Likeliest Explanation

The raised serum acid phosphatase is virtually diagnostic of *carcinoma of the prostate*. Re-examination of the x-ray pictures will probably confirm that the bone has fractured through a secondary deposit (that is, a pathological structure). The raised blood urea may be related to the primary tumour. The marginally raised serum calcium may be due to bony secondaries (which are not always 'osteosclerotic' from a prostatic primary).

Treatment

The abnormalities can be expected to respond to *oestrogen therapy*. The serum protein changes probably reflect old-standing rheumatoid arthritis.

11a

Likely Reasons for Chest Pain

The most likely diagnosis is *myocardial infarction*, but the radiation of the pain to the back should alert the wary to the possibility of a *dissecting aneurysm*. In view of the recent oesophagoscopy a *ruptured oesophagus* must be considered while another possibility is a *massive pulmonary embolism*.

Additional Physical Signs to be Looked For

The physical signs which should be noted specially are the *peripheral pulses;* inequality or absence of these would suggest 'dissection' of the aorta with occlusion of one or more of its branches. An *aortic early diastolic murmur* would likewise point to dissection with damage to the aortic ring.

A ruptured oesophagus is a possibility and physical signs are likely to be sparse — support for the diagnosis would be provided by the finding of *surgical emphysema in the neck.*

The absence of jugular venous congestion makes pulmonary embolism unlikely, but no examination of the cardiovascular system is complete without looking at the legs for signs of *venous thrombosis* although many cases of pulmonary embolism are not associated with overt thrombosis.

Investigations

The crucial investigations will first be an ECG — this might support the diagnosis of myocardial infarction although the absence of evidence of infarction would not exclude either a very recent myocardial infarction or dissecting aneurysm. Elevated *serum enzyme levels* (SGOT + LDH) would be of value in supporting the diagnosis of myocardial infarction and excluding dissecting aneurysm. A *straight and left lateral x-ray of the chest* might show broadening of the aortic shadow and this is the only way of positively diagnosing a dissecting aneurysm in the absence of vascular obliteration. The x-ray should also be examined carefully for signs of mediastinal emphysema which would suggest a diagnosis of ruptured oesophagus.

Comment

The subsequent development of a right hemiplegia followed by death now makes the diagnosis of dissecting aneurysm the most probable. Sometimes the fall in blood pressure which occurs following a myocardial infarct, especially in those with preceding cerebrovascular disease, can cause focal cerebral signs. Embolic cerebrovascular disease following a myocardial infarction is well-recognized, but the interval between the cardiac and cerebral episodes is usually at least a week; this allows time for the intraventricular thrombus to form.

12a

Causes

This girl demonstrated the signs of true *precocious puberty:* breast enlargement, increased growth, and oestrogenization of the vagina. She started menstruating within 4 weeks of first being seen. The presence of numerous café-au-lait patches on the body suggested *neurofibromatosis* (von Recklinghausen's disease). This condition is known to be associated with midline intracranial tumours.

Investigation

An *air encephalogram* demonstrated an inoperable midline tumour in the region of the hypothalamus, which is probably a hamartoma which is resistant to radiotherapy. When the father visited the child he was found to have numerous café-au-lait spots and a number of small mobile tumours under the skin along the course of the cutaneous nerves.

Index

Abdominal examination in heart
   disease, 20
Acantholytic bullae, 265, 267
Acid phosphatase, 280, 283
Adherent pericardium, 6
Adrenal gland tumours, 87
Adrenergic beta-blocking drugs in
   disorders of heart beat, 68
Adrenocorticotrophic hormones,
   Guillain Barré syndrome, in,
   212
   rheumatic disease, in, 232
Adreno-genital syndrome, 93
Aerosols, death from asthma and,
   187
Alanine transferase, 284
Albright's syndrome, 91
Alkaline phosphatase, 279
   bone disease, in, 282
   intestinal, 280
   levels following fractures,
   276
   liver, in, 284
Allergic reactions
   drugs, to, 182
   types of, 183
Alport's syndrome, 174
Amino acid metabolism in colon,
   120

Aminorex, pulmonary embolism
   and, 187
Ampicillin, reactions to, 184
Amylase levels in pancreatitis,
   277, 280
Amyloidosis, 138, 168
   rheumatoid disease, in, 245
Amyotrophy in diabetes mellitus,
   107
Anaemia, 82
   heart disease and, 2
   rheumatoid disease, in, 244
Anal lesions in Crohn's disease,140
Androgens, excess production, 91
Angiitis, hypersensitivity, 191
Angina pectoris, 22
   smoking and, 33
   tachycardia causing, 58
Angiokeratoma corporis diffusum,
   175
Anhidrosis, 111
Ankle, arthrodesis of, 241
Ankylosing spondylitis, 224
   diseases of the colon and, 137
Anorexia nervosa, 81
Antibiotics in nephrotic
   syndrome, 177
Antinuclear antibodies in
   rheumatoid disease, 225

315

INDEX

Antireticulin antibodies, 270
Anuria, 153, 278
Aortic regurgitation, 4, 10, 17, 18
Aortic stenosis, 82
    heart sounds in, 15, 16
    pulses in, 3
Apex beat, 7, 8, 11
Arethylcarb-amazine, reaction to,
    196
Argyll Robertson pupil, 107
Arrhythmias (*see* Cardiac
        arrhythmias and Heart beat
        disorders)
Arterial pulses, 3
Arthritis,
    gonococcal, 224
    psoriatic, 223
Arthrodesis, 239
Arthrography, 238
Ascites in heart disease, 20
Aspartate transaminase, 281
    liver disease, in, 284
Aspirin in rheumatoid disease,
    228, 244
Aspirin asthma, 190
Asthma,
    drug-induced, 189
    pressurized aerosols and, 187
    retarding stature, 82
Atherosclerosis, diabetic, 99
Atlanto-axial subluxation, 243
Atrial extrasystoles, 54
Atrial fibrillation, 10, 18, 55,
    60, 61
Atrial flutter, 60
Atrial myxoma, 3
Atrial septal defects, murmurs
    in, 18
Atrial tachycardia, 58
    non-paroxysmal, 59
    paroxysmal, 68
Atrio-ventricular node, 46, 47
Auscultation, 4
    heart disease, in, 9
Auto-immunity,
    pemphigoid and, 267
    pemphigus and, 265

Azathioprine,
    Goodpasture's syndrome, in,
        172
    Guillain–Barré syndrome, in,
        213
    malarial nephropathy, in, 173,
        174
    pemphigoid, in, 268
    pemphigus, in, 266
    systemic lupus erythematosus,
        in, 169

Bacterial endocarditis, 2
    heart sounds in, 16
    subacute, 171
Baker's cysts, 238
Barber's chair sign, 205
Barbiturates, reactions to, 258
    259, 264
Benorylate, 228
Bernheim syndrome, 3
Beta-carotene, 263
Black fat, 195
Bladder dysfunction in diabetes,
    110
Blalock operation, 18
Blood pressure (*see* also
        Hypertension), ischaemic
        heart disease and, 31, 42
Bone development, assessment of,
    79
Bone disease,
    alkaline phosphatase in, 282
    rheumatoid disease, in, 247
Bonnevie–Ullrich syndrome, 82
Breast cancer, 283
Broadbent's sign, 6
Broad beta disease, 30
Bromides, skin reactions to, 261
Bronchial neoplasms, peripheral
        neuropathy in, 214, 215,
        217
Bronchodilator aerosols, dangers
    of, 188

Bullous dermatoses, 253–272
   classification, 254
   congenital, 263–264
   definitions, 253
   diabetes, in, 263
   diagnosis, 255
   drug-induced, 257, 260–261
   idiopathic, 264
   infections causing, 255
   metabolic abnormalities, in,
      261
   physical agents causing, 255
   unconscious states, in, 264
Bundle branch block, left,
   heart beat in, 55
   heart sounds in, 12, 13
Bundle branch block, right, 68,
   73
   heart beat in, 44, 58
   heart sounds in, 11, 12
Bundle of His, role of, 47, 50
Busulphan lung, 192

Capillary changes,
   diabetes, in, 99
   rheumatoid disease, in, 246
Carbohydrate intolerance,
     ischaemic heart disease and,
     26
Carcino-embryonic antigen, 129
Carcinomatous neuropathy, 202,
   213, 214
Cardiac amyloidosis, 3
Cardiac arrhythmias, 45–73 (see
     also Heart beat disorders)
   diagnosis, 4, 48, 50, 51
   electrocardiography in, 48
   sinus, 4
   supraventricular, 68
   Wenckebach phenomenon, 48,
     51
Cardiac neurosis, 54
Cardiac tamponade, 6

Cardiomyopathies, 2, 23
Cardiomyopathy, hypertrophic
     obstructive (see Hyper-
     trophic obstructive cardio-
     myopathy)
Cardioversion, 67
   atrial fibrillation, in, 61
   atrial flutter, in, 60
Carotid stenosis, 18
Carpal tunnel syndrome, 205, 238,
   248
Cataract in diabetics, 117
Cerebral thrombosis, contra-
     ceptive pill and, 186
Cerebrospinal fluid examination,
     carcinomatous neuropathy, in,
      215, 217
     Guillain–Barré syndrome, in,
      211
     peripheral neuropathy, in, 202
Ceremide trihexosidase, 175
Chagas' disease, 2
Charcot–Marie–Tooth disease, 201,
   203
Charcot's joints, 111
Chest disease,
   drug reaction and, 179–197
     allergic, 182
     epidemiological studies,
      185
     intolerance, 181
     overdose, from, 180
     toxic, 180
   oxygen-induced, 195
Chest examination in heart
     disease, 6
Children,
   growth and development,
     assessment, 75
     disorders in, 75–95
   nephrotic syndrome in, 87, 159
   rheumatoid disease in, 223,
     232, 246
   serum enzyme levels in, 282
Chloroquine,
   rheumatoid disease, in, 230

Chloroquine, (*cont.*)
  side effects, 249
Cholesterol levels,
  ischaemic heart disease, in,
      24, 26, 28, 29, 30, 34,
      35, 36
  nephrotic syndrome, in, 150
  reduction of, 36
Cholestyramine, prevention of
    ischaemic heart disease, in,
    30
Cholinesterase, 285
Chromosomal abnormalities causing
    short stature, 82
Clofibrate,
  diabetic retinopathy, in, 115
  reduction of cholesterol
      levels, in, 30, 36, 41
Cockayne's syndrome, 90
Coeliac disease, 81
  dermatitis herpetiformis and,
      270
Colitis,
  aetiology and pathogenesis,
      136
  ischaemic, 122, 131–136, 137,
      138
    diagnosis, 135
    disease state associated
        with, 132
  ulcerative (*see* Ulcerative
      colitis)
Collagen diseases, 209
Colon,
  absorptive mechanism, 120, 121
  blood supply to, 122
  carcinoma of, 135, 142
  Crohn's disease of, 119
  disorders of, 119–142
  diverticular disease of,
      127–130
    diagnosis, 130
    disease states associated
        with, 128
    terminology, 127
  function and structure, 120
  gangrene of, 131, 133, 136

  ischaemic disease of, 131–136
    disease states associated
        with, 132
  necrosis, 133
  non-specific, inflammatory
      disease, 136
  spastic, 123, 125
  transit through, 121
  water and electrolyte
      absorption in, 120
Complement in glomerulonephritis,
    147, 156
Conducting system,
  anatomy, 45
  physiology, 47
Conduction
  concealed, 55
  disturbances of impulse, 48
  retrograde, 63
Connective tissue disease, in
    peripheral neuropathy, 209
Constrictive pericarditis, 6
Contraceptive pill,
  herpes gestationis and, 268
  thromboembolism and, 186
Conus medullaris lesions, 206
Corn oil diet in diabetic
    retinopathy, 115
Coronary artery disease,
    definition, 22
Coronary thrombosis in diabetes,
    102
Corrigan's sign, 4
Corticosteroids,
  erythema multiforme, in, 260
  nephrotic syndrome, in, 159,
      177
  pemphigoid, in, 268
  pemphigus vulgaris, in, 266
  rheumatoid disease, in, 230–234
    local injections, 233
  secondary effects, 182
  side effects, 231
Cranial nerves, 213
Cretinism, 84
Crohn's disease, of colon, 119,
    130, 131, 135, 136–142

Chrohn's disease, (*cont.*)
   aetiology, 137
   complications, 142
   differential diagnosis, 141
   incidence of, 137
   symptoms of, 139
Cushing's syndrome, 87
Cyclophosphamide,
   Goodpasture's syndrome, in,
      172
   malarial nephropathy, in, 174
   nephrotic syndrome, in, 177
   rheumatoid disease, in, 234
   systemic lupus erythematosus,
      in, 169

Dapsone in dermatitis herpeti-
      formis, 269
Deficiency syndromes, 209
Déjérine neuropathy, 201, 203
Delta-amino laevulic synthetase,
      261
Dermatitis herpetiformis, 269
Dermatomyositis, 226
Diabetes insipidus, 81, 168
Diabetes mellitus,
   aetiology of, 98
   amyotrophy in, 107
   arteriolar sclerosis in, 99
   atherosclerosis in, 99
   bladder dysfunction in, 110
   bullous dermatoses in, 263
   calcification of media in, 99
   capillary changes in, 99
   cataract in, 117
   chronic complications of,
      97–118
     neurological, 98, 100,
       105–112, 207, 208
     renal, 102–105, 165–167
     retinopathy, 103
     skin lesions, 117
     vascular, 99
   chronic pancreatitis in, 109
   gangrene in, 101

   gastric emptying in, 108
   glomerulonephritis in, 165–167
   growth disorders in, 88
   impotence in, 110
   intermittent claudication in,
      100, 101
   ischaemic heart disease and,
      26, 102
   malabsorption in, 109
   necrobiosis lipoidica in, 117
   papillary necrosis in, 105
   peripheral neuropathy in, 105,
      106
   pyelonephritis in, 104, 110
   rubeosis iridis in, 116
   vasomotor instability in, 111
Diabetic dermopathy, 117
Diabetic diarrhoea, 108
Diabetic enteropathy, 108
Diabetic nephropathy, 102–105,
      165–167
Diabetic neuropathic arthropathy,
      111
Diabetic neuropathy, 98, 100
      105–112, 207, 208
Diabetic retinopathy, 103, 115
Diarrhoea,
   diabetic, 108
   diverticular disease, in, 127
   ischaemic disease of colon, in,
      131, 132, 135
   nervous, 125
   spastic colon, in, 123
   ulcerative colitis, in, 137
Dibucaine, 286
Diet,
   cholesterol-lowering, 37
   irritable bowel syndrome, in,
      126
   ischaemic heart disease and,
      34
   nephrotic syndrome, in, 176
Digitalis,
   heart beat disorders, in, 60,
      61
   overdose, 59, 62
Digoxin, 180

INDEX

Disseminated intravascular co-
    agulation, 173
Disodium cromoglycate, 189
Disulphuram, reactions to, 208
Diuretics,
    diabetic nephropathy, in, 103
    nephrotic syndrome, in, 176
Diverticular disease, 125
    diagnosis, 130
    disease states associated with,
        128
    incidence of, 127
    terminology, 127
Diverticulitis, 128, 135, 138
Diverticulosis, 127
Donahue's syndrome, 90
Down's syndrome, 1, 83
Drug addiction, 196
Drug eruptions, 260
Drug reactions,
    chest disease and, 179–197
        allergic, 182
        asthmatic, 189
        epidemiological studies in,
            185
        intolerance, 181
        overdose, from, 180
        toxic reactions, 180
    secondary effects, 182
    side effects, 182
Duchenne hereditary dystrophy,
    281
Dwarfism, 79
    nutritional, 81
Dystrophia myotonica, 2

Ebstein's anomaly, 11
Ectopic heart beats, 53
Ejection clicks, 15
Elbow, synovectomy, 237
Electrocardiography,
    cardiac arrhythmias, in, 48
    intra-cardiac, 50
    ischaemic heart disease, in,
        27
    WPW syndrome, in, 68

Electromyography,
    carcinomatous neuropathy, in,
        215, 217
    Guillain-Barré syndrome, in,
        212
    peripheral neuropathy, in, 202
Encephalomyelitis, associated
    with carcinoma, 217
Endocrine disorders, short stature
    caused by, 76, 84
Endogenous creatinine clearance in
    glomerulonephritis, 155
Enteropathy,
    dermatitis herpetiformis and,
        269
    diabetic, 108
Enzymes in serum (see Serum
    enzymes)
Epidermal necrolysis, toxic,
    257
Epidermolysis bullosa, 263
Epiphyses, premature fusion of,
    88
Erythema multiforme, 258, 259,
    268, 269
Erythema nodosum, 137
Erythropoietic porphyria,
    congenital, 261
Erythropoietic protoporphyria,
    262
Escape heart beats, 53
Ethacrynic acid in nephrotic
    syndrome, 176
Exercise, ischaemic heart
    disease and, 33, 42
Exocardial sounds, 19
Extrasystoles, 53
Eye in rheumatoid disease, 249

Fabry's disease, 145, 175
Facial palsy, 200
Fatty acids in aetiology of
    ischaemic heart disease,
        28
Felty's syndrome, 245
Fibrocystic disease, 81

Finger, arthroplasty, 241
Fludrocortisone, 111
Flufenamic acid, 229
Folic acid deficiency in
    rheumatism, 244
Fowler's operation, 241
Fractures, alkaline phosphatase
    levels following, 276
Friedreich's ataxia, 2
Framingham study of ischaemic
    heart disease, 24
Frusemide in nephrotic syndrome,
    176
Furocoumarins, 255

Ganglioradiculitis, 216
Gangrene,
    colon, of, 131, 133, 136
    diabetes, in, 101
Gastric emptying in diabetes, 108
Gaucher's disease, 175
Gibson murmur, 18
Gigantism, 93, 94
Glaucoma, 116
Glomerular disease, 143–178
    (*see* also Glomerulonephritis)
Glomerulitis, 145
Glomerulonephritis,
    acute renal failure in, 153
    amyloidosis, in, 168
    anti-GBM antibodies, due to,
        148
    antigen–antibody complexes,
        due to, 147
    chronic, 166
        renal failure in, 153
    classification, 143–144
    clinical features, 148
    diabetes mellitus, in, 166
    diffuse exudative (*see*
        Glomerulonephritis, post-
        streptococcal)
    endogenous creatinine clearance
        in, 155

focal, 152, 162, 170, 172
    'embolic', 171
    idiopathic, 165
    rheumatoid disease, in, 246
Goodpasture's syndrome, in, 172
haematuria in, 151
Henoch-Schönlein purpura,
    in, 170
hereditary and metabolic, 174
hypertension in, 152, 153,
        154, 162, 165, 177
immunological factors, 147, 160
intercapillary, 166
investigations in, 154
lupus, 169
malaria, in, 173
management of, 175
membranous, 158, 160–161
minimal change, 155, 157, 158,
        159–160, 177
pathogenesis, 147
polyarteritis nodosa, in, 171
post-streptococcal, 147,
        161–162
    complicating impetigo, 257
    diagnosis, 162
    mesangial sclerosis
        following, 162
    serum complement in, 156
    symptoms, 151
primary, 158
proliferative, 158, 161–166,
        171
protein excretion in, 155
radiology in, 156
rapidly progressive, 163
renal biopsy in, 157
renal failure in, 153, 162
secondary, 166
serum complement in, 156
subacute, 163
subacute bacterial endocarditis,
        in, 171
systemic lupus erythematosus,
        in, 169
thrombotic thrombocytopenic
        purpura, in, 172

Glomerulonephritis, (*cont.*)
   types, 158
   urinary infections in, 178
   urinary microscopy in, 154
   with epithelial crescents, 163
Glomerulosclerosis, 103, 159
Glomerulus,
   damage to, 147
   normal structure, 145
Glucocorticoid, excess of, short
      stature caused by, 87
Glucose tolerance and ischaemic
      heart disease, 31
Glutamic oxalo-acetic transaminase,
      281
Gluten sensitivity, 109
Glycolipid lipoidosis, 175
Gold nephropathy, 229, 246
Gold therapy,
   reactions to, 191, 193, 229,
      246
   rheumatoid disease, in, 229
Golfer's elbow, 233
Goodpasture's syndrome, 144, 163
   glomerulonephritis in, 148,
      152, 172
Gout, 224
Graham Steell murmur, 9
Growth and development in children,
      75–95 (*see* also
      Stature)
   assessment of, 75
      height and weight, 78
      sexual, 79
      skeletal, 78
   delayed, 88
   parental role, 78, 89
   percentile charts, 77
Growth hormone, 81
   deficiency, 86
   treatment with, 90
Growth spurt, 80
Guillain-Barré syndrome,
      200, 202, 207 210–213

Haematuria,
   Alport's syndrome, in, 174

glomerulonephritis, in, 151,
      154, 165
Haemochromatosis, 113
Haemodialysis, 143
Haemolytic–uraemic syndrome, 153,
      172
Hand–Christian–Schüller
      disease, 85
'Harris lines', 82
Heart,
   atrio-ventricular node, 46
   conducting system,
      anatomy of, 45
      physiology of, 47
   conduction,
      abnormal pathway, 68
      concealed, 55
      intraventricular disturbances, 70
      retrograde, 63
   electrical axis of, 49
   enlargement of, 6
   haemosiderosis, 2
   monitoring, 51
   sino-atrial node, 46
Heart beat disorders, 52–73
   atrial fibrillation, 60
   atrial flutter, 60
   ectopic beats, 53
   escape beats, 53
   extrasystoles, 53
   intraventricular conduction, 70
   non-paroxysmal atrial
      tachycardia, 58
   parasystoles, 57
   pre-excitation syndrome, 68
   sinus irregularities, 52
   supraventricular, 68
   treatment, 56, 57, 68
   ventricular flutter and
      fibrillation, 67
   ventricular tachycardias, 63
Heart block, 70–73
   congenital, 72
   first degree, 70
   Mobitz type, second degree,
      71, 72
   signs of, 73
   third degree, 72

Heart disease,
  beriberi, 2, 23
  congenital, 1
  diagnosis, 1–6
  examination in, 1–20
    abdominal, 20
    auscultation, 9
    exocardial sounds, 19
    heart murmurs, 16
    heart sounds, 10
    inspection, 6
    lungs and pleura, 19
    method, 6
    palpation, 7
    percussion, 7
  ischaemic (*see* Ischaemic
      heart disease)
  pulmonary oedema in, 19
  stature and, 82
Heart failure,
  congestive, 5, 19, 73
  ischaemic heart disease, in, 23
  tachycardia causing, 58
Heart murmurs, 16–18
  continuous, 18
  delayed diastolic, 17
  diastolic, 17
  Gibson, 18
  Graham Steell, 9
  loudness of, 10
  systolic, 16
  transmission of, 9
Heart sounds, 10–16
  ejection clicks, 15
  exocardial, 19
  first, 10, 11
  fourth, 11, 13
  rapid ventricular filling, 13
  second, 10, 12
  snaps and clicks, 14
  third, 8, 13
  transmission of, 9
Heberden's nodes, 223
Height, assessment of, 78
Henoch–Schönlein purpura,
    152, 163, 164, 170–171
Hepatitis, 283

Hereditary coproporphyria, 262
Heroin, 196
Herpes gestationis, 268
Herpes virus infection, 259, 260
Hexamethonium lung, 192
Hip joint, replacement of, 236, 241
Homocystinuria, 94
Hydantoins, reactions to, 191, 197
Hydrallazine, 209
Hydrocortisone in rheumatoid
    disease, 233
5-Hydroxy-tryptamine, 122
Hypercholesterolaemia in
    ischaemic heart disease, 30
Hyperchylomicronaemia in ischaemic
    heart disease, 29
Hyperglycaemia, complications
    caused by, 97
Hyperglycaemic neuropathy, 106
Hyperlipidaemia, 27, 150
Hyperlipoproteinaemia, 29
Hypertension,
  benign, proteinuria in, 149
  glomerulonephritis, in, 152,
      153, 154, 162, 165, 177
  heart sounds in, 13
  ischaemic heart disease, in,
      27, 31, 42
  malignant, 154
  nephritic syndrome, in, 154
  polyarteritis nodosa, in, 171
  pulmonary, 9, 12, 13, 15, 16, 187
  systemic lupus erythematosus,
      in, 169
Hyperthyroidism, 93
Hypertrophic obstructive cardio-
    myopathy,
  heart murmurs in, 17
  pulses in, 3
Hypoalbuminaemia in nephrotic
    syndrome, 149
Hypoglycaemia, 86
Hypoglycaemic coma, 264
Hypolactasia, 126
Hyponatraemic syndrome, 218
Hypophysectomy in diabetic
    retinopathy, 115

INDEX

Hypopituitarism, short stature
    caused by, 85
Hypotension, orthostatic, 111
Hypothyroidism, short stature
    caused by, 84

Ileitis, backwash, 138
Immunoglobulins,
    deposition in glomerulus, 147
    glomerulonephritis, in, 160
    Henoch-Schönlein purpura,
      in, 170
    rheumatoid disease, in, 235
Impetigo, 255
    complications of, 257
Impetigo neonatorum, 256
Impotence in diabetics, 110
Indomethacin, 229
    asthma from, 190
    side effects, 244
Insulin production, failure of, 98
Intensive coronary care, 22
Intermittent claudication in
    diabetes, 100, 101
Intra-articular injections of
    corticosteroids, 233, 234,
      235
Iodides, reactions to, 185, 191,
    261
Irritable bowel syndrome, 123–127
Ischaemic heart disease,
    aetiology, 23–35
      age and sex factors, 25
      broad beta disease, 30
      cholesterol levels in, 24,
        26, 28, 29, 30, 34,
        35, 36
      cigarette smoking, 32, 42,
        43
      diabetes and potential
        diabetes, 26
      diet in, 34, 37
      difficulties, 25
      familial hyperlipoprotein-
        aemia in, 29
      family history of, 27
      hypercholesterolaemia, 30
      hyperchylomicronaemia, 29
      hyperlipidaemia, 27
      hypertension, 27, 31, 42
      irreversible causes, 25
      obesity in, 33
      personality and mental
        stress, 27
      physical exercise, 33, 42
      potentially reversible
        factors, 27
      racial factors, 23, 25, 29,
        34
      social class and, 33
      stature, 35
    angina, 22
    chest wall inspection in, 7
    definition, 22
    diabetics, in, 102
    electrocardiogram in, 27
    Framingham study, 24
    heart failure in, 23
    heart sounds in, 12, 15
    major causes, 24
    mortality, 21
    myocardial infarction, 23
      atrial fibrillation
        following, 61
      extrasystoles following,
        54, 56
      monitoring, 51
      tachycardia following, 62
    prevention, 35–43
      'anti-coronary club', 38
      blood pressure, 42
      cigarette smoking, 42, 43
      physical activity in, 42
      reduction of cholesterol
        levels, 36
      trials, 38
    sudden death in, 23
Ischio-rectal abscesses, 140
Isocitric dehydrogenase, 281, 284
Isoenzymes, 279
Isoniazid, reaction to, 181, 208
Isoprenaline, 188

Janaway's spots, 3
Jugular venous pulse, 4, 12, 20
Junctional extrasystoles, 55
Junctional tachycardias, 62

Keratoconjunctivitis sicca, 249
Kidney (*see* also Renal failure,
    Glomerulonephritis, etc)
    endstage, 153
    rheumatoid disease, in, 246
Kimmelstiel—Wilson lesion, 103,
    166, 167
Knee, synovectomy, 238
Kussmaul, pulsus paradoxus of, 4

Lactate dehydrogenase, 280, 281
    isoenzyme, 281
Lentiginosis, 1
Leucopenia, 245
Lhermitte sensation, 205, 206
Lichen planus, 271
Lignocaine in heart beat disorders,
    57
Lipid metabolism, disorders of, 2
Lipids in aetiology of ischaemic
    heart disease, 27
Lipoid nephrosis (*see*
    Glomerulonephritis, minimal
    change)
Lipoid pneumonia, 194
B-lipoprotein, 30
Liver,
    alkaline phosphatase in, 284
    carcinoma, 284
    enlargement in heart disease, 20
Liver disease,
    peripheral neuropathy in, 208
    serum enzymes in, 283
Lungs,
    disease, oxygen induced, 195
    examination in heart disease, 19
    rheumatoid disease, in, 247

Lupus erythematosus, systemic
    (*see* Systemic lupus
    erythematosus)
Lyell's disease, 257
Lymphangiography, oil embolism
    from, 195

Macroamylasaemia, 278
Macroglobulinaemia, 215
Malabsorption syndrome, 78, 209
    diabetes, in, 109
    rheumatoid disease, in, 244
Malaria, nephropathy in, 147, 173
Malignant disease, peripheral neuro-
    pathy and, 213—217
Malignant melanoma, 267
Malnutrition, 81
Marfan's syndrome, 1, 94
Masugi nephritis, 147
Meadow dermatitis, 255
Measles with pneumonia, 182
Media, calcification of, 99
Median nerve compression, 201
Mefenamic acid, 229
Mental stress, ischaemic heart
    disease and, 27
Mesangial sclerosis, 162
Methotrexate in pemphigus, 266
Methysergide, 196
Mitral stenosis, heart sounds in,
    12, 13, 14, 17
Mobitz type heart block, 48, 72
Monckeberg's sclerosis, 99
Mononeuropathy, 199, 207
Mononucleosis, infectious, 207
Motor neurone disease, 199, 206
Multiple myeloma, 168
Multiple sclerosis, 205
Muscles, rheumatoid disease and,
    250
Muscle biopsy, 204
de Musset's sign, 4
Myelomatosis, 157, 215

INDEX

Myocardial infarction, 23
  atrial fibrillation following,
    61
  diabetics, in, 102
  extrasystoles following, 54, 56
  heart sounds in, 15
  monitoring in, 51
  serum enzymes in, 281
  tachycardia following, 62
Myocarditis, in rheumatoid
    disease, 246
Myopathic–myasthenic syndrome
    214, 218
Myopathies, 204

Necrobiosis lipoidica in diabetes,
    117
Nephritic syndrome, acute, 151
Nephritis, 145
  acute, 152
  hereditary, 165, 174
  Masugi, 147
  potassium-losing, 211
  shunt, 156
Nephropathy,
  definition, 145
  obstructive, 149
Nephrotic syndrome, 149–151
  amyloidosis, in, 168
  causes of, 150
  children, in, 87, 159
  diabetes, in, 167
  glomerulonephritis, in, 149,
    160, 163
  idiopathic (*see*
    Glomerulonephritis,
    minimal change)
  management of, 175
  polyarteritis nodosa, in, 171
  proteinuria in, 155
  radiology, 156
  renal biopsy in, 157
  symptomatic treatment, 176
Nerve biopsy, 204

Nervous system, involvement in
    rheumatoid disease, 248
Neuropathic ulcers in diabetes,
    112
Neuropathy, carcinomatous, 202,
    215
  diabetic, 207
Neuropathy, peripheral (*see*
    Peripheral neuropathy)
Nikolsky's sign, 265
Nitrofurantoin, pulmonary
    eosinophilia from, 190
Nodal extrasystoles, 55
5-Nucleotidase, 281, 284, 285
Nutritional dwarfism, 81

Obesity, ischaemic heart disease
    and, 33
Obstructive airways disease, 6,
    9
Oedema,
  erythema multiforme, in, 259
  glomerulonephritis, in, 161
  nephrotic syndrome, in, 149
  post-streptococcal glomerulo-
    nephritis, in, 162
Oesophageal motility, 108
Oestrogens, excess production, 91
  thromboembolism and, 186
Oil embolism, 194
Orciprenaline, 188
Osler's nodes, 3
Osteo-arthrosis, 223
Osteomalacia, 282
Oxygen-induced lung disease, 195

Pacemakers, 57, 58
  artificial, 67, 70, 73
  role of, 53
  wandering, 52
Paget's disease, 2, 282
Palpation in heart disease, 7

Pancreatitis, 276
  acute, 277
  chronic, 113
    diabetes, in, 109
Papillary necrosis in diabetes, 105
Para-aminosalicylic acid, reactions to, 190, 193, 197
Paraffin, lipoid pneumonia from, 194
Parasystoles, 57
Patent ductus arteriosus, 12, 18
Pemphigoid, 260, 267, 269
Pemphigus vulgaris, 265
Penicillamine in rheumatoid disease, 232
Penicillin reactions, 183, 193
Percentile charts, 77
Percussion in heart disease, 7
Pericardial effusion, 19
Pericardial friction rub, 19
Pericardium, adherent, 6
Pericolic abscess, 129, 130
Peripheral nerves, malignant infiltration, 213
Peripheral neuropathy, 199–219
  cerebrospinal fluid examination in, 202
  classification, 206
  conditions simulating, 204
  deficiency syndromes causing, 209
  diabetes mellitus, in, 105, 106
  electromyography in, 202
  investigation of, 201
  malignant disease and, 210, 213–217
    cerebrospinal fluid in, 215, 217
    non-metastatic, 215
    pathology, 216, 217
  metabolic and endocrinological, 208
  nerve and muscle biopsy, 204
  rheumatoid disease, in, 248
  symptoms, 199, 200
  toxic, 208
Peritonitis, 131
Personality, ischaemic heart disease and, 27
Phenothiazines, reactions to, 191
Phenylbutazone,
  reactions to, 193, 197, 258, 259
  rheumatoid disease, in, 229
Phosphocreatine kinase, 281
Phospholipids in aetiology of ischaemic heart disease, 28
Photocoagulation in diabetic retinopathy, 116
Pickwick syndrome, 187
Piperazine, asthma from, 189
Pituitary, ablation in diabetic retinopathy, 115
  eosinophil adenomas, 93
  gigantism, 93
Pituitary snuff, reactions to, 184
Plasma expansion in nephrotic syndrome, 176
Pleura, examination in heart disease, 19
Pleurisy,
  rheumatoid disease, in, 247
  systemic lupus, in, 194
Pneumothorax, spontaneous, 182
Polyarteritis nodosa, 152, 171, 199, 226
  drug reaction, as, 185, 191
  idiopathic, 191
Polyneuropathy, post-infective, 210
Polyostotic fibrous dysplasia, 91
Polyradiculopathy, 210
Porphyria, 200, 207, 211, 261–262
Portal pyaemia, 129
Practolol, 189
  heart beat disorders, in, 56, 59
Prednisolone,
  erythema multiforme, in, 260
  nephrotic syndrome, in, 177
  pemphigus vulgaris, in, 266

Prednisolone, (*cont.*)
    rheumatoid disease, in, 233
Pre-excitation syndrome, 68
Procainamide, 209
    reaction to, 193
Pronethalol, 189
Propantheline, 130
Propranolol, 189
Prostaglandins, 122
Prostate, carcinoma of, 275
Protein excretion in glomerulo-
      nephritis, 155
Protein malnutrition, 20, 151
Proteinuria,
    amyloidosis, in, 168
    diabetic nephropathy, in, 103,
      167
    glomerulonephritis, in, 154,
      162, 165, 177
    Henoch-Schönlein purpura,
      in, 170
    nephrotic syndrome, in, 149,
      155
    symptomless, 149, 157, 160
Pseudocholinesterase, 285
Pseudopolyposis, 133, 134, 138
Pseudo-tabes, 107
Puberty,
    delay in, 88
    precocious, 91
    stages of, 79, 80
Pulmonary embolism,
    acute, 19
    contraceptive pill and, 186
Pulmonary eosinophilia, drug-
      induced, 190
Pulmonary hypertension,
    aminorex and, 187
    diagnosis, 9
    heart murmurs in, 16
    heart sounds in, 12, 13, 15
Pulmonary oedema in heart disease,
    19
Pulmonary regurgitation, 17, 18
Pulmonary stenosis, 15, 82
    heart murmurs in, 16

Pulmonary systolic murmurs in
      pregnancy, 12
Pulsus paradoxus of Kussmaul, 4
Purapen, 183
Purpura, allergic, 170
Pyelonephritis,
    Alport's syndrome, in, 174
    chronic, 149, 157
    diabetes mellitus, in, 104,
      110, 167
Pyoderma gangrenosum, 137
Pyridoxine, 94

Quinidine in tachycardia, 59
Quinine, intolerance, 181

Rectal bleeding in diverticular
    disease, 129
Refsum's disease, 201, 208
Reiter's syndrome, 224, 246
Renal biopsy,
    amyloidosis, in, 245
    contra-indications, 158
    glomerulonephritis, in, 157
Renal failure,
    acute, 152
    chronic, 153
    glomerulonephritis, in, 162, 163
    renal biopsy in, 157
    serum enzymes in, 278
Renal glycosuria, 151
Renal transplantation, 143
Renal vein thrombosis, 160
Respiratory distress syndrome, 195
Retinitis proliferans, 114
Rheumatic fever, 223
Rheumatoid disease, 221–251
    aetiology, 221
    amyloidosis in, 245
    anaemia in, 244
    antinuclear antibodies in, 225
    auto-immunity in, 221
    cardiovascular system, in, 246
    children, in, 87, 223, 232, 246

Rheumatoid disease, (*cont.*)
  chloroquine in, 230
  corticosteroids in, 230, 232,
     235
  diagnosis, 223, 225
  gold therapy, 229
  heat in, 227
  immunological factors, 221
  immunosuppressive drugs in,
     230, 234, 235
  local treatment, 227
  management of, 221–251
  natural history in relation to
     treatment, 226
  nervous system involvement, 248
  ocular lesions, 249
  penicillamine in, 234
  renal lesions in, 246
  rest in, 227
  skin and bone lesions in, 247
  surgery in, 235
  systemic drug therapy, 228
  systemic features, 244
  voluntary muscle and, 250
Rheumatoid factor, 225
Rickets, hypophosphataemic
     vitamin D resistant, 79, 84
Ritter's disease, 256
Rubella, growth anomalies caused
     by, 90
Rubeosis iridis, 116

Salbutamol, 188
Scabies, 269
Schistosomiasis, 2
Scleroderma, 152
Sensory impairment, 200
Serum enzymes, 273–286 (*see*
     also under specific enzymes)
  cause of increased molecular
     turnover, 275
  children, in, 282
  fate of, 278
  function of, 273
  liver disease, in, 283
  myocardial infarction, in, 281
  names and units, 279
  origin of, 274
  quantity versus activity, 276
  raised, mechanism of, 274
  skeletal muscle disease, in,
     281
  tests, 277
Sexual development, 79
Sexual precocity, 88, 90, 92
Shier's prosthesis, 241
Sick sinus syndrome, 53
Sigmoid colon obstruction, 129
Silicone oil, 234
Silver's syndrome, 90
Sino-atrial node, 46, 47, 52
Sinus bradycardia, 53
Sinus irregularities, 52
Sjögren's syndrome, 249,
     250
Skeletal muscle disease, serum
     enzymes in, 281
Skeleton,
  abnormalities causing short
     stature, 76, 83
  development of, 75, 79
Skin lesions (*see* also
     Bullous dermatoses)
  diabetes, in, 117
  rheumatoid disease, in, 247
Smoking, ischaemic heart disease
     and, 32, 42, 43
Social class, ischaemic heart disease
     and, 33
Sodium absorption in colon, 120
Souffle aspiratif, 18
Spinal lesions simulating
     peripheral neuropathy, 205
Splenomegaly in heart disease, 20
Spondylotic myelopathy, 203
Staphylococcus pyogenes, 256
Stature,
  short,

Stature (*cont.*)
  short, (*cont.*)
    causes of, 76
    chromosomal disorders
      causing, 76, 82
    endocrine disorders
      causing, 76, 84
    familial and racial causes,
      89
    glucocorticosteroid excess
      causing, 87
    hypopituitarism causing, 85
    hypothyroidism causing, 84
    nutritional causes, 76, 81
    skeletal reasons, 76, 83
    systemic disease causing,
      82
  tall, 90–95
    causes of, 91
    cerebral gigantism causing,
      94
    constitutional, 95
    homocystinuria causing, 94
    hormonal causes, 90
    Marfan's syndrome, in, 94
    pituitary lesions causing,
      93
    thyroid disease causing, 93
Steatorrhoea, 81
Steroids,
  carcinomatous neuropathy, in,
    216
  Goodpasture's syndrome, in,
    172
  Guillain–Barré syndrome,
    in, 212
Stevens–Johnson syndrome, 258,
  259, 260
Still's disease, 87, 223, 232,
  246
Stokes–Adams attacks, 53, 68, 73
Streptococcus, causing glomerulo-
  nephritis, 161 (*see*
  also Glomerulonephritis,
  post-streptococcal)
Streptomycin, reactions to, 193
Strictures in Crohn's disease, 142

Subacute combined degeneration of
  the cord, 209
Subclavian stenosis, 18
  the cord, 209
Sulphonamides, reactions to, 191,
  258, 259
Supraventricular tachycardias, 57
Synovectomy, 236
Syphilis, congenital, 264
Syringomyelia, 203
Systemic lupus erythematosus,
  169–170, 235
  arthropathy in, 224
  drug-induced, 193, 209
  renal lesions, 144, 160

Tachycardias, 55
  atrial, 58
    non-paroxysmal, 59
  diabetes, in, 111
  junctional, 62
  paroxysmal supraventricular,
    68
  supraventricular, 57
  treatment, 59
  ventricular, 63, 65
Tennis elbow, 233
Terbutaline, 188
Tetracycline in diabetic entero-
  pathy, 109
Thiamine deficiency, 209
Thiazide diuretics, 103
Thromboembolism, contraceptive
  pill and, 186
Thrombotic thrombocytopenic
  purpura, 153, 172
Thyroid-stimulating hormone, 86
Thyrotoxicosis, 61, 93
Transaminase, 275, 277
Triamcinolone hexacetonide, 234
Tricuspid stenosis, heart murmurs
  in, 17, 18
Tricuspid valve disease, 3

Triglycerides,
    aetiology of ischaemic heart
        disease, in, 28, 31
    nephrotic syndrome, in, 150
Triorthocresyl phosphate, 207
Tubular necrosis, acute, 152
Turner's syndrome, 82
Tzanck test, 265

Ulcerative colitis, 131, 135, 136
    aetiology, 137
    complications, 142
    differential diagnosis, 141
    immunological aspects, 137
    incidence of, 137
    malignancy and, 138
    symptoms, 139
Ulnar nerve lesions, 201, 248
Uraemia, 153, 169, 208
Urinary infections in glomerulo-
    nephritis, 178
Urine examination in glomerular
    disease, 154
Urticaria pigmentosa, 271

Vasomotor instability in diabetes,
    111
Venous congestion,
    causing hepatic swelling, 20
    heart disease, in, 19
Venous pulses, 4, 12
Venous thrombosis,
    contraceptive pill and, 187
    ischaemic colitis, causing, 136

Ventricles,
    aneurysm, 7
    hypertrophy, 50
Ventricular dyskinesia, 8
Ventricular extrasystoles, 55
Ventricular failure,
    left, 3, 19
    right, 3
Ventricular flutter and fibril-
    lation, 57, 67
Ventricular hypertrophy, 27
Ventricular septal defect, heart
    murmurs in, 16
Ventricular tachycardia, 63, 65,
    67
Verapamil in heart beat disorders,
    59, 61
Vitamin B_6 deficiency, 208
Vitamin B_{12} deficiency, 209
Von Recklinghausen's disease, 91

Water absorption in colon, 120
Wegener's granulomatosis, 152, 171
Weight, assessment of, 78
Wenckebach phenomenon, 48, 51, 72
Wernicke's encephalopathy, 209
Wolff—Parkinson—White syndrome,
    58, 68
Wrist,
    arthrodesis, 239
    synovectomy, 237

Xanthoma, 29, 30

Yttrium implantation, 93, 115